ENVIRONMENT, HEALTH AND POPULATION DISPLACEMENT

As this book goes to print, a new cholera epidemic is expanding in Mozambique. Due to being a very recent reappearance, an evaluation of the extent, nature and context of this latest event has not been possible here.

The Making of Modern Africa

Series Editors: Abebe Zegeye and John Higginson

Environment, Health and Population Displacement

Development and change in Mozambique's diarrhoeal disease ecology

ANDREW E. COLLINS
Division of Geography and Environmental Management
School of Behavioural and Environmental Sciences
University of Northumbria at Newcastle

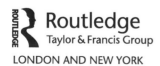
Routledge
Taylor & Francis Group

LONDON AND NEW YORK

First published 1998 by Ashgate Publishing

Reissued 2018 by Routledge
2 Park Square, Milton Park, Abingdon, Oxon OX14 4RN
711 Third Avenue, New York, NY 10017, USA

Routledge is an imprint of the Taylor & Francis Group, an informa business

Publisher's Note
The publisher has gone to great lengths to ensure the quality of this reprint but points out that some imperfections in the original copies may be apparent.

Disclaimer
The publisher has made every effort to trace copyright holders and welcomes correspondence from those they have been unable to contact.

ISBN 13: 978-1-138-31912-7 (hbk)
ISBN 13: 978-1-138-31914-1 (pbk)
ISBN 13: 978-0-429-45391-5 (ebk)

Contents

List of Figures

List of Tables

Preface

The status of human health in geographically defined space is a product of the interplay of pathogenesis with changing biological, physical environmental, social structural and behavioural phenomena. Most research has endeavoured to understand the determinants of ill-health and disease through the strengthening of disciplines that explain disease infection from particular disciplinary perspectives. However, much important information also remains to be known about complexes of environmental, socio-behavioural and demographic factors that influence the pattern of incidence of specific diseases. Rapid expansion of anthropogenic influences on the biosphere, and coincident persistence or increase of some diseases through modifications to their ecology, is occurring at a time of increasing vulnerability amongst the majority of the world's population. Meanwhile, infrastructural development and policy aimed at combating ill-health to varying degrees has fallen short of counteracting these processes. Interdisciplinary enquiry and applied research can assist in understanding patterns of disease incidence emerging from a dynamic infectious disease ecology. Effective and appropriate preventative strategies are more likely to be produced out of such an approach, particularly in ongoing endemic and epidemic situations of the Third World. Such a rationale provided the ontological basis for the research that produced this book.

One methodological gap in our understanding of contemporary health phenomena has come about through lack of analysis of spatial and temporal variations in incidence of infectious diseases. In particular, little research has focused on the relative influence of environmental, demographic and socio-economic factors in rapidly changing areas of the developing world. *Environment, Health and Population Displacement* provides key information on the nature and context of cholera and bacillary dysentery in Mozambique, a country undergoing major demographic and political changes. Focusing predominantly on the centre of the country, in particular on three major contrasting urban centres, the book provides important new information on how pathogens, people and places shaped an emerging ecology of health. The book emphasises that environmental health management and wider development policy can best tackle complex disease phenomena through understanding individual disease ecologies in changing locales.

Mozambique is a particularly relevant location within which to analyse the complex and multidimensional causes of health and well-being. During the first part of the 1990s the country suffered some of the highest disease incidence in the world, much of which was attributable to cholera and bacillary dysentery. This coincided with significant developments in micro-biological knowledge enabling a better understanding of the ecology of *Vibrio cholerae* and inference about other pathogens, such as *Shigella dysenteriae*. However, a disease epidemic is not just a biophysical event, but also what happens when physical and biological changes coincide with and respond to a vulnerable society. This book shows how Mozambique's recent history of destabilising war, and subsequent structural changes linked to internationally financed adjustment programs, caused changes in vulnerability to emergent disease.

Population displacement was a major impact of the war, and had many implications for health. There were large scale movements of people from the rural areas to urban zones, along major transport routes, to internal displacement centres, and to refugee camps across international borders. There has been a variable degree of post-war resettlement to areas of origin and increase in movement for small scale trading of produce. Besides this, recent policy shifts involving adjustments to local infrastructures and the role of the state in welfare have also led to changes that have significant implications for health. The sum of these processes is that spatial coincidence of diarrhoeal disease incidence during the early 1990s has been open to explanation in a number of ways. Despite the recent increases in incidence of cholera and dysentery in many parts of the world, a clearer picture of the extent of influence of environmental, demographic or structural factors has hitherto been limited by a lack of empirically based information.

Preliminary research and pilot fieldwork in Mozambique during the early 1990s confirmed the lack of detailed research on recent epidemics of cholera and dysentery, two ongoing diseases affecting the region, and identified key study areas in central Mozambique as suitable for investigating contrasting influences on their distributions. This was partly guided by work that had identified specific physical characteristics of local environments as influential on the distribution of incidence of cholera in Quelimane in Zambézia province (Collins 1991, 1992, 1993). The extensive fieldwork on incidence of cholera and dysentery that followed in field locations in Sofala and Zambézia provinces is described in this book. This research investigated how the distribution of the two diarrhoeal diseases, with different micro-ecological characteristics, were affected by varying environmental, socio-economic and demographic conditions. Specific questions related to the role of environmental reservoirs for pathogens, the role of population displacement, and the influence of structural changes in the post war period. The objective was to understand a changing disease ecology and assist policy making in sustainable preventative health.

The book uses analyses of recent discoveries in microbiology, the space-time distributions of incidence of cholera and bacillary dysentery, measures of variation of physical environmental conditions, and socio-behavioural enquiry, to understand the influence of environment and population displacement on health in central Mozambique. This leads to assessment of the relative role of development policies and their influence on local environmental health issues. The book shows how the changing vulnerability of different communities to diarrhoeal disease is associated with past and present development contexts. Specific disease ecologies influence the distribution of ill-health and physical environmental changes are proving to be important in this relationship. Analysis of the changing physical and social influences on incidence of individual diarrhoeal diseases is able to indicate the most appropriate management strategies for individual areas.

The book draws out several key principles that are of wider interest to studies on changes in infectious disease incidence. This includes affirming through detailed primary research that, endemic and epidemic disease foci are variously phenomena greater than the sum of their constituent pathogenic and non-pathogenic causes. An important point is that patterns of emergent and resurgent diseases have become less a function of diffusion of disease, as emphasised in many traditional approaches to spatio-temporal patterns of ill-health. Instead they should be considered a function of coinciding windows of opportunity between disease ecology and the human condition in changing places.

A practical aspect of the book is that it shows how understanding of the inter-relationship between pathogen ecology and human vulnerability in the context of environmental and structural change can provide guidance for appropriate environmental health management. In particular it emphasises a 'bottom up' approach to research and development in environmental health issues. It demonstrates how insights gained from local ecological analysis are of broader relevance to wider development policy. As such patterns and processes of change in disease are a function of changes in disease ecology at micro level and changes in the political ecology of health affective at a macro scale. Progress in sustainable prevention can be best achieved through localised research that increases understanding of diseases and environmental health care in changing places. The case of Mozambique suggests that reducing human vulnerability to infection and ill-health will require a reawakening of the role of informed and empowered communities in preventative health care.

The book is divided into nine chapters. The first provides an introduction to spatial perspectives in infectious disease incidence, the ecology of cholera and bacillary dysentery, and to incidence of these diseases in Mozambique. Chapter 2 provides an account of how human vulnerability has been associated with incidence of cholera and bacillary dysentery. Particular attention is paid to seasonal changes in well-being, locational vulnerability, forced displacement and the structural context of epidemics of these diseases. Chapter 3 discusses methodological issues, presents the systems approach that accompanies this research and details a range of appropriate methods and techniques for gathering data. Emphasis is made of how distributions of cholera and bacillary dysentery are able to illuminate an understanding of the influence of environment and population displacement on health in Mozambique. Chapter 4 describes three disease locales in central Mozambique with particular reference to the physical environment, demographic changes and development context. Chapter 5 uses primary field data to investigate specific environmental influences associated with the distribution of incidence of cholera and bacillary dysentery in each area. Chapter 6 uses primary field data to determine the role of resettlement at these locations with specific reference to forced displacement, susceptibility and environmental change. Chapter 7 uses further data to assess how structural and behavioural changes are influential on people-environment interactions and disease incidence at the different locations. Chapter 8 addresses the theoretical, methodological and policy issues resulting from the research in Mozambique. The importance of a focus on health ecology in wider issues of environmental management and sustainable development is emphasised.

Acknowledgements

I am grateful to many people in Mozambique and the U.K. Particular thanks to Dr. Richard Black (Sussex University) for his expert supervisory skills and belief in this project. Thanks also to all at King's College, London who took an interest in this work, in particular to Dr. Martin Frost. Thanks to Professor B. S. Drasar (London School of Hygiene and Tropical Medicine) for taking an early interest in my approach to diarrhoeal diseases. Thanks to Professor David Phillips and Dr Deborah Potts for comments on the PhD thesis that preceded this book.

Many people in Mozambique made this research possible. In particular, thanks to Professor Manuel Araújo (Universidade Eduardo Mondlane) for providing essential endorsement of field work; Desiderio, Moravia, Paulo and Director Marcelino (Centro de Higiene Ambiental e Exames Medicos, Beira), Joaquim Arrota (Conselho Executivo da Cidade de Beira), Gracinda Abreu (Laboratorio Provincial das Águas, Quelimane), Marcos Mulalo (Direcção de Saúde da Zambézia), and Gonçalves Mirione (Direcção de Saúde de Gorongosa) for assistance with field work; governmental departments who approved research activities and/or provided data (fieldwork was co-ordinated with nine local government structures); The British Embassy, Maputo for funding 2 portable water testing kits and supplies of disposables that were donated to the Beira and Quelimane water laboratories.

I also acknowledge ESRC (Economic and Social Research Council) for a full time research award No. R00429234054 and funding of fieldwork; NERC (Natural Environment Research Council) for the loan of 2 Global Positioning Systems; Quaker Peace and Service and Skillshare Africa for financial assistance, Oxfam for equipment loans, and the Rovins Institute for skills training for preliminary fieldwork. Thanks to Wendy Payne for donating funds towards follow up work in Mozambique in 1997.

Figure 2.1 is reprinted from *Social Science and Medicine*, vol. 26:1, Bhardwaj, S.M. and Rao, M.N., 'Regional development and seasonality of communicable diseases in rural Andhra Pradesh, India', pp. 15-24, (1988), with kind permission from Elsevier Science Ltd, The Boulevard, Langford Lane, Kidlington OX5 1GB, UK. Figures 1.1, 1.2, 1.3, 1.4, 1.5, 4.5 are reproduced with the kind permission of the World Health Organization.

Thanks to Gabinete de Epidemiologia, Ministério da Saúde, Maputo for Figures 4.1, 4.2 and 4.3 which have been redrawn from Figures first appearing in *Noticiário Epidemiológico* 3:12, (1993), and to Comissão Provincial do Plano de Sofala for Figures 4.10 and 4.11 which have been redrawn from Figures first appearing in *Boletim Estatístico: Provincia de Sofala* (1993). Thanks to Roma Beaumont (Kings College London) for help with reproducing several of the figures. All other figures and tables used in this book are the original work of the author based on primary data through extensive field research.

Finally, thanks to my parents and family for ongoing support. Engela and Maria (now 5yrs) accompanied me in Mozambique despite hazardous journeys and difficult living conditions. Engela worked as a volunteer in the front line of Mozambique's national health service (Sofala Province) during some of its darkest hours in the mid to late 1980s. The book is dedicated to her and to the people of Mozambique who so often contributed through insight, friendship and hospitality.

1 The Ecology of Cholera and Bacillary Dysentery

Introduction

The effect of infectious disease on human health is an ongoing concern, both in terms of magnitude and unpredictability. Whilst earlier, this century it was expected that many 'old' diseases would diminish as development progressed, as they had done in most of Europe the reality has been that infectious diseases remain the world's leading cause of death (WHO 1996). The 1990s have experienced overall increases in incidence of diseases such as tuberculosis, malaria, dengue fever, cholera, dysentery and HIV/AIDS. This period has also been accompanied by resurgence, emergence, or recognition of new pathogens, including strains of cholera, bacillary dysentery and E. Coli. diarrhoea, with particularly severe consequences for much of the 'developing world'. There are many more known diseases and others that remain undetected or are still evolving. 'Waterborne diseases' make a particular contribution to mortality, the United Nations Environment Programme (1993, p231) estimating that they are responsible for about 4 million child deaths alone each year and the World Health Organization (1996, p38) attributing 3 million deaths to diarrhoeal diseases classified as water related in 1995. One estimate is that as much as eighty per cent of all reported disease outbreaks are caused by waterborne organisms or can be traced to a water-borne source (Epstein *et al*. 1994, p14), though the role of food is also increasingly recognized (WHO 1996, p38).

Cholera and dysentery are just two examples of evolving diseases that to a varying extent fit the above descriptions. They form the focus of this book because findings from recent laboratory and field research have indicated the need for further analysis of a multiplicity of possible influences. However, an even more poignant reason has been because of their ongoing magnitude and unpredictability in Mozambique and other parts of the developing world. Meanwhile, because there is a unique ecology associated with these two diseases, focused research has provided

1

an additional opportunity for conceptualisation and validation around the theme of environmental change, health and development.

An increase in infectious disease incidence has occurred at a time when the world is experiencing large scale environmental and social changes. This has been accompanied by a growing interdisciplinary awareness of both evolution and adaptation of pathogens (Wilson and Levins et al. 1994, New York Academy of Sciences) and the development context of health (Phillips and Verhasselt 1994). Despite decades of research progress on pathogenic and socio-economic causes of ill-health, and improved medical remedies for sickness, there is still an inadequately understood prevalence of ill-health associated with emergent and resurgent infectious disease. However, improved detection of contamination by pathogens and awareness of environmental influences on human susceptibility to infection is increasingly assisting in understanding the association of certain environments with particular pathogens.

As the micro-ecology of specific pathogens has become better recognised, the influence of environmental conditions in explanations of disease distributions can be more precisely specified. Population settlement is fundamental to this association since change in the number, composition, status and distribution of people alters patterns of exposure to disease and anthropogenic impacts on the disease environment. Urbanisation is a major aspect of population settlement with significant implications for health. Disease urbanisation is occurring as increasingly large percentages of the population of the Third World is concentrating in and around cities. Whereas over half the world's population currently resides in rural areas, it has been predicted that in 35 years time over 60 per cent will be inhabitants of urban agglomerations (UNEP 1993, p201).

Urbanisation in developing countries often combines communicable diseases of high density poverty, such as cholera, dysentery and TB, with relative increases in degenerative illnesses associated with the urban 'developed' world, such as circulatory diseases and cancers. However, whereas transition to higher incidence of some of the latter is observable in parts of south-east Asia (Phillips and Verhasselt 1994a), it has been the upward trend in incidence of 'old' infectious diseases that remains a major concern in most of South Asia, Africa and South America. Though, accurate statistics are not available, it is clear that the global death rate from infectious diseases outweighs that of chronic diseases. Further to this there is inconclusive evidence of a simple linear correlation between 'greater development' and 'better health' (Phillips and Verhasselt 1994b, p301).

Population resettlement resulting from conflict, unrest or environmental catastrophe has increasingly become associated with communicable disease outbreaks (Shears and Lusty 1987; Toole and Waldman 1993). Between 1990 and 1993 the global number of refugees and internally displaced people grew from approximately 30 million to 43 million with approximately 16 million internally displaced living in Africa (UNHCR 1992; Refugee Policy Group 1992; US Committee for Refugees 1993). With currently about 50 million refugees and internally displaced civilians in the world the association between population displacement and health is an increasingly important issue (Toole 1995). In these circumstances congestion of people into disease-conducive environments, often combined with increased human vulnerability through having been forcibly displaced, can accompany negative stresses on local disease ecologies. One way in which this can occur is when large numbers of internally displaced populations (figures are unknown) seek refuge in urban areas. Displacement also sometimes causes the creation of new urban areas that are not based on pre-existing settlements, such as occurred in Mozambique at strategic points along the Beira Corridor during the 1980s. However, to date little detailed research of these circumstances has determined if and how there might be higher incidence of specific diseases amongst displaced people in comparison to existing residents living in the same areas. In these circumstances the role of being 'displaced' in influencing incidence of disease, and general standards of health, remains largely theoretical and speculative.

Whereas population displacement invokes change borne out of forced mobility, modifications to infrastructure and policy may similarly 'displace' the well-being of people in their place of residence. Whilst there is evidence of a correlation between economic development and reduced incidence of communicable disease in some areas (World Bank 1993), there is mounting contrary evidence that contemporary macro-development strategies may also exacerbate ill-health in others (Brinkmann 1994). This book explores how displacement may be considered an influential process on health through creation of physical environments that are more favourable to disease, through social differentiation that exacerbates poverty amongst some sectors of a population; and through disruption of local community cohesion that causes a breakdown of local survival strategies.

Figure 1.1 shows the increase in number of countries reporting cholera and number of cases reported by year for the period 1984-1993. The total number of cases throughout the world between 1990 and 1993 was in excess of 1.5 million. The highest overall number of cases for this period was in South America (954,501). However mortality rates were highest in Africa and more than three times (13,998) that of South America (4,002) in 1991. Figures 1.2-1.4 show the global distribution of cases of cholera for the period 1990-1993. The strain of *Vibrio cholerae* 01 that was most responsible for this widespread increase belongs to the El Tor subgroup which had been spreading from its origin in Indonesia since 1961. However of particular importance during 1993 (Figure 1.4) was the emergence of epidemic cholera produced by a non-01 cholera serogroup. *Vibrio cholerae* 0139 (Bengal) was first identified in 1992 as the causative organism of large outbreaks in India and in 1993 was isolated in 7 countries in Asia (WHO 1994a, p205). This continued to spread with later reports recording 11 countries affected and estimating in excess of 100,000 cases (MMWR 1995). At least 19 countries were experiencing the impact of this new threat in 1996 (Drasar and Forrest 1996). Global figures for bacillary dysentery caused by *Shigella dysenteriae* type 1 are much harder to obtain since it has not been a WHO notifiable disease. However the

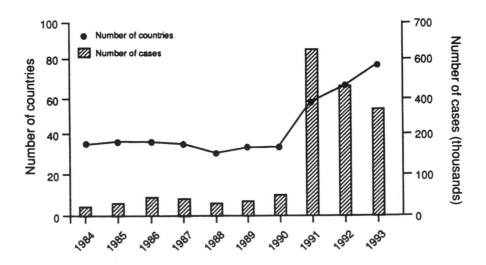

**Figure 1.1   Number of countries reporting cholera and number of
cases reported by year, 1984-1993**

Source: WHO, 1994a, p.208

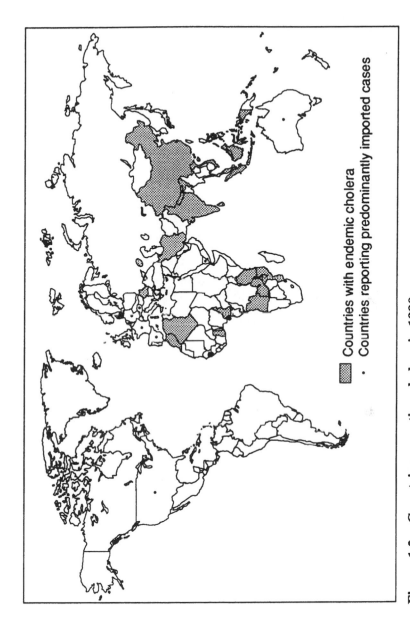

Figure 1.2   Countries reporting cholera in 1990
Source: WHO, 1991c, p.134

▨ Countries with endemic cholera
·   Countries reporting predominantly imported cases

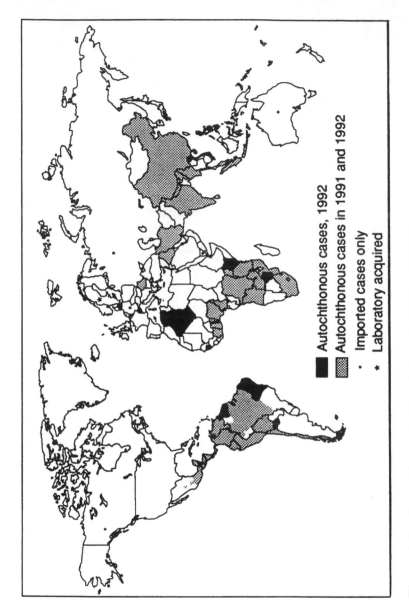

Figure 1.3 Countries reporting cholera in 1991 and 1992
Source: WHO, 1993a, p.150

Legend:
- ■ Autochthonous cases, 1992
- ▦ Autochthonous cases in 1991 and 1992
- · Imported cases only
- * Laboratory acquired

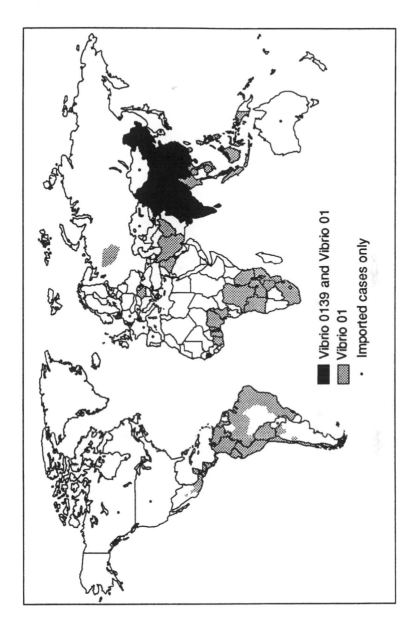

Figure 1.4   Countries, or areas within countries, reporting cholera in 1993
Source: WHO, 1994a, p.206

Vibrio 0139 and Vibrio 01

Vibrio 01

Imported cases only

7

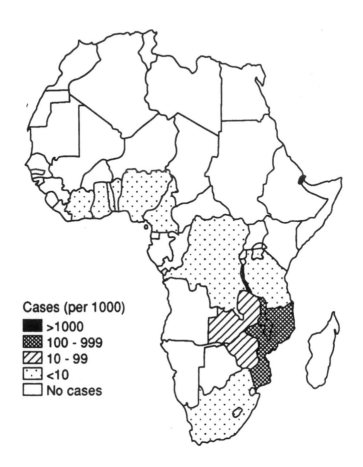

Figure 1.5   Incidence rates of cholera in Africa, 1993
Source: WHO, 1994a, p.210

recent pandemic is thought to have been responsible for hundreds of thousands of cases and tens of thousands of deaths in Africa alone (CDD 1994).

Mozambique has suffered particularly badly from both of these diseases. In 1992 it had the highest notified incidence of cholera in Africa with 30,802 cases and 726 deaths, taking second place to Malawi in 1993 (Figure 1.5; WHO 1993a, 1994a). Incidence of bacillary dysentery in Mozambique has also been amongst the highest with official sources reporting 11,783 cases and 426 deaths for one short part of the epidemic in

1993 (WHO 1993b), and others, a total of 47,483 cases and 199 deaths for the entire year (Aragón and Barreto *et al*. 1995). Despite its severity, and some indication of the contexts within which disease incidence occurs, specific mechanisms behind this changing magnitude and pattern are not yet fully understood and require further attention. This is essential for the development of more appropriate policy aimed at preventing further disaster regions. Despite its massive recent epidemics, Mozambique in particular presents a case where very little research has been attempted on complex environmental and socio-demographic processes that influence disease incidence.

In this book, specific urban areas within the worst affected central third of Mozambique have been selected. Analyses of the space-time distributions of incidence of cholera and bacillary dysentery, measures of variation of physical environmental conditions, and socio-behavioural enquiry are used to understand the influence of environment and population displacement on health. The relative role of broader contextual factors that are interconnected with causation at the local scale are also examined. In each instance the work promotes a geographical perspective on infectious disease incidence as a basis for both understanding health ecology and determining appropriate preventative action. This includes identification of priority action and development policy to curb the development of the diseases in susceptible areas and amongst susceptible communities.

Specific objectives with the Mozambican case studies were firstly, to examine the extent of spatial association between incidence of cholera and environmental factors identified by laboratory experimentation as being favourable to the 'success' of *Vibrio cholerae* 01. This had two parts; first, to replicate initial work carried out on this question in 1991 using varied environments, in order to confirm its reliability (Collins 1992); and second, to distinguish patterns of infection related to two distinct serotypes of *Vibrio cholerae* 01, which occur in Mozambique. Questions concerning possible patterns of endemicity and the relative importance of an environmental reservoir in determining levels of incidence of cholera are addressed with respect to each of the two. They are serotype Inaba and Ogawa of the biotype El Tor (Figure 1.6).

This is followed by an examination of the extent of spatial association between environmental factors and the distribution of bacillary dysentery. In this case, greater host adaptability of *Shigella dysenteriae* 1 have suggested that human populations are its principal reservoir in endemic areas. However, comparison of the patterns of incidence of bacillary dysentery with that of cholera, has been designed to not only contribute to assessing the reliability of findings on health-environment relations for the latter based on background knowledge of *Vibrio cholerae*, but also the relative importance of biological and social causality of diarrhoeal disease in general.

This research material is also used to try to identify the role of population movements in influencing incidence of cholera and bacillary dysentery. This could be expected to operate either through changes to local environments caused by the resettling of displaced people (such as in the creation of physical conditions more conducive to disease pathogens), or through changes in the environmental circumstances experienced by displaced people which make them more susceptible to health problems

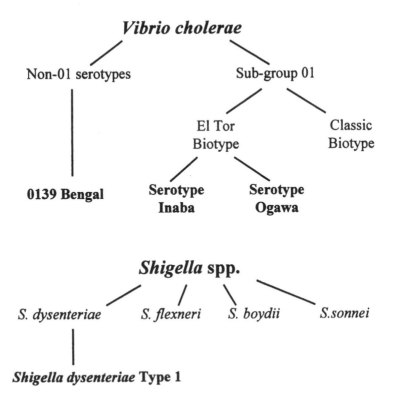

Figure 1.6 Cholera and bacillary dysentery pathogens

(such as increased exposure to disease risks and/or increased susceptibility to infection caused by a lowering of living standards).

Building on insights gained from this first hand research, the book goes on to assess the extent of influence of structural changes and policies in Mozambique on disease hazards and vulnerability. This is particularly relevant since high incidence of cholara and bacillary dysentery during the early 1990s has coincided with the health implications of a controversial structural adjustment programme. A wider purpose in using this case study material is to contribute to understanding the nature of current association, interactions, and contexts that influence ill-health in developing countries, and generate new perspectives to assist appropriate policy making in primary environmental health care. The book identifies 'health ecology' research applications in environmental health management and highlights important ongoing questions about emergent diseases and sustainable development.

A secondary, and largely methodological aspect of research described in this book has been to consider the potential development of appropriate applications for GHIS (Geographical Health Information Systems) for assisting planning in disease susceptible areas of developing countries. Though ultimately limited by its intrinsic concern with spatially defined phenomena, the implications of its further incorporation in health and development related research need to be considered. GIS and GPS applications may be of increasing use in the surveilance of emergency environmental health situations including those that accompany large scale population displacement.

Background to Spatial Perspectives in Disease Incidence with Specific Reference to Cholera

Work relating to geographical dimensions of disease incidence pre-dates the laboratory orientation of scientific and clinical medicine which was emerging around the time that Robert Koch discovered the cholera *Vibrio*. Distributions of diseases, of which cholera serves as an excellent example, have been utilised to both explain disease occurrence by elucidating causal mechanisms, and to provide guidance in prevention and the administration of health services.

Studies of disease incidence with an essentially spatial perspective traditionally emphasise both the search for non-uniformity in disease distributions and the search for association with factors responsible for the pattern displayed. These approaches may be accredited with the titles of medical cartography and disease ecology respectively. Good examples of both are the early and well known studies by John Snow who successfully isolated a contaminated hand pump water supply as the cause of a cholera epidemic in London in 1857. It was Snow in his publication *On the mode of communication of cholera* (1855) who showed that those administrative areas served by the Southwark and Lambeth water-works were associated with the high rates of death from cholera. He had noted that five years on from the initial outbreak a change in pattern had come about in that the Southwark and Vauxhall Company water supply was still associated with high cholera mortality, but the Lambeth supply was not and that they had moved their waterworks to a point higher up the Thames, thus obtaining a supply of water free from the sewage of London. A less helpful association had been made by William Farr (1852) who made the mistake of postulating a direct relationship between cholera cases and altitude. The error of Farr in attributing cholera mortality directly to residence at low altitude illustrates in a simple way a fundamental problem in ecological associative studies in general, namely that influences on a disease distribution may be mis-interpreted due to inter-related factors. In this case there was correlation but no causative mechanism had been identified.

The theory that there is a natural tendency for zoonotic diseases to become localised in a specific habitat still carries much weight in modern epidemiology and may in particular help in explaining distributions of cholera now that the micro-ecology of the organism is better understood. It is a perspective that has been referred to as 'landscape epidemiology' by Pavlovskiy *et al.* (1955) in Soviet work carried out in the 1950s. This delimits the foci of infectious, zoonotic diseases by analysing the associations of factors such as vegetation, animal and insect life, soil type and acidity, precipitation regime, and other elements of the natural landscape. More well known (in western countries) is the similar perspective adopted by Jacques May (1950) who described the epidemiological constraints of various diseases as requiring the coincidence of two, three or four factors, identifying geographical elements, or 'geogens' as fundamental to determining their existence and distribution. Merson *et al.* (1980, p43) in their epidemiological study of cholera and enterotoxigenic *Escherichia coli* diarrhoea in Bangladesh asked the question, 'are we dealing with a phenomenon that is related to the biology of the organism or the host or simply to a difference in exposure to contaminated vehicles?' Interestingly, this echoes an early concept captured by Pasteur on his death-bed in the 19th century who remarked that 'the microbe is nothing; the terrain is everything' (Learmonth 1988 title page). A geographical understanding of 'terrain', somewhat different to Pasteur's principally biological context, would include factors pertaining to the physical and to the human environment and provides a good framework for understanding distributions of communicable diseases such as cholera and dysentery.

Also particularly significant in the development of medical geographical thinking was the inclusion by May of the role of culture as a buffer between disease agents and human infection. Behaviour, which may be considered as the observable aspect of culture, often has spatial expression and may create some of the environmental conditions which are linked to disease and health. Increased awareness of social and behavioural aspects of health come through further consideration of processes determining health, such as the location of health care, rather than simple descriptions of a particular disease and its distribution. It should also be emphasised that behavioural and socio-economic factors often become confounding variables when carrying out studies in search of a straight environmental link (Stephens and Harpham 1992). For example, investigations into links between water quality and incidence of cholera or dysentery may be seriously flawed if consideration is not given to factors such as water storage, hygiene behaviour, socio-economic status, and provision and use of health services. Outcomes determined by macro-economics, settlement pattern, human inter-relationships, cost of transport, or concentrations of health care provision are generally visible and spatially definable phenomena and therefore of major importance to surveillance of disease distributions. Since diseases such as cholera and dysentery spread selectively across space and through people, understanding of specific locations and their inhabitants are very important.

Generally, a broader understanding of 'environment' must be included if our understanding of 'health' is to include the full parameters of the WHO's 1948 definition of 'a state of complete physical, mental and social well being and not merely the absence of disease or infirmity' (WHO 1948). Something of the synthesis that is required in viewing the complexity of health outcomes is expressed by Learmonth (1988) who describes 'a holism that extends to consider community health as a whole, ultimately to put health and disease into a community and societal context, always - ideally at least - with respect for and conservation of the ecological balance of people, plants and animals in a particular setting' (Learmonth 1988, p 263). The concept of balance is also echoed by Howe (1982) who has suggested that health equates with ecological equilibrium while ill-health may be considered a state of maladjustment, disharmony or ecological disequilibrium. The main spatial perspective of this approach is that individual biomes or regions may broadly categorise the conditions under which a wide variety of well-being or ill-health may flourish. Changes in the balance of these ecological systems, whether in a physical environmental or socio-economic sense, are influential factors in bringing about new patterns of disease. A simplified systems approach to analysis of the geography of infectious disease, indicating the main interconnected factors constituting the balance referred to above, is represented in Figure 1.7.

Because of its added emphasis on environment and society, disease ecology requires contextual understanding, the term 'environment' taken as inclusive of external economic and social phenomena that influence the functioning of the local system. The 1992 World Bank Development Report in a section entitled 'Environmental Priorities for

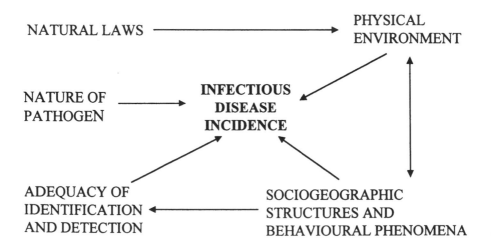

Figure 1.7 A simplified systems approach to an analysis of infectious disease incidence

Development' to some extent joins in with this perspective stating that 'too little is known about how risks and diseases are distributed and interact with each other, and uncertainty remains over the extent to which modest changes in infrastructure account for long-run health improvements' (p49).

Disruption of ecosystems can result in new disease distributions and higher rates of incidence for affected areas. For example, with regard to direct disruption of the physical environment, Egunjobi (1994) suggests that higher mortality in the central/northern zone of Nigeria is explained by large scale dam construction that has enhanced the spread of water-borne and water-related disease. Changes in disease prevalence downstream from the Aswan Dam subsequent to its construction has been well documented. Hughes and Hunter (1970, p479) wrote about the 'hidden costs' of ecologically-naïve development projects in Africa and how often ecological disruption had negative health outcomes. During the present decade this could be extended to the emergent issues of political and economic change, structural adjustment policies, a changing world order, and their impact on environment and health in many parts of the world. Stock (1986) describes a study strategy that involves looking at 'the political economic nature of ill-health occurring in particular ecological niches ...' 'In other words, a fully-developed holism, oriented toward understanding the underlying as well as immediate causes of ill-health' (p698).

With these advances in medical geographical perspectives, spatial association remains fundamental. For example, the failed aspects of structural adjustment policies in many Third World countries have been expressed in the form of greater regionalisation of resources and an accentuated urban to rural division of wealth (Timberlake 1985; Reed 1993; Rich 1994). Additionally, the effects of changing emphases in development policy is apparent in terms of spatial differentiation of well-being within the urban areas of the same countries (Harpham and Lusty *et al*. 1988; Bergstrom and Ramalingaswami 1992; Rich 1994, pp1-24). Bergstrom and Ramalingaswami (1992) estimate that 80 per cent of urban health problems are connected with the environment, and that the poorer conditions of crowding and microbial flourishing lie at the root of this health crisis. However, whilst confirming the impact of physical and social factors on the health of the urban poor, the WHO (1991) confirm that our understanding of the way in which they interact with the urban development process is incomplete and imprecise, partly due to inadequate information. Part of the explanation is contained in the 1995 World Health

Report (WHO 1995) which maintains that increasingly the poor pay the price of social inequality with their health. It is demonstrated in this book that this poverty-disease nexus can be defined through varying complexes of local environmental factors and human vulnerability.

Variation in exposure to contaminated environments, often degraded through human poverty, forms the theme of many existing commentaries on the spatial distribution of cholera and dysentery, though opinion as to the most significant cause is varied. Typically this type of associative environmental approach focuses on secondary transmission, correctly highlighting the importance of factors such as congestion, socio-economic and behavioural disruption, and poor provision of appropriate health care. For example, Meade (1987, p79) comments on how diseases, particularly those found in the tropics, display an occurrence heavily modified by activities that promote economic development for some areas. Certainly, the 1991 spread of cholera through Latin America has cruelly exposed areas with deteriorating social conditions, the legacy of widespread economic stagnation.

Connection has been made between cholera and 'policies of hard-nosed foreign financiers' (Donovan 1991), the breakdown of government infrastructure resulting in inadequate housing and sanitation (Robinson 1991), and lack of personal hygiene and education (Pan American Health Organization 1991), overcrowding, lack of adequate and safe water supplies, and insanitary disposal of excreta (WHO 1991a). Other suggested links have been an over-burdened medical service and poor communications (Ferguson 1975), and peoples' lack of commitment to maintaining a sanitary environment in post colonial areas, the maintenance of which they consider to be the sole responsibility of the Government (Adesina 1987). Rapid increase in incidence of gastrointestinal infections, such as cholera and dysentery, has also been linked to the importation of pathogens by migrants from rural areas where disease is endemic (WHO 1986), or amongst groups of newly arriving refugees to camps, such as has been described by Mulholland (1985) in an account of a cholera epidemic in a refugee camp in eastern Sudan in 1985.

However, the last few years have also thrown up extensive new information on the nature of some diseases and their terrains demanding a further extension of geographical research on health. In particular, in the case of cholera, this relates to the role of primary transmission of the pathogen from its ecological niche in environmental reservoirs (Colwell and Huq 1994; Drasar and Forrest 1996), a feature which is thought to influence the distribution of the disease (Collins 1993, 1996). Indication of key mechanisms involved in this process would help explain some of the recent surges of incidence linked to the massive seventh pandemic affecting South America and Africa and the appearance of the new *Vibrio cholerae* 0139 strain in India. In contrast the role of environmental reservoirs has been rarely studied for dysentery, for which the human body is still believed to be the only reservoir. Though some recently emerged microbiological information on dysentery (Islam *et al.* 1993a) suggests this assumption may be an oversimplification, there is no evidence of the role of specific physiological stresses and optima in the environment, as has been indicated for cholera.

Geoecology of Cholera and Bacillary Dysentery

Interest in the changing biology of cholera, the continued and widespread suffering it causes, and its importance as a global issue has rightfully been reflected by a recent increase of both specialist and non-specialist academic papers published in a wide range of journals. Some generalised reviews on the current state of knowledge of cholera, that include accounts of recent discoveries on pathogen ecology, are provided by Barua and Greenough (1992), Shears (1994), and Nalin (1994). In terms of output of published material, bacillary dysentery has not been so heavily represented, though this has started to change with the recent onset of epidemics associated with *Shigella dysenteriae* 1. It has therefore not been clear to what extent results from research on the changing status of cholera are important to investigations on incidence of bacillary dysentery and other bacterial diseases. Part of the strategy of this research is to compare the known nature of one in contrast to that of the other in the situation of epidemics of both in Mozambique. This is to determine if the known differences in the nature of the respective pathogens is a distinguishable feature explaining distributions of incidence in affected sub-regions.

Environmental Reservoirs and Vibrio Cholerae

One of the more significant recent developments in the study of cholera relates to information derived from laboratory research carried out in the 1980s. This has pointed to the existence of aquatic environmental reservoirs in which *Vibrio cholerae* survives for prolonged periods of time and from which a toxigenic form, under certain conditions of temperature, alkalinity and salinity, may emerge to support epidemic conditions (Miller *et al.* 1984, 1985, 1986; Barua and Greenough 1992). The need for attention to be paid to the possibility of these pools existing in nature was suggested after laboratory investigation into the impact of physio-chemical stress on *Vibrio cholerae* 01 (Miller *et al.* 1984, 1986). Work by Miyaki *et al.* (1967), Pandit *et al.* (1967), and Prescott and Bhattacharjee (1969) had earlier suggested survival times dependent on factors such as temperature, pH, osmotic pressure, moisture content, salt or carbohydrate concentration, and the presence of organic matter and bacterial flora as key factors in determining survival times in different foodstuffs. Alkaline mediums are widely used for laboratory culturing of *Vibrios*. Experimental studies have shown that gastric acid is one of the body's main lines of resistance against cholera (Cash *et al.* 1974) and *Vibrios* are known to be unable to survive in carbonated water due to its low pH (WHO 1986).

Other investigations carried out on water suggested the key factors to be temperature, pH, salt, bacterial and organic content (Singleton *et al.* 1982; Colwell and Spira 1992). Shellfish have often been suspected of spreading cholera and several recent studies in coastal areas of the USA have served to reawaken the possibility of the non-human animal reservoir (Kaysner *et al.* 1987; Doran *et al.* 1989). The aquatic reservoir and the non-human animal reservoir theories are open to convergence, in that the feature of a brackish environment can be considered common to both circumstances. This has recently been emphasised further by the isolation of *Vibrio cholerae* 01 from intestines and skin of fish in polluted coastal waters along the coastline of Peru (Tamplin and Parodi 1991) and *Vibrio cholerae* 01 and 0139 in plankton in Bangladesh (Tamplin and Gauzens *et al.* 1990; Islam and Miah *et al.* 1994; Huq and Colwell *et al.* 1995).

However, survival in aquatic environments with favourable conditions has been only part of the accumulated findings from research on *Vibrio cholerae*. It is also now believed that toxigenic isolates of *Vibrio cholerae* 01 and other *Vibrios* are able to enter a period of dormancy in unfavourable environments (Xu *et al.* 1982; Colwell *et al.* 1985, 1992). If in addition to nutrient depletion, the cells are subjected to reduction in temperature and/or elevation in salinity, the cells rapidly go nonculturable but remain viable and potentially pathogenic (Colwell *et al.* 1985). This would mean that in the past potentially toxigenic pathogens capable of causing major epidemics of cholera have remained hidden in the natural environment. New techniques of isolation which use fluorescent antibody or gene probes help overcome this problem of evasion, meaning that an entirely new appreciation of the space-time distribution of *Vibrio cholerae* and incidence of cholera is possible. There are also possibly new implications for understanding the distribution and behaviour of many other bacterial enteric pathogens.

Linked to these developments, Martins *et al.* (1993) partly explain a low number of positive samples from sewage water in Brazil between 1974 to 1983 in terms of the ability of *Vibrio cholerae* 01 to undergo environmental adaptation and be non-culturable. Martins *et al.* conclude that *Vibrio cholerae* 01 was therefore likely to be already present in the aquatic environment of Sao Paulo prior to the present outbreak of cholera in that country. However, Wachsmuth *et al.* (1993) state that there is still no real evidence of a nontoxigenic precursor for the toxigenic Latin American isolates and that the neighbouring isolates found along the U.S Gulf Coast are not directly related to them. The Latin American isolates are considered more likely to be a clonal variant of the 7th pandemic that has been described elsewhere as being introduced by travellers. Wachsmuth (1993) and Vugia *et al.* (1994) also draw attention to a shift from Inaba to Ogawa serotype within the Latin American clone between 1991 and 1992 (Figure 1.6). The high number of cases associated with each phase suggest some form of selective pressure but little further insight on this is available yet.

The findings of Salazar-Lindo (1993) suggest that the Latin American isolates are clonal but distinct from the other three clones; the seventh pandemic, the US Gulf Coast, and the Australian isolates. He suggests that the toxigenic cholera *Vibrio* organism was introduced into the aquatic environment of the Peruvian coast long before the outbreak flourished and long enough to evolve into a different clone. Further to this, instability in the *ctx* genes in the chromosomes of the recently appeared 0139 isolates in Bengal and Bangladesh has been reported as unusual (Lida *et al.* 1993, p926) and 'could be key to understanding the genetic mechanism for the sudden appearance of 0139 strain' (Figure 1.6). Waldor and Mekalanos (1994a, 1994b) point to possible evolutionary aspects of the genetic structure and virulence factors, including the similar chromosomal organisations of the *ctx* element, as proof of the close relationship between serotype 01 and 0139. Questions of gradual evolution or genetic instability leading to 'spontaneous appearance' of the toxigenic form of the organism are likely to contribute to an ongoing debate on the biogeography of *Vibrio cholerae* into the future.

Some key points to bear in mind when considering microbial evolution in general are that because of their relatively short generation times, as compared to higher organisms, changes in the genetic information of micro-organisms can be widely and rapidly disseminated. Genetic information may be changed in a favourable way for the micro-organism introducing information into the gene pool that can make an organism more fit for competing with other organisms and for surviving in the environment. Also, overspecialisation in the gene pool can lead to temporary success of a population under a single set of conditions but ultimately may lead to nonadaptation. Therefore some micro-organisms possess features that make them better adapted for survival in a particular ecosystem (Atlas and Bartha 1993, p30).

A further topic of major interest is environmental change that impacts on the nature of the organism. Drasar (1992, p368) has stated that 'survival is only part of the story' and that the implication of an aquatic reservoir is that 'they form an essential component of the ecosystem'. Interaction takes place between the dormant/starved non-toxigenic *Vibrios* and the environmental reservoir, and between hypertoxigenic strains and people who become cholera patients. He also draws attention to possible continuity in the action of cholera toxin in these reservoirs and the intestine. The ecosystem hypotheses opens up much insight to distributions of *Vibrio cholerae* at micro and macro scale and forms a good basis from which to begin an analysis of the role of environmental change.

Environmental Change and Cholera

There now exists background information to indicate that different biotypes and serotypes of *Vibrio cholerae* inhabit distinct zones determined by a combination of spatially defined environmental preferences and the relative immunity of the population that occupy an area.

Craig (1988) signalled caution in making generalisations in comparing epidemics of different biotypes when analysing time-space clustering of cholera in Matlab, Bangladesh. Spatial differentiation between biotypes has been demonstrated in Bangladesh during the epidemics of 1988-1989 (Siddique *et al.* 1991), where there was clustering of the classic biotype in the southern region and of the El Tor biotype in all other regions. Whilst the reason for the interplay between *Vibrio cholerae* 01 biotypes in Bangladesh was not entirely clear, the ecological changes in various regions, caused by soil erosion and construction of barrages and dams in the river system were thought to be possible associating factors. This was because the appearance of the El Tor biotype coincided with increasingly severe flooding in the north-eastern and middle-belt regions. Siddique reasons that since El Tor is hardier and more viable in water than the older classic biotype, it may have found a more suitable habitat in those areas. Also, a drastic reduction of fresh water flow caused by the Farakka barrage in the catchment area changed the dry season hydrodynamics in southern Bangladesh and resulted in an increase in salinity and incursion of brackish water deeper inland. Siddique suggested that the classic biotypes in the south may have become adapted to this changing environment.

Interestingly, *Vibrio cholerae* 0139 may be even hardier with a survival advantage over *Vibrio cholerae* 01. Islam *et al.* (1993b) note that whereas *Vibrio cholerae* 01 is normally isolated from less than 1 per cent of water samples during epidemics, 12 per cent of water samples in his study of 92 water samples from ponds, lakes, rivers, and canals in rural Matlab and urban Dhaka, Bangladesh yielded *Vibrio cholerae* 0139. Also, attention is drawn here to the much higher toxigeneity of the new serogroup (Islam *et al.* 1993b). A reciprocal seasonal pattern in prevalence of *Vibrio cholerae* 0139 with *Vibrio cholerae* 01, identified by Jesudason and Jacob John (1993) also implies a tendency for one strain to fill the niche of the other in response to a controlling environmental factor. However, it can also be noted that *Vibrio cholerae* 0139 has been reported as having an overall similarity with *Vibrio cholerae* 01 El Tor (Higa *et al.* 1993; Mahalanabis *et al.* 1994).

The replacement of the classical biotype by the El Tor biotype in the Bay of Bengal in 1991 and the subsequent displacement of the El Tor biotype by the new 0139 strain has prompted further speculation on the role of pollution of major rivers with agricultural and industrial waste (Siddique 1994). Adverse effects on the organisms caused by the pollution may have given a selection advantage for the new strains. Observation of the nature of previous pandemics of cholera should now warn us that the distribution of the more recent serogroup is unlikely to be explained solely in terms of the biology of the organism or the host but indeed also through differences in exposure to its habitat. Two factors stand out as particularly important. First, non-01 serotypes are known to be widely prevalent in natural aquatic environments (Mandal 1993) and secondly, previous infection with the El Tor serotypes does not provide immunity to infection from *Vibrio cholerae* 0139 (Bhattacharya *et al.* 1993; Mahalanabis *et al.* 1994).

Reports from the cholera epidemic in Angola also present a situation of shifting serotypes (Colombo *et al.* 1993). In 1988 all strains were Ogawa, and by 1991 the prevalent epidemic strain was also Ogawa, but by 1992 this had changed to Inaba, identified both in patients and in the Bengo river which serves the Luanda piped water system. As in the case of Mozambique, this pattern might relate to environmental and/or demographic change caused by major instability.

Global changes in distribution may also be partly dependent on *Vibrio cholerae* being able to survive in coastal waters with other salt water organisms, such as algae and plankton. The association with plankton has become increasingly apparent, though survival without active proliferation occurs in its absence (Huq and Colwell *et al.* 1995, p1249). Since successful multiplication of *Vibrio cholerae* is dependent on temperature, pH, salinity and available nutrients, it is reasonable to postulate changes in distribution similar to that displayed by some oceanic algal and plankton blooms. Epstein (1992) has suggested that the recent pattern of cholera in the Americas may represent the first detectable impact of climatic change on the distribution of water-based and vector-borne diseases. Some evidence for this is that unusually large algae and plankton blooms were reported at sea at the same time as plankton in the harbour near Lima, Peru was found to be contaminated with *Vibrio cholerae* (Tamplin and Parodi 1991). Epstein points out that the unexpected intensity of the outbreak, which penetrated cities and towns along the Pacific coast in January and February, 1991, was consistent with multiple entry points from marine life blooms, with fish, molluscs, and crustacea as vectors.

Environmental change at the global scale may affect cholera pandemics due to *Vibrio cholerae* being sensitive to the physical parameters of temperature, alkalinity, and salinity. In addition to changes in the salinity of aquatic reservoirs, salinization of a surface environment in some regions can occur through continual addition of water, lack of drainage, and high evaporation rates. Excess compounds such as sodium chloride, magnesium and calcium carbonate, and sulphate are precipitated on the soil surface or in the soil pores and then raised to ground level by capillary action. In time this process becomes evident in a white surface, characteristic of 'white alkali' soils (Tivy and O'Hare 1989, p134). Additionally, where there is a high concentration of free sodium chloride in the soil, downward leaching produces compounds of sodium with either carbonates or hydroxides, both of which make the soil solution excessively alkaline. As organic matter is dispersed and goes into solution, when the soils eventually dry out they become highly compacted and impermeable. They become covered with a black surface scum of very alkalinized organic matter, known as 'black alkalis', which are practically sterile (Tivy and O'Hare 1989, p135). A correlation between these zones, reservoirs of higher quantities of *Vibrio cholerae* and incidence of cholera has never been investigated, but white and black alkalis are often a part of the landscape of urban and semi-urban environments in cholera endemic areas.

A further factor relating to global climate and environmental change is a link between agricultural productivity, nutritional well-being and incidence of cholera, since malnutrition predisposes to higher rates of infection (Cash *et al.* 1974; Nalin *et al.* 1978; Thomason *et al.* 1981). Also, where there are reduced amounts of clean fresh water due to lowered rainfalls, people can be forced to drink from fewer and more contaminated sources. These issues are dealt with in more detail later in this book.

Bacillary Dysentery

The term dysentery was used by Hippocrates to indicate a condition characterised by frequent passage of stools containing blood and mucus accompanied by straining and painful defecation (DuPont 1990). At the end of the last century amoebic dysentery, caused by *Entamoeba histolytica*, was differentiated from the bacillary form caused by *Shigellae* organisms, now known to be some of the most highly communicable enteric pathogens. The higher prevalence of the bacillary form has lead to the term shigellosis and bacillary dysentery being almost interchangeable. *Shigellae* are gram-negative rods that are members of the family *Enterobacteriaceae* and as such virtually indistinguishable from certain strains of enterohemorrhagic *Escherichia coli*. Approximately 40 serotypes of *Shigella* are divided into four groups depending on serologic similarity (Figure 1.6). The subgroup of strains that is particularly virulent, has caused widespread morbidity and mortality both in the past and present, and which affects the regions focused upon in this book is *Shigella dysenteriae* 1, sometimes referred to as the classical Shiga bacillus. It is distinguished by high case fatality and extreme debility in survivors (WHO 1988).

The microbial ecology of *Shigella dysenteriae* 1 has some distinct differences to that of *Vibrio cholerae*. To date *shigellae* have been found to have a uniquely low infective dose requiring only 10 to 500 organisms to cause dysentery (WHO 1988; DuPont *et al.* 1989; Lima and Lima 1993) as opposed to 10^8 for *Vibrio cholerae* and 10^5 - 10^{10} for *Salmonella* species (Cash *et al.* 1974; Blaser and Newman 1982). As a better host adapted organism, it is widely understood that humans are the only important reservoir and that the major mode of transmission is person to person (WHO 1988; Keusch and Bennish 1989). Persistence of *Shigella dysenteriae* in human communities was demonstrated by Ferreccio *et al.* (1991) who found that the pathogen could be isolated from one or more of a sample group of 360 children, in Santiago, Chile throughout 99 of 120 calendar weeks surveyed. This was considered as indicating existence of a detectable human reservoir in that area.

The search for evidence of environmental reservoirs of *Shigellae* has been given much less attention than for cholera, although in Bangladesh epidemiological work has shown that surface water sources such as ponds, lakes, wells, and rivers can act as sources of infection (Khan *et al.* 1979; Islam *et al.* 1993a). Ebright *et al.* (1984) reported that cultures from two of three surface water sites in north-east Zaire grew gram-negative enteric organisms but no *Shigellae,* though at the same time suggested contamination of these sites could be one of the causes of dysentery in that region. Part of the reason that environmental reservoirs have generally been classified as insignificant in the case of bacillary dysentery may be due to the difficulty of isolating small infective doses in large quantities of media, but also that *Shigellae* may have been capable of a viable but nonculturable state, and therefore evaded detection. The development of polymerase chain reaction and fluorescent-antibody techniques for detection of nonculturable but viable *Shigella dysenteriae* 1 (Islam *et al.* 1992, 1993a) is now providing some evidence of previously misunderstood survival.

The inference of the laboratory work carried out by Islam *et al.* (1993a) on microcosms containing water collected from various surface waters is that *Shigella dysenteriae* 1 may also survive for extended periods in natural aquatic environments after deposition by humans. This however still varies from the case of *Vibrios* for which there is strong evidence that they are autochthonous to the aquatic environment. Studies by Bratoeva and John, Jr. (1994) support the hypothesis that R-plasmid transfer may occur between non-pathogenic, faecal strains and pathogenic *Shigellae,* but in comparison with the recently emerged information for cholera *Vibrios,* little clear information on interactions of this kind has been established.

Little work has been carried out on the influences of possible environmental stresses on survival time and toxigeneity of *Shigella dysenteriae* because of the notion that environmental reservoirs were not important to dysentery ecology. However, the organisms are generally known to be more acid resistant in the stomach than cholera. Gorden and Small (1993) suggest that survival at low pH is a stochastic characteristic of the population rather than a result of the presence of genetically altered variants, but that they are primed for ingestion and survival through the stomach. However, the particular case of *Shigella dysenteriae* 1 does not seem to have been clearly included in this analysis. DuPont *et al.* (1989) suggests the resistance of *Shigellae* to acid is due to its ability to rapidly invade the gastric epithelial cells.

Explanations for the interplay between endemic and epidemic situations also remain unclear, though secondary transmission mechanisms are more identifiable than in the case of cholera. It is likely that Shiga bacillus subsisted at a very low level in Central America prior to the epidemic that affected 100,000 people there in 1969 (Mata *et al.* 1970). Also, molecular epidemiologic techniques reveal that recent Mexican isolates of *Shigella dysenteriae* 1 were chromosomally similar to earlier Central American isolates and distinct from Asian and African strains. This indicates that the 1988 outbreak in Mexico was caused by strains present in Central America since at least 1962 (Strockbine *et al.* 1991). Two isolates of *Shigella dysenteriae* 1 in Zaire (Ebright 1984) were found to be of the same strain but different to isolates obtained from Indonesia at that time. However Haider *et al.* (1988) using plasmid analysis of *Shigella dysenteriae* 1 obtained from widely scattered cross continental locations suggested there may be one genetically related group of strains with plasmids which appear to constitute a stable gene pool and which has persisted over several years.

Data produced by Blaser *et al.* (1992) also supported the hypothesis that the Central American epidemic was not caused by introduction of a new more virulent strain from elsewhere and that the South Asian clone of *Shigella dysenteriae* 1, which has existed in several parts of the world during three decades, is responsible for both epidemic and endemic situations. This is confirmed by Bhattacharya *et al.* (1994) in India who note that *Shigella dysenteriae* 1 has now become the predominant endemic cause of dysentery in Calcutta although it did not appear there before the 1984 epidemic which was caused by the same pathogen. However increased incidence resulting from the introduction of new strains from the same clone is a significant factor for some areas, as was shown in the case of Thailand where the disease was endemic until the late 1960s and then virtually disappeared until 1986 when a large epidemic took place due to the new variation (Taylor *et al.* 1989).

As with *Vibrio cholerae,* questions of evolution of pathogens *in situ* or importation of new or modified versions from elsewhere to zones with less resistance is important in assessing the relative importance of local environmental changes, processes of transferability and vulnerability of people. Generally, despite decades of research, uncertainty remains over whether it is microbial factors or changing host variables that leads to the development of dysentery. Cruz *et al.* (1994) favour the former after researching Guatemalan children and finding that age, gender, nutritional status and feeding habits did not affect the outcome of *Shigellae* infection, though agreeing that immunity of the host to specific *Shigellae* serotypes may be functional for prolonged periods after natural exposure. However, the sample used did not include sufficient cases of all strains, and does not necessarily apply to the case of *Shigella dysenteriae* 1. By way of contrast, Blaser *et al.* (1992) dismiss the theory of a change in the organism as being the more significant causal factor in the Central American epidemic. They suggest rather that the epidemic was due to the endemic strain, changes in socio-economic or hygienic conditions, or changes in the specific herd immunity of the population.

The current state of knowledge of *Shigellae* supports less of a direct link with specific physical environmental changes and ecology than is becoming apparent for the case of cholera, though indirectly environmental changes that impact on human-well-being are implicated. Significant direct associating factors that may influence the disease organism appear to be more a function of the human body as reservoir and behavioural factors that relate to infection from diarrhoeal disease in general. However broader principles of diversity reduction are likely to apply. For example, widespread use of standard drugs for treatment of dysentery is causing universal contrary reactions from the pathogen through emergence of drug resistant strains (Table 1.1). Increased homogeneity, in this case combined with the apparent inability of the medical establishment to counteract fast enough with new drugs, could signify an increasing struggle to effectively treat infection. Resistance to antibiotics as a treatment for infected people, can be considered as similar to adaptation and survival in an environmental reservoir. It is possible that this has played a major role in the well documented diminishing efficacy of a series of drugs for treating bacillary

Table 1.1 Reports of resistance of *Shigellae* to antibiotic treatment

Author	Location of study
Khan, *et al.* (1979)	Dhaka urban area, Bangladesh
Ebright, *et al.* (1984)	Rural north-east Zaire
Eko and Utsalo (1991)	Calabar, Nigeria
Taylor, *et al.* (1991)	Bangkok, Thailand
Paquet (1992)	Lisungwi refugee camps, Malawi
Bennish *et al.* (1992)	Bangladesh
Lima and Lima (1993)	Multiple locations
Bhattacharya *et al.* (1994)	Calcutta, India
Ries *et al.* (1994)	Burundi
Lijima, *et al.* (1995)	Kenya

dysentery.

Classifications of diarrhoeal diseases often group dysentery with those which are water-washed, as opposed to water-borne diseases such as cholera (White *et al.* 1972; Bradley 1977). However, differentiation between diarrhoeal diseases on the basis of water quality for consumption and water quantity for washing can be inappropriate as contamination occurs between the two regardless of availability. Further to this it should be borne in mind that several studies, such as those of Sandiford *et al.* (1990) and Gorter *et al.* (1991) have found greater correlation between diarrhoeal disease and a range of other associations, such as the proximity of a water supply, owning a latrine, and a mother's level of schooling. These results reflect some of those of Daniels *et al.* (1990) in a case-control study of the impact of improved sanitation on diarrhoea morbidity in Lesotho. The following sub-section includes further assessment of the combined roles of both water quality and quantity with specific reference to the seasonality of cholera and dysentery.

Seasonality of Cholera and Bacillary Dysentery

There are two main aspects of seasonality and disease. One relates to changes in climate and local environments that influence pathogens, the other to the well-being and behaviour of people who become more vulnerable at certain times of year. Whilst each factor may be capable of causing disease, the spatial and temporal coincidence of the two multiplies the probability of a major outbreak. For example, reduced water supply can mean simultaneous increases in exposure to pathogen laden drinking water and reduced nutritional well-being through loss of crops. The dichotomous nature of seasonal influence, dependent on changing environmental aspects of disease pathogens and the vulnerability of people, varies for different diseases and at different locations.

Seasonality of Cholera and Vibrio Cholerae

Whereas the WHO reported in 1970 that not much was known about the seasonality of cholera (WHO 1970), we are well informed on the seasonal role of estuarine salinity, climate, water availability and quality, agricultural output, and human mobility all of which, it has been suggested, may influence cholera. Miller *et al.* (1982) have shown how the salinity of estuaries fluctuates in accordance with seasonal variation in river flow and, with reference to Calcutta and London in the nineteenth-century, suggested this may explain the seasonality of cholera in estuarine cities. Colwell and Spira (1992) suggested the seasonality of cholera in Bengal may be explained by primary transmission controlled by environmental factors such as temperature, salinity, nutrient concentration, and zooplankton blooms; as well as by seasonal variations in seafood harvesting and consumption, and in direct water contact. Salinity in estuarine zones is likely to relate to cholera incidence both directly and indirectly. Firstly, salinity may be a direct environmental control on survival times and toxigeneity of *Vibrio cholerae*, as has already been described. Secondly, it will affect the availability of potable water supplies, as occurs when a freshwater pumping site becomes too saline during a drought, or when wells are made inactive by a change in the balance of fresh and saline groundwater in a zone of wells.

Many studies on cholera incidence include the role of rainfall in seasonal variation. However, these have revealed a variety of patterns between the epidemic curve and monthly rainfall pattern and a variety of explanations are given of principal causal mechanisms. Two patterns of incidence in relation to patterns of rainfall are broadly;

- the epidemic curve steeply rising during the rainy season and dropping off with the coming of the dry season; and

- the epidemic curve taking off in the driest period of the year and being sustained throughout the rains before tailing off.

An example of the first pattern has been provided by Mbwette (1987) for Tanzania and of the second by Utsalo *et al.* (1992) in Calabar, Nigeria. For different locations in Bangladesh the pattern has been reported as variable by McCormack *et al.* (1969) who noted that in Dhaka, the cholera season was during the dry winter months (December and January), but in nearby rural areas a second epidemic occurred during May-July. Moe *et al.* (1991) explain their result of no significant seasonal difference of diarrhoea in the Philippines, as being due to a lack of seasonal differences in rainfall. Meanwhile Sandiford *et al.* (1989) found that, whilst there was an overall correlation between higher rainfall and faecal contamination in rural Nicaragua, protected wells had higher average levels of contamination than others during the dry period, presumably due to intense usage of a diminished quantity of water.

These differences may support the view that patterns of faecal contamination which increases during the wet season do not serve as definitive indicators of cholera seasonality if *Vibrio cholerae* is controlled by an additional range of environmental stress factors. This is supported by the findings of Ventura *et al.* (1992) who, in monitoring non-01 *Vibrio cholerae* in Lima sewage lagoons, show that a seasonal variation in incidence of cholera was distinct but that there was no correlating seasonal variation of faecal coliforms. Moe *et al.* (1991) conclude that quantification of indicator bacteria such as faecal coliforms may mislead in that only beyond a certain threshold will they correlate well with incidence of diarrhoea. In some instances better directed attention may be towards important factors in transmission subsequent to collecting water. For example, sampling of stored household water often reveals that contamination with bacteria continues to take place after collection. This has been shown by Awad el Karim *et al.* (1985), Deb *et al.* (1986), Lindskog and Lindskog (1988), and Swerdlow *et al.* (1992). A seasonal pattern to post collection contamination is more likely to be related to varying ability to care for personal hygiene with the seasonal abundance or scarcity of water. However, with respect to rainfall and the environment, consideration might also be given to the implications of more favourable reservoirs for *Vibrio cholerae* as wells become more saline but still potable during the dry season. This combined with lower water levels and increased concentration of *Vibrios* might account for surges of cholera in coastal areas during a dry period.

Temperature has also been considered to be a direct controlling factor on cholera. In the nineteenth century, there were summer outbreaks of cholera between the isotherms of 60°F and 80°F and limits of 2-4 inches per month of rain (May 1960). We are now able to consider the mechanisms behind this correlation, such as the possible role or synonymous behaviour of large algal and plankton blooms which increase with higher temperatures. The seasonal variation in nutrient levels in aquatic reservoirs caused by increased use of fertilisers and runoff from irrigation may also play a role here. Should both factors be operative, natural seasonal cycles and human activities have combined to produce a potential vector for cholera. Seasonal difference in sunlight is a relevant factor if *Vibrio cholerae* in drinking water is reduced by direct ultraviolet irradiation (Acra *et al.* 1989). However a study by Mackenzie *et al.* (1992) carried out in Ecuador found that there was only a reduction in *Vibrios* for bottled water at the high altitude site of Quito and little change at the low altitude site of Santo Domingo. The affects of U.V. radiation in the natural cholera reservoirs of the world is a complex factor not only of season but of altitude, availability of shade, and depth of penetration into the epilimnion of water bodies. The complexity of sunlight patterns most likely renders its relevance as only minor as an identifiable controlling factor.

The variability and contrasts of accounts outlined above indicate that seasonal physical changes affecting the survival and virulence of *Vibrio cholerae* are inconclusive, and that on their own they are unlikely to explain the temporal patterns of incidence at all locations. Rather, they are part of a wider equation which includes variation of human well-being and behaviour that affect susceptibility to disease. Further examination of these influences is presented in Chapter 2.

Seasonality of Bacillary Dysentery

Though seasonality of dysentery has also been recorded in relation to changes in rainfall and temperature, a lack of any clear evidence of significant biogeophysical stress on the bacteria, other than the case of pH in the stomach, means the role of geophysical seasonal processes outlined for cholera are not considered important.

Reported correlations of dysentery with seasons are also varied. Hossain *et al.* (1990) report an endemic situation all year round but a distinct epidemic peak in the monsoon season of July and August, with a smaller one in November, for the Teknaf coastal area of Bangladesh. Ferreccio *et al.* (1991) draw attention to significant increases in incidence during the warm months of the year for Santiago, Chile whilst Taylor (1991) reports a clear increase with the hot dry season in Thailand. In Africa, Eko and Utsalo (1991) draw attention to a 74 per cent isolation rate during the dry season in contrast to 25.9 per cent in the wet season for Calabar, Nigeria. Ries *et al.* (1994) refer to a sharp seasonal increase in cases of dysentery that has occurred in Burundi between September and December every year since 1980, when surveillance began. Interestingly, Ebright *et al.* record no apparent effect of the change from dry to rainy season for nearby north-eastern Zaire. Keusch and Bennish (1989) mention seasonal patterns that vary from place to place referring to peak infection in the hot dry season for Bangladesh and Egypt and peak infection in the monsoon season for India, whilst in Guatemala just before and during the first part of the rains.

Because only small quantities of *shigellae* cause infection there is more evidence that they are conducive to transmission by flies than there is for cholera. One study in the specific circumstance of army camps in Israel, where open latrine trenches were in use, reports that reduction of houseflies using traps caused a 42 per cent drop in clinic visits for diarrhoeal diseases and an 85 per cent drop for shigellosis (Cohen *et al.* 1991). Consistent with this, Levine and Levine (1991, p693) draw attention to the historical documentation of correlation between seasonal prevalence of flies and incidence of dysentery, though this association lacks evidence of a singular causative link. A seasonal convergence of factors is implicit in conclusion to their own research which says that 'in some geographical areas where sanitation is poor, in certain seasons, houseflies can play an important role in transmitting Shigella dysentery.'

It is not entirely clear to what extent some explanations that have been promoted for increased cholera in wet and dry seasons apply for bacillary dysentery or vice versa. However, risk of transmission due to water contamination after collection could be a greater factor for dysentery since less organisms are capable of increased transmissibility.

Conclusion

Health status with respect to enteric disease, such as cholera and dysentery, is associated with systemic processes of environmental, demographic and developmental change, effecting both the ecology of the pathogen and people who become infected. Though spatial perspectives on disease incidence have progressed from seeking association of singularly defined phenomena, there is a need for greater understanding of the influence of complexes of factors that interact at a variety of scales.

Recent microbiological advances on the nature of *Vibrio cholerae* reveal new information on its ecology. However, the role of this in shaping incidence of cholera has not been adequately included in field investigations of affected locations. There is less detailed information and understanding of the ecology of bacillary dysentery, typically associated with *Shigella dysenteriae,* but sufficient to indicate less of a role for environmental reservoirs than for the case of *Vibrio cholerae.* Field studies are able to compare and contrast patterns of incidence and association for the two diseases to confirm or negate the influence of environmental reservoirs on incidence of cholera and its relative non-influence on dysentery. This in turn can contribute to better understanding of the variable role of biological, environmental, and social causality for each.

The seasonal dimensions of water quality and water quantity have been found to be relevant in explaining temporal patterns of diarrhoeal disease. However, less emphasis has been given to understanding individual diseases in terms of spatial and temporal differences in human vulnerability and localised risk ecology. Clarification is needed on how and why factors relate to the host and to the terrain.

2 Human Vulnerability to Cholera and Bacillary Dysentery

The previous chapter has predominantly examined how biological and physical environmental factors may control the ecology of cholera and dysentery. This chapter examines the role of socio-economic and demographic factors that influence human vulnerability to incidence of cholera and dysentery. Subsections focus on the implications for human vulnerability to disease of seasonal change, population movement, forced displacement, and changing structural contexts.

Seasonality of the Host

The correlation of incidence of cholera with poverty has been well documented and is referenced in the previous chapter. Seasonal poverty relates to factors such as predisposing conditions of malnutrition and insufficient access to clean water at certain times of year. Since coping mechanisms are affected at these times of crisis, standards of personal and household hygiene can also be reduced. Further behavioural factors that are not necessarily linked to poverty might also include changes in diet, and cultural practices that occur at specific times of year. Some of these factors are well covered by Chambers *et al.* (1981) writing on seasonal dimensions to rural poverty. Support for the Chambers thesis that the existence of pronounced seasonality in morbidity is an indication of a lower level of overall development is demonstrated by the work of Bhardwaj and Rao (1988). They found that the seasonal changes in dysentery cases in rural Andhra Pradesh were more pronounced in the least developed region where sanitation was poorest, dropping below average for areas classified as high or moderate development for the greater part of the year, but surging above average with the rains (Figure 2.1).

At one level, the predisposing conditions of malnutrition are associated with immunologic responses to infection modified by

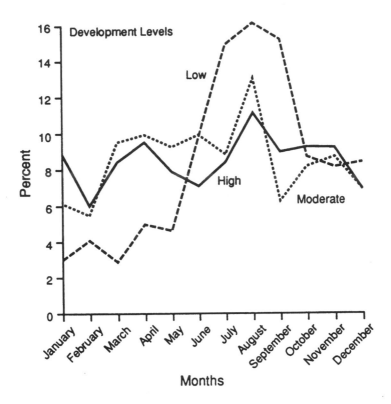

Figure 2.1 **Seasonal changes of dysentery cases by development regions of rural Andhra Pradesh**

Source: Bhardwaj and Rao, 1988, p.22

nutritional status (Scrimshaw *et al.* 1968). Hypochlorhydria through loss of gastric acids, which are one of the body's main lines of resistance against cholera, predisposes to higher incidence (Cash *et al.* 1974). If the evidence of Thomason *et al.* (1981) that acute malnutrition predisposes to hypochlorhydria is correct, then it is reasonable to suspect that this is the mechanism by which cholera selectively attacks the malnourished (Nalin *et al.* 1978). The patterns of infection take on a seasonal dimension because there is a direct association between agricultural productivity and biological vulnerability for communities dependent on primary subsistence.

Given that there is an interaction between malnutrition and cholera infection through the pathophysiology of the lower intestine, there can be further environmental and socio-economic factors that are related to nutrition. In a multivariate study of association of malnutrition and diarrhoea in children aged under five years in a rural Sudanese community, El Samani *et al.* (1988) found factors such as rainy season operated together with a general socio-economic effect. Arnold (1993) has illuminated how the seasonal onset of famine in nineteenth-century India resulted in the 'breakdown of normal social relations and produced a series of often dysfunctional behavioural responses' that influenced the spread of epidemic diseases such as cholera and dysentery. Survival strategies such as use of 'famine foods' and migration in search of food and work, facilitated disease in that the poor people's resistance was further weakened. Weakening came about by the extra outlay of energy necessary to gather enough marginal foods and because these were coarse and unpalatable or poisonous unless thoroughly cooked. Interestingly, a rice based diet, the indigenous staple diet of some of the world's enteric disease prone regions is indicated as highly effective in the management of persistent diarrhoea in terms of improved nutrient absorption (Roy *et al.* 1994). An extension of this discussion leads to a fundamental concept in holistic medicine in general, that the cause and remedies of sickness are found in the same place. Extraneous interference with this balance, such as occurred with the subsistence crises of nineteenth-century India, caused a breakdown of the relative protection to certain communicable disease epidemics provided by local ecologies and subsistence norms.

Non-availability of water is a major constraint in food hygiene and makes hand washing during food preparation and feeding a less frequent practice (Utsalo *et al.* (1992). During the dry season, contaminated surface streams and rivers often become the main sources of household water. This has been reported as a factor in Argentina near to the Bolivian Border (Chaudhary 1992) and by Utsalo *et al.* (1992) in Calabar, Nigeria. Utsalo (1992) suggests an intensification in fishing and trade in fishery products carrying increased *Vibrio* loads occurs in the hot dry season when estuarine waters are shallow, and that this is a factor in the seasonality of cholera. In Trujillo, Peru a multivariate study found that going to a fiesta was one of the associating factors as El Tor *Vibrio cholerae* 01 can grow rapidly in many of the cooked foods (Swerdlow *et al.* 1992). Increased seasonal mobility at planting and at harvest time and religious ceremonies that attract large numbers of people into a small area have been further factors correlating with general communicable disease transmission. Risks associated with spiritual sites on the Ganges and migration to Mecca are well known epidemic hazards of this type. A dramatic surge of cholera in

February 1992 in the Camiri area of Cordillera Province, Bolivia was found to be favoured by the mass gathering of Guaranì native Indians to commemorate the centenary of their last genocide (Guglielmetti *et al.* 1992).

Diffusion and Locational Vulnerability

The spread of disease cannot be explained without understanding the spatial variation of any one moment. There are no simple diffusion models that can be easily applied to communicable diseases, such as cholera and dysentery, which spread across space and through people. Non-uniformity of space guiding the diffusion of cholera and dysentery includes differences in environmental influence on *Vibrio cholerae* and possibly *Shigellae* spp., and variations in climate, settlement patterns, social and economic well-being, and culture.

Biological differences between people who are exposed to the pathogens constitute a further non-uniformity guiding cholera and dysentery transmission. For example, infants and the young are particularly susceptible to infection since they have established less immunity. Whilst immunity increases for adults exposed to a local pathogen, they have little resistance to new diseases, biotypes or serotypes introduced from elsewhere. There is evidence that biological differences, considered as risk factors in contracting cholera, also include lowered levels of gastric acid, not breast feeding, and presence of O blood group (Glass *et al.* 1985, 1991, 1992; Van Loom 1993; Swerdlow *et al.* 1994). In the case of shigellosis not breast feeding, exposure to the pathogen in the first years after breastfeeding, and immunity from previous infection have all been suggested (Ahmed *et al.* 1992, 1993; Huskins *et al.* 1994).

The local environment can influence differences in spread of cholera and dysentery since there is variation in the relationship between pathogens and diverse physical environmental and human biological conditions. The magnitude and direction of an epidemic may therefore be considered as being determined by predisposing, biological, socio-demographic and environmental circumstances. Against this background, more complex vectors are generated by human mobility between environmental zones with varying disease ecologies. This effect is particularly pronounced in situations of forced population displacement where the balance between infection and protection, sensitive to local environment and social organisation, is disrupted.

As the location and persistence of cholera and dysentery is determined by a combination of physical environmental phenomena, people, and pathogenesis, change to any one of these elements is likely to alter the distribution of cases. Diffusion of the disease therefore occurs against a backdrop of spatially defined environmental risk factors, a dynamic distribution of susceptible, infective and immune people, and the changing biology of the organism responsible. As mobility in the late 20th century has increased globally, potential opportunity for communicable disease transmission has broadened so that it is increasingly difficult to screen for disease carriers. Consequently, more can be learnt from identifying the nature of the terrain that forms the path of the disease and the sites in which it becomes established, than can be derived from individual cases of transmission. Further to this, an emphasis solely on processes of secondary transmission in explaining diffusion and distributions of cholera and dysentery is confounded by additional problems of identification and detection.[1]

The controlling effect of the aquatic environment on cholera diffusion has been hinted at by Marsden (1992) commenting on the spread of cholera down the Amazon basin. He suggests that the river Negro might be inimical to cholera as it has passed through large amounts of decomposed vegetable matter and is therefore acid in the range of pH 5-6, not suitable to *Vibrio cholerae*. The importance of surface water in transmission in rural Bangladesh has been recorded by Hughes *et al.* (1982). However, diffusion of diarrhoeal disease is also guided by areas with more vulnerable communities, the stakes being raised over time as the pathogen

---

[1] The ability of *Vibrio cholerae* to remain dormant in the environment and the problems this causes in detection of natural reservoirs has been outlined earlier. However, there is a further limitation if monitoring diffusion of the disease through routes of secondary transmission due to the high proportion of symptom-free carriers. This is particularly prevalent with the El Tor strain. Symptom-free infections, and mild to moderate cases of diarrhoea, have been known to outnumber severe cases by as much as 100 to 1, particularly where the disease is endemic (Woodward and Mosley 1971). The numbers of carriers of shigellae not displaying signs of infection has been recorded as up to 55.5% for above 10 age groups decreasing to 0% for descending age groups in Dacca, Bangladesh (Khan *et al.* 1979). In the Guatamalan epidemic up to half the infectives were believed to be symptomless (Gangarosa 1970). Routine public health strategies aimed at controlling the diffusion of the two diseases via infected persons are not effective as many infected travellers are probably symptom-free.

becomes more virulent and/or the herd immunity of a population decreases. Intensification of human vulnerability can relate to a decline in nutritional status through less productive soil and general land degradation. It can also be caused by habitation in marginalised low lying areas, increases in population density, deteriorating housing conditions, and the interactions between people and places that create more favourable disease niches.

The evidence of an association of high incidence of blood group O with high attack rates of cholera, as discovered in Trujillo, Peru illustrates that predisposition to ill-health could be genetic in some instances. Since blood group O is very prevalent in South America compared to other parts of the world, it may be significant in understanding rapid dispersal of the disease there (Swerdlow 1994). Meanwhile, further widespread evidence shows that localised socio-economic and behavioural factors determine the selectivity of disease amongst communities. In addition to the role of hypochlorhydria in famine situations detailed earlier, there are further recorded examples of how the body's metabolism can predispose to infection. These include alcoholism, which causes a loss of the resistant acids in the stomach (Hospedales 1992), and gastric hypoacidity from surgery, disease, or medication (Baine *et al.* 1974). Although investigations have shown that cholera can be transmitted by a variety of seafoods, lowering the pH during consumption of these same foods could inhibit transmission. Some evidence for the effectiveness of this strategy is provided by St Louis *et al.* (1990) who identified a lower risk of cholera in Conakry, Guinea when people ate the food with acidic tomato sauce (pH 3) rather than a neutral peanut-based sauce (pH 7). A similar approach is suggested by Mujica *et al.* (1994) who maintain that promotion of the consumption of toronja drink, which has a pH of 4.1, may be a useful cholera prevention strategy for the Amazon region of Peru, a theme which has also been upheld by Anand (1995) commenting on the use of lime juice in northern India.

Importantly, breast feeding has been demonstrated as beneficial in protecting children up to the age of 36 months against cholera in work carried out by Clemens *et al.* (1990) in rural Bangladesh. However, a study conducted by Bhattacharya *et al.* (1992) established that, in the cholera endemic area of Calcutta, about one-third of the admitted children up to the age of two years could have cholera and that even children below the age of 6 months were not spared, despite the fact that the average duration of predominant breast feeding was about 4.7 months since birth. Ahmed *et al.* (1993) and others have pointed out that higher risk of shigellosis during the weaning process could be due to either greater exposure to contaminated foods or to a decline in the intake of immune and non-immune antidiarrhoeal protective factors in breast milk, or both.

An additional public health problem caused by shigellosis is its impact on host nutritional status (Keusch and Bennish 1989; Henry 1991; Rahman *et al.* 1992). This may perpetuate infection or predispose to reinfection through malnutrition (Struelens 1990; Heikens *et al.* 1993). The synergistic nature of combinations of malnutrition and dysentery is the basis for a call by Henry (1991) for essential collaboration of social and biomedical scientists and more effective control programs. With respect to complexes of preconditioning host factors Fauveau *et al.* (1991) suggest a move away from a policy that solely emphasises use of the remedy Oral Rehydration Therapy (ORT) to a more multifaceted approach. The main challenge can be considered as the breaking of the cycle of susceptibility and infection that ensures persistence and concentration of ill-health in disease prone environments and amongst vulnerable people. High density slum areas in rapidly expanding Third World cities and concentrations of displaced people present high levels of risk resulting from the combination of living in inappropriate environments and reduced biosocial resistance. Once well established, there are numerous additional pathways through which secondary transmission can occur. Particularly virulent strains of disease, such as *Shigella dysenteriae* 1, easily spread to better off areas and social sectors, as was noted by Bernardino *et al.* (1993, p495) in Luanda, Angola. Increase in dysentery was suggested as being 'exacerbated by the season and the concentration of war refugees' but quickly spread to the better-housed families living towards the centre of the city normally spared from cholera.

Only a brief account of modes of diffusion of diarrhoeal disease through secondary transmission is presented here as literature on these is extensive elsewhere. They include factors such as drinking water contaminated during storage, unhygienic sanitation practices, going to festivals where food and beverages are prepared by multiple food-handlers, consumption of vegetables from farms irrigated by untreated sewage, and the transportation and sale of contaminated seafood. They are factors dependent on local cultures and on the behaviour of individuals and this accounts for the diversity of emphases that have been highlighted by different studies. For example, Traoré *et al.* (1994) found that in a study on diarrhoea in Burkina Faso it was not where the child defecates, but how the mother then deals with the child's stool that was the critical factor in transmission. Aziz *et al.* (1990) report reductions in incidence of diarrhoea, including dysentery, in a case control exercise in rural Bangladesh where modifications were made to environment and behaviour. Living closer to hand pumps and modification of sanitation habits were outlined as key changes. Other research in rural Bangladesh concluded that the simple presence of a latrine showed no evidence of decrease in paediatric shigellosis and that use of hanging latrines significantly affected risk (Ahmed *et al.* 1994).

Conteh *et al.* (1990) report that the supply of household water from a river or stream was associated with a 30 per cent higher risk of childhood mortality and that the effect of differential access to toilet facilities was unimportant once water supply was considered. However, other studies have suggested that improving sanitation has more impact than improving water supply (Feachem *et al.* 1983; Esrey and Habicht 1986; Esrey *et al.* 1985). Khan (1982) highlighted the positive interruptive effects of handwashing, even in insanitary environments. Taylor *et al.* (1991) suspected the young age of cooks, boiling water, use of storage containers and hand washing as key epidemiological aspects in spreading *Shigella dysenteriae* type 1 in a village epidemic in Ubon province, Thailand. Indices for overall cleanliness and kitchen hygiene, but not for more general living conditions, were associated with severe childhood diarrhoea in Manila, Philippines (Baltazar *et al.* 1993). Of interest here is that the general living conditions are suggested as having been below a level where socio-economic status showed enough variation to make any difference. This is a theme which is returned to for the case of urban Mozambique in Chapter 6.

Behaviour conducive to secondary diffusion of cholera and dysentery is also subject to the influence of cultural landscapes determining people's perceptions and expectations. For example, in the Muslim/Hindu context Zeitlyn *et al.* (1991) have shown how perceptions of cleanliness are not based on germ theory but rather in a larger socio-religious context of purity and spiritual need. Stemming from this area of enquiry, Nichter (1991) points out the need for gaining a knowledge of cultural contexts in understanding bloody diarrhoea and Kunstadter (1991) the importance of traditional etiologic models in promoting appropriate behaviour to reduce transmission.

Two key issues in behavioural studies on incidence of diarrhoeal diseases, mentioned by Pelto (1991), are useful in unravelling this complex of associations and are consistent with the approach to behavioural aspects represented in this book. Firstly, that behavioural risk factors are not only related to cultural practices but also to behaviours influenced or constrained by environmental conditions; and secondly, the need for identification of the antecedent factors that explain the distribution of positive or negative behaviours. These are factors which are relevant to spatial approaches to communicable diseases in that they are intrinsically and directly related to the underlying terrain that determines their distribution and spread.

Population Movement and Forced Displacement

The spread of cholera and dysentery through and across nations by mobile populations is dependent on who, when and why people travel. For example travel by people from developed countries into and out of endemic areas in the Third World has been proven to be relatively insignificant in terms of transmission, as such travellers are generally socially and economically less susceptible. One report put the risk of cholera to US nationals travelling to affected areas at one per 500,000 travellers (Snyder and Black 1982). In contrast, amongst the people living in the suburbs of Quelimane, Mozambique in 1991, many of whom were forcibly displaced from war affected rural areas, the rate was more typically 200 per 10,000 people. Identification of particular groups of mobile people, their varying characteristics, and associated activities is as important as identifying individual causal pathogens (Prothero 1977). Prothero identified a matrix of mobility in tropical Africa by time and space, indicating the associated health hazards in terms of physical or psychological stress and contact with new ecological zones and different groups of people.

Migrants to endemic areas may be exposed to pathogens to which they have little or no resistance. The same return migrants or new migrants from endemic areas may introduce new pathogens to areas previously unaffected by the disease or where a different strain has been endemic. Also migrants to new areas may be unfamiliar with appropriate behaviour that protects against disease in particular places. A good example of this is where rural people in Third World countries move to urban areas and do not adhere to the more rigorous sanitation behaviour needed to prevent disease in higher population densities. The length of a migrant's stay in a new area is therefore important in terms of both biological and cultural adaptation. A further factor relates to a migrant's socio-economic status as this determines the ability to defend against infection in terms of nutrition and acquiring facilities such as housing, water and safe sanitation. This is particularly the case with people from rural areas who are attracted to a perceived opportunity in a rapidly swelling Third World city, but who end up scraping a living in a poorer neighbourhood.

A further important factor in determining susceptibility to diseases such as cholera and dysentery may also be the degree to which migration is voluntary or forced, partly since this is often a reflection of how rapid the transition from one place to the next has been made. In the last two decades forced population movements have become part and parcel with epidemics of cholera and dysentery in Africa and Asia with a marked increase in the first part of the 1990s. Toole and Waldman (1993) report that diarrhoea and other enterically transmitted diseases routinely cause between 30 per cent and 50 per cent of deaths in displaced populations. High rates of malnutrition which often become the focus of attention in international assistance programs are sometimes associated with diarrhoeal disease rather that absolute food shortages. If forced population displacement occurs across borders, the displaced technically become refugees and may be moved into camps, where they are more exposed to the risks of disease and especially diarrhoeal disease, through environmental hazards and reduced personal resistance (Table 2.1).

The processes which cause high incidence of disease in the context of forced displacement are not yet fully understood and support a range of explanations. Whilst drawing attention to the importance of forced movements of population in tropical Africa, Prothero (1994, p657) concludes that they constitute a 'more exaggerated version of health hazards already experienced by most people in tropical Africa' and that 'unintentionally movements of all kinds create and exacerbate health hazards.' Relative similarity between migration and refugee movements is demonstrated by Dick (1984) who adapted existing typologies of migration factors relevant to disease for the specific case of refugees as follows: the pre-refugee situation, causes, the displacement period, arrival and initial responses, the camp, long term problems of adaptation, and the final settlement outcome.

The main factors leading to higher rates of incidence of communicable diseases in the refugee camps are outlined by Shears and Lusty (1987) as, a breakdown of health services, movement to new ecological zones,

Table 2.1   Studies reporting diarrhoea as the highest, or amongst the top few causes of morbidity and mortality in refugee situations

Author(s)	Location
Mulholland (1985)	Ethiopian refugee camp, eastern Sudan
Sørensen & Dissler (1986)	Ethiopian refugee camp, eastern Sudan
Shears & Lusty (1987)	Ethiopian refugee camps, eastern Sudan
Toole &Waldman (1988, 93)	Multiple locations cited
Moren & Bitar *et al.* (1991)	Mozambican refugee camps, Malawi
Moore & Marfin *et al.* (1993)	Somali camps, Somalia
Yip & Sharp (1993)	Kurdish refugee camps, Iraq border
Marfin *et al.* (1994)	Bhutanese refugee camps, Nepal
Goma Epidemiology Group (1995)	Rwandan refugee crisis, Zaire

malnutrition, crowding and the poor sanitation of camps. Meanwhile, Moore *et al.* (1993) highlight the pre-displacement period as vital to understanding post migration health status, pointing out that displaced persons may migrate because of pre-existing poor health, nutrition, and socio-economic conditions. Whilst there is good evidence of post-migration increases in morbidity and mortality in refugee camps, the weighting of influence of pre-migration and post-migration factors still lacks empirically based research, for these and other destinations of forcibly displaced people.

Increased susceptibility is likely to be a characteristic of forcibly displaced people since they generally experience deteriorated socio-economic conditions after surviving a period of pronounced instability. Survival systems of primary production and consumption which may have selectively adapted over long periods are disrupted. For example, people forced to migrate due to war or famine, such as in the case of Mozambique, may require several growing seasons to re-establish adequate levels of food production to become self sufficient again. Morbidity and mortality has been shown to be higher amongst displaced populations than for local resident populations in some instances. Toole and Waldman (1988) estimate that figures can be up to 40 times higher amongst refugees than for non-refugee populations in host countries.

Moore *et al.* (1993) found in comparing displaced and resident populations in central Somalia during the 1992 famine that, in towns, displaced people were at higher risk of dying than residents, and that displaced people in temporary camps were at the highest risk. Interestingly, dysentery caused by *Shigella dysenteriae* 1 was indicated as the biggest killer disease in their study. However, Bradford and Gessner (1994) report that the displaced and resident populations of Kabul, Afghanistan displayed a similar crude mortality rate apart from the younger than 5 age group. This was interpreted in terms of exceptional factors concerning the displaced people's employment achievements, previous residence in the city, support from non-displaced relatives and positive discrimination in the locating of health posts by aid agencies. Further to this, Van Damme (1995) draws attention to the fact that there were indications that Rwandan refugees in Zaire who settled outside camps and mixed with the local population fared better than those in the camps, and that refugees in Guinea suffered similar levels of illness to their host communities. These few reports demonstrate that ratios of displaced/non-displaced morbidity varies for different contexts and that model outcomes are not easily observable.

Little background information on differential patterns of health for the condition of being displaced or non-displaced in urban zones is available despite 58 per cent of all forced migration being to areas of existing habitation (US Committee for Refugees figure provided by Toole and Waldman 1993). Further to this, Dodge *et al.* (1987) complain of an associated lack of attention in the form of aid for disease stricken internally displaced people in Khartoum. They calculate that these people benefited from about US$2.50 per capita in comparison to US$73.00 per capita in refugee camps assisted by UNHCR. Despite intrinsic concern for the case of concentrations of displaced people selectively disadvantaged in urban areas, these situations have the potential to become the endemic focus of diseases such as cholera and dysentery. Suspicion of endemicity in the region was already raised in Eastern Sudan in the mid 1980s since two sources of cholera were responsible for epidemics, one caused by El Tor Inaba and the other by El Tor Ogawa (Mulholland 1985; Sørensen and Dissler 1986). Serotype Inaba was consistent with the main global epidemic strain at that time, but El Tor Ogawa extended from previously formed endemic areas of high population concentration in lowland areas of Ethiopia.

Forced Displacement and Environmental Change

The need to understand issues relating to refugees and environmental change has become increasingly important (Young 1985; Leach 1991; McGregor 1993; Black 1994a, 1994b; RPN 1995). It is maintained in this book that this extends to the need to understand issues of forced population movements and environmental health in and around existing urban areas. Dick (1985) suggests that the presence of refugees may cause impacts on the biological environment (including water and sanitation), and to the socio-economic environment (including unemployment and food prices altered as a result of incoming aid), with the result that health is affected. However, these interconnections, which are also apparent in some other accounts (Dick 1984; Prothero 1994), lack concrete field investigation for individual health problems. Also, in the light of recently emerged microbiological and epidemiological information, factors relating to the ecologies of high incidence diseases, such as cholera and dysentery, need to be specifically taken into account.

This book proposes that the identification of geographically defined risk areas and processes of change, such as those associated with resettlement and being displaced, are important to environmental health management. There can be changes in environmental location experienced by displaced people that expose them to increased disease hazards and/or make them more susceptible to health problems, and impacts on local environments that create more favourable conditions for disease, or variable combinations of these. Also, behavioural differences between displaced and host communities and behavioural changes associated with the prevailing conditions at different resettlement locations may be influential on health outcomes. Finally, the environmental context of settlement and disease, as with other health and environment issues, can be viewed with respect to wider issues of human development.

The Structural Context of Cholera and Bacillary Dysentery

In addition to proximate determinants of disease incidence, a number of elements of wider context are important. Structural phenomena determine the quality of water supply and sanitation, settlement patterns, population density, economic activity and environmental risks that impact on the distribution of cholera and dysentery. The environmental properties of climate, soil, rainfall, temperature, altitude and seasonality that have been listed as possible proximate determents of child mortality by Mosley and Chen (1984), and the added features of slope of terrain, population density and crowding within households listed by Blacker (1991), which affect disease distributions in particular ecological settings, are also influenced by wider structural changes. Meanwhile, health care structures and the effects of economic adjustment are further aspects of context that are relevant to incidence of cholera and bacillary dysentery.

Water and Sanitation as Infrastructure

If the provision of basic infrastructures were good enough the world over, it would be reasonable to imagine little opportunity for the faecal-oral route of *Vibrio cholerae* transmission and other pathogenic contamination. Incidence of diarrhoeal disease would be much more contained. However, a brief *résumé* of the state of the world's water and sanitation supply indicates that contamination through this route is not likely to be eradicated in the immediate future. In 1980 WHO estimated that only 20 per cent of the world's population had access to totally safe drinking water, that 80 per cent of all sick were suffering from diseases related to poor water and sanitation, and that 6 million children every year die from diarrhoeal diseases primarily associated with bad water. Cholera and dysentery account for just some of the pathogens responsible.

Infrastructural developments during the United Nations Drinking Water and Sanitation Decade of the 1980s increased access to uncontaminated water, a trend that has largely continued in the 1990s. WHO figures suggest that between 1980 and 1990 more than 1.6 million additional people were provided with access to water of reasonable quality (WHO 1992b; World Bank 1992). However, though commendable this barely kept pace with population growth and about 1 billion people still lacked an adequate water supply with 1.7 billion people lacking adequate sanitation facilities (World Bank 1992, p47; Briscoe 1993). It was estimated the implementation rates of the 1980s for urban water and sanitation and rural water would have to be increased by two and a half times and rural sanitation about forty four times during the 1990s if 100 per cent coverage were to be attained by the year 2000 (UN Children's Fund, 1989). There is also the harsh reality that many of those registered as officially having access to clean water still drink polluted water. Improvements have also been dependent on key areas of the developing world being relatively free of war. Overall statistics tend to therefore ignore major regional differences, reflecting genuine improvements in some areas but not the deterioration in others.

Control of Diarrhoeal Disease Programmes (CDD's) in many countries have also fallen short of their goals. For example, Babaniyi (1991) reports that in Nigeria an analysis of community-based CDD survey data revealed minimal, and insignificant impact on diarrhoeal disease incidence and diarrhoeal treatment practices from 1986-1989. In this case the suggestion was made that as oral rehydration therapy becomes established as a major component of CDD's for the reduction of mortality, more emphasis could be put on primary prevention aimed at reducing initial morbidity, such as immunisation, promotion of breast-feeding, improving water supply, and promotion of domestic and personal hygiene. The daunting scale of the effort required to eradicate the world's water and sanitation problems must mean that any additional preventative action that can be taken to reduce incidence should be explored in detail and with urgency. One emphasis of this book is that greater understanding of the role of micro-ecology and human vulnerability in wider ecological contexts can assist in finding additional and more sustainable solutions for limiting cholera and dysentery.

Health Care Structures and Structural Adjustment

In addition to direct physical impacts on disease, quality of health care and education determine people's ability to contain secondary transmission of disease once an epidemic is established. The decision of individuals to only use clean water, observe basic sanitation standards and take the appropriate treatments, should they be available, is dependent on the provision of affordable health and education. However, health education schemes on their own have sometimes proved to have limited success in changing knowledge and attitude to diarrhoea and dysentery (Akogun 1992). One possible explanation comes through a study carried out by Dargent-Molina (1994) in Cebu, Philippines who suggested that the protective effect of maternal education on infant diarrhoea varies according to the socio-economic environment in which the mother lives. The contention is that knowledge is only effective if appropriate means and resources allow people to take action, and therefore incidence of the disease is associated with wider reaching economic considerations. The rate of morbidity from cholera and dysentery in any population may therefore be considered the result of hazards present in the environment and the ability of the population to acquire the necessary resources and support to defend itself against those hazards.

The greatest dilemma facing health care programmes in many developing areas at present is how to reconcile dependency on global institutions and top down models of economic development, as precursors to health for all (World Bank 1993), with the hard learned principles of Primary Health Care (PHC) in the community. The success of 'bare foot doctors' versed in PHC principles was rarely doubted in the past and its positive legacy is still recognisable in the health policies of many countries. Accounts of grass roots approaches, and its successes and shortcomings, are covered by Walt and Melamed (1984) for the case of Mozambique, by Garfield and Williams (1989) for the case of Nicaragua, and more thematically by Phillips (1990). The success of Primary Health Care, or Preventative Health Care, is dependent on organisation and mobilisation of communities at grass roots level. A current shortcoming is that the commodification of health care and increasing inequalities in many developing areas are making this approach difficult to achieve, whilst the more recent health through economic growth strategy falls short of making up the deficit.

It can be argued that it is possible to maintain the economic growth models, but overcome the *top down* dilemma, by facilitating greater participation in health (Morgan 1993). However, as Morgan has illustrated, participation is not the same as encouraging empowerment and consequently fundamental ideological differences are back on the agenda, reminiscent of the colonial era. Cutbacks in public spending orchestrated by the IMF have left many African countries streamlining their approach, for example by use of selective primary health care (SPHC), where those causes of mortality perceived as most important are targeted (Stock 1995, p268). This implies that general aspects of particular diseases take precedence over the specific complexity of places, as policies are conceived and evolve in remote cultures. As such, the remedies run the risk of failing to address health issues that result from unique combinations of localised phenomena.

There is a concern that multinational financial institutions have gradually become dominant influences on development policy in many developing countries, and that areas of social policy such as health are often major casualties of the restructuring that accompanies these. Structural adjustment policies aimed at picking up the economies of the

Third World are criticised as failing to give priority to grass-roots local concerns, and that they have caused a general downward trend in health and education standards in some countries (Anyinam 1989; Tumwine 1992; Asthana 1994). UNICEF in Zimbabwe (1989) have stated that 'adjustment programmes are rending the fabric of African society. Of the estimated half a million child deaths in 1988 which can be related to the reversal or slowing down of development, approximately two thirds were in Africa' (UNICEF 1989 quoted in Loewenson 1993, p717). Loewenson (1993, p717) argues that 'Structural Adjustment Programs have been associated with increasing food insecurity and undernutrition, rising ill-health, and decreasing access to health care in the two-thirds or more of the population of African countries that already lives below poverty levels'. The loss of a proactive health policy framework, a widening gap between the affected communities and policy makers, and the replacement of the underlying principle of equity in and social responsibility for health care are outlined in the same study.

Specific hazards for the prevention and treatment of diarrhoea may emerge with transitions in infrastructure and health care provision towards the private sector if the poorer sectors of communities, often representing the foci of infectious diseases, are priced out of obtaining facilities and treatment, and ostracised from participating in decision making. Though most areas are reached eventually, once an epidemic is established and campaigns offering emergency treatment get under way, the restructuring process can become synonymous with a shift from preventative health care to curative medicine with profit making an underlying factor. This may be particularly the case with shigellosis where updated antibiotics increasingly need to be a part of the treatment and have to be purchased. Though there is an obvious difficulty if infected people are unable to pay for such treatments, there are additional complex issues that concern the non-material impact on the integrity of communities and their effectiveness in preventative health programmes.

At the wider scale questions still remain as to whether the new economic approach, linked to both financial restructuring and to comprehensive principles of 'Health for All by the Year 2000' is compatible with sustainable development. Environmental stresses caused by attempts to generate capital through inappropriate agricultural and industrial programmes, partly to pay for the interest on debt, can produce negative impacts on health and well-being for many sectors of society. In particular, poorer countries' attempts to re-establish credit-worthiness with the International Monetary Fund, the World Bank and the international finance community after debt accumulation is associated with a tightening of public expenditure. Consequently, Peru's expenditure on health fell from U.S$18.4 to U.S$13.4 per head between 1980 and 1985 (Donovan 1991). Average daily caloric intake dropped almost 30 per cent since 1982, to well below accepted minimum standards, and in 1992 malnutrition rates approached 60 per cent (Labonte 1992). Meanwhile, the cost of cholera to Peru in 1991 was about 25 per cent of its total budget. These authors suggest that as cholera developed Peru's population had little resistance as it was weakened by economic restructuring, and that policymakers had paid little attention to the public health impact of their policies.

Conclusion

In addition to the pathogenic and physical environmental factors which affect incidence of cholera and dysentery, it is important to take into account socio-economic, demographic and structural factors which can influence their ecology, and provide the context in which individuals and communities are susceptible to disease. In this chapter, it has been argued that forced population displacement is associated with higher incidence of cholera and dysentery. Questions remain however concerning the linkages between the socio-economic processes and the physical environmental changes that influence incidence of these diseases. It also remains to be examined how environment and health interactions for the case of cholera and dysentery are caused and/or experienced by displaced people, especially as increasing numbers are becoming displaced.

The wider contexts of infrastructural development and shifts in political economy impact on health outcomes at local scale. However the isolation of specific changes in ecology and behaviour associated with these processes and policies is rarely understood for specific health problems and places. Analysis of environmentally determined causality needs to be weighed against and integrated with analysis of these wider influences. Whilst incidence of ill-health from diarrhoeal disease may variably relate to changing environmental and societal factors affecting the ecology of disease, changes in infrastructure and development are influencing the nature of local environments and human vulnerability.

3 Epistemological Challenges and Health Ecology Research Methodologies

The ontological basis of the research described in this book spans traditions from both the natural and social sciences. This has been stimulated by the diverse physical and human nature of the phenomena under observation. As such, the methodology draws on an integrated framework born out of earlier approaches to disease ecology and enhanced by contemporary perspectives on the geography of health and disease. Cohesion is maintained in that different aspects of health and diseases are analysed around the central issue of incidence of cholera and dysentery in Mozambique. Building on discussion in the previous chapters, it is proposed that environment and population displacement influence the distribution of incidence of cholera and bacillary dysentery, and that specific factors relating to these diseases and their terrain are dynamically interrelated. Pathogens are opportunistic of these interrelationships that are associated with both changes in nature and humanity, can be identified for different scales of analysis, and vary in influence at different times and places.

The main theoretical approach involves the conceptualisation of dynamic and open systems as a framework within which individual hypotheses relating to environment-health-population displacement interactions for the case of cholera and bacillary dysentery can be quantified. Three main areas of enquiry were identified, based on the following broad hypotheses:

- Incidence of cholera and bacillary dysentery are variably influenced by environmental factors relating to the ecology of their respective pathogens.
- There is an association between population displacement, environmental change, and higher incidence of these diseases.
- Wider structural changes have influenced disease hazards and human vulnerability.

The initial aim is to assess the role of an environmental reservoir of *Vibrio cholerae*, patterns of diarrhoeal disease endemicity, and the relative importance of biological and social causality in the field sites. A key area of exploration here concerns the role of the environment and human vulnerability. The wider theoretical context of environment, health and population displacement is also addressed from a *realist* perspective. In doing so, a central tenet of this research as a whole is therefore that understanding of health and disease can only be approached successfully through pluralistic endeavour.

Fieldwork tested the specific hypothesis that there is spatial association between disease incidence caused by two serotypes of *Vibrio cholerae* 01, dysentery caused by *Shigella dysenteriae* type 1, and environments with higher faecal contamination, salinity and/or pH. Further analysis tested the hypotheses that there is a spatio-temporal relationship between these diseases and rainfall, and that specific local environmental factors influence the spatial persistence of disease incidence. Primary fieldwork data also focused on examining the association between different levels of incidence of these diseases and areas with higher percentages of migrants. This required analysing whether forcibly displaced migrants experience higher incidence of disease and whether migration contributed to high disease incidence through its influence on the existing environment. Specific hypotheses were that forced migrants were more susceptible to diarrhoeal diseases than established residents and that forced migrants became more susceptible to diarrhoeal disease following resettlement, through changes in water supply, sanitation, fuel, cultivation and economic activity. Further analysis evaluates the hypothesis that higher rates of incidence are associated with behavioural differences, such as lower levels of internal community assistance. Finally, the role of structural adjustment in these processes is also addressed.

Disease Ecology Revisited

One of the major historical aims of Disease Ecology within Medical Geography has been to integrate environmental, economic, social and biological knowledge of disease causation for individual places, as epitomised by the work of May (1950, 1958, 1970). This approach has often been synonymous with the development of Regional Geography in the broader realm of Geography. The emergence of new paradigms in

Human Geography during the quantitative and post quantitative eras have also been reflected in the Medical Geography sub-discipline.

In recent years, critical perspectives have succeeded in broadening the scope of Medical Geography by using themes from mainstream social and behavioural sciences. This is epitomised through work on health care and the mechanisms of its delivery (Eyles and Woods 1983; Jones and Moon 1987). Recent debates within the discipline have also been extended to the social construction of health status and the concept of place as centre of lived meaning, social position and sickness in this instance being a combination of behaviour in illness and disease process (Eyles 1985; Kearns 1994). There has been contention that the adjective 'medical' before geography and 'disease' before ecology determine these subjects as ultimately contingent on the medical professions to the detriment of the broader subject (Kearns 1993, 1994). The recent change in the name of the 'Canadian Study Group in Medical Geography' and the name change of the 'RGS-IBG Medical Geography Study Group' to the 'RGS-IBG Study Group for the Geography of Health' (MGSG 1995) reflect this concern.

Differences of opinion in the wider debate on the role of Medical Geography are mainly between those who see geographical perspectives on health issues as more centred on social theory (Kearns 1994; Dorn and Laws 1994) and those who feel that social theory can be developed from within the existing parameters of the discipline (Mayer and Meade 1994, p105). The debate serves as a good example of how differing perceptions of relevance encourage varied methodological approaches. Despite these differences in emphasis, the need for further diversity of approach has emerged as a common theme (Jones and Moon 1993; Mayer and Meade 1994; Kearns 1994). For example, Jones and Moon (1993, p520) write:

> Research in medical geography needs to be sensitive to spatiality...and temporality...comprehensive enough to understand a complex interplay of forces, yet sufficiently focused to get valid and meaningful results. We need a methodology that recognises that 'people make a difference and places make a difference' (Gregory, 1985, p74). People should not be reduced to statistical aggregates, and places should not be reduced to generalisations. We need micro- and macroscales, structure and agency, intensive and extensive approaches, qualitative and quantitative methods...all need to be considered together.

Though the development of research that answers these demands is rare, initiatives are increasingly being taken to advance interdisciplinary enquiry for some aspects of health and disease, such as those discussed by the Harvard Working Group on New and Resurgent Disease (Wilson and Levins *et al.* 1994).[1]

A further point that can be added to recent perspectives on Medical Geography is that, with applied research addressing major disaster issues, consideration of policy relevance should be important. The framework devised by Feachem *et al.* (1989, p136) considers five types of research that may arise from health problems in developing countries; health problem research, aetiology research, intervention research, operational research, and health services research. Although they refer to an 'unacceptable ignorance' of four of these, particular attention is paid here to their assessment of the state of *intervention research.*

> There is unacceptable ignorance of interventions or measures against the health problems that are efficacious. This may require epidemiological, sociological and demographic research to define further the important risk factors and to test the efficacy of interventions to reduce the magnitude and/or prevalence of these risk factors.

Despite varied perceptions of relevance, in disaster situations the subject under observation more typically plays a part in determining the methodology employed for a study. Thus, where environmentally endemic pathogens are evolving in response to physical environmental changes, it is reasonable to develop a more bio-physiological approach to a disease problem than would be suitable in health studies of localities grappling with the issue of institutional control and the medical profession. However, in the real world, where causality is the result of a complex mix of phenomena, there is considerable advantage in the use of several approaches, modifiable for specific times and places.

---

[1] During their work on 'Global Changes and Emergence of Infectious Diseases' the Harvard Working Group on New and Resurgent Disease have brought together a range of disciplines, including among others, ecology, entomology, epidemiology, infectious diseases, population biology, mathematical modelling, international health, evolutionary biology, climate, environmental analysis, and marine ecology.

The Use of Systems and a Holistic Understanding of Diarrhoeal Disease Incidence

A fundamental question in the use of systems as a research methodology is, at what point of inclusion of variables does the system significantly represent a portion of reality? Should human elements be involved, then the answer in most instances is likely to be never. However, it is maintained here that development in understanding of a human-environmental system, typified by many infectious disease problems, can be obtained through open systems analysis.

The use of systems in the analysis of human phenomena has developed substantially since its early presentation as *General Systems Analysis*. Of the use of these closed systems in dealing with human phenomena Chisholm (1967, p45) wrote 'General systems theory seems to be an irrelevant distraction', a theme later echoed by Langton (1972) and Huggett (1980). Kennedy (1979) contended that an over emphasis on the analysis of environmental systems leaves many basic questions concerning the nature of environmental complexity unanswered, and therefore that prior and usually qualitative information about the earth's landscapes was equally valid.

The successful use of systems analysis in approaching human phenomena has by necessity been through the open system within which flows to and from its environment are hypothesised. Largely evolving out of ecosystems analysis and the role of human impacts on natural systems through analysis of feedback mechanisms, this has often been given a sociological and economic extension. For example Garcia and Escudero (1972) described a socio-ecosystem in their analysis of the relationship between drought and anthropogenic activity and similarly Pearce and Turner (1990) for the case of both Indonesian uplands erosion and resource interconnections in developing countries. The broader use of ecological systems questions the point of disciplinary boundaries, not so much because of the categorisation of subject matter, but because of differing theoretical traditions. Approaches such as human ecology and political ecology have as a consequence emerged from theoretical origins in several subjects. A key research area addressed by political ecology that embraces different social and ecological scales is the contextual sources of environmental change. This is concerned with environmental impacts of the state and its policies, interstate relations, capitalism and interdependence (Black 1990; Bryant 1991, 1992). A good practical example of the political ecology framework was provided by Harris (1982) who identified the structural determinant of inequality in land and water distribution as the determinant of underdevelopment of an entire village agricultural system in North Arcot District, Tamil Nadu. The health component of these approaches can represent a major area of research in itself.

The emergence of these emphases strengthens the role of Ecology as earlier identified by Cook (1973, p27), who described it as a frame of reference that anticipates theory, rather than theory itself. In this sense the main potential of ecological systems analysis becomes not in attempting to model the unmodelable but rather as a background for analysis. The process involved here is to conceptualise and isolate a system or a segment of a system defined by the problem being studied (Susser 1973). Morgan (1981, p221) refers to this as 'soft system methodologies' and their role as a 'problem-solving framework'. Krebs (1995, p11) aptly refers to 'phenomenological models that give an impressionist insight into the behaviour of a system and extract underlying principles'. Something of the balance between what should and should not be attempted specifically for the case of identifying health problems and health research priorities in developing countries is well put by Feachem *et al.* (1989, p138).

> Models of the larger system must, at this stage in our understanding, operate in broad conceptual terms that are both specific enough to be useful as a guide to data collection, analysis and policy formation, but general enough to preserve clarity in the face of potentially limitless detail. The trees are important but they must not obscure the wood.

Figure 3.1 represents the way in which a systems approach is used to provide a methodological framework for the research described in this book centring around the issue of incidence of cholera and dysentery in Mozambique. The curved edged boxes represent the elements of a sub-system that are hypothesised as being proximate influences on incidence of cholera and dysentery at the scale of the research project. Early definition of the broad themes of physical environment, sociogeographic/behavioural condition, and population displacement were derived through examination of existing facts and hypotheses, including preliminary fieldwork on environmental influences on cholera in one of the field sites (Collins 1993), and a pilot investigation in all the sites. Answers to the hypotheses defined at the beginning of this chapter were sought through confirmation or negation of the interdependence of these elements. The unshaded rectangular boxes depict phenomena that define the open aspects of the system requiring a second level of analysis. 'Nature of pathogen' and 'natural laws' are hypothesised here as phenomena relating to wider theories of genetic evolution and the dynamics of chaos and complexity in the physical world respectively. The other element, 'development and structural adjustment' is analysed at secondary level through a more structural approach. The open ends, as defined above, are proposed as

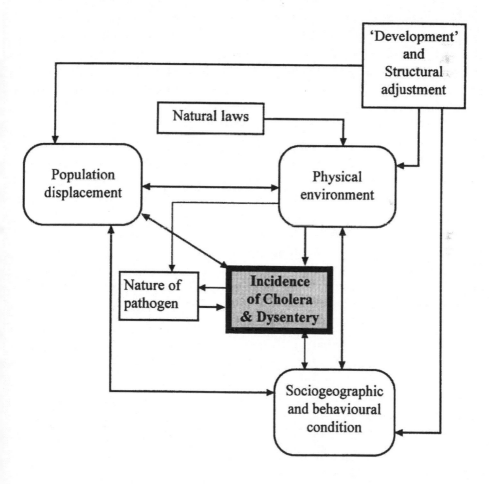

Figure 3.1   A systems approach to analysis of incidence of cholera and dysentery

being the underlying forces influencing incidence of cholera and dysentery and determine the essentially dynamic nature of the overall system.

The Disease Context: The Need to View both Structure and Nature

The dynamic open system proposed for analysis of incidence of cholera and dysentery is flexible in that it can be combined with other theoretical approaches. This is necessary since disease incidence is caused by social and physical factors. Though it may be maintained that theories have limited practical application, their existence influences the way in which all phenomena are perceived, observations being interpretations of observed facts in the light of theories (after Popper 1968). This principle is relevant to the role of theory in the study of environment, health and population displacement since an improved theoretical approach will ultimately lead to improved action in reducing disease.

Concerning social factors Ellen (1982, p276) asserts that 'ecological approaches and data can only ever constitute part of a substantive analysis of a particular social formation, which must also be grounded in methodology and theory drawn from other than ecological precedent.' The relationship between systems concepts and other theories has been noted by Williams (1983) who identifies links with structuralism. A structuralist approach is relevant to this research in that 'development' and structural adjustment are proposed as influences on health (Figure 3.1). However, on its own a structuralist approach to health is limited both because it excludes human agency (important to understanding some behavioural approaches to health), and because disease may also be partly a function of 'natural' evolutionary processes. The first of these shortcomings is reminiscent of perspectives addressed by Anthony Giddens whose 'structuration theory' has explored the reciprocal role of human agency in wider social systems and social structures (Johnston 1986; Holt-Jensen 1988; Clark and Modgil *et al.* 1990).

Theories on underlying influences in nature are also difficult to define and open to varied interpretation in the light of recent genetic discoveries. For example, the scientific idea of *complexity* in environmental systems includes both the concept of *chaos* where systems unpredictably spin off, and the crystallisation of order from within a system, sometimes called the 'vital force' (Lewis 1993). This is relevant to genetic aspects of the emergence of bacteria if DNA can cause complex changes due to its ability to self propagate in millions of different ways (Dawkins 1996). Based on these principles it would be possible to consider biology 'the production of order from chaos' and evolution as 'chaos with feedback' (Pellegrino 1994, p332). The implication of these processes in understanding disease is worth consideration, for if self-organisation is the root source of order (Kauffman 1995), there are grounds to propose that complexity in emerging disease epidemics may not be fully explainable in terms of environment and/or society.

Interconnections between human and natural systems are particularly well demonstrated by disease ecologies. At microbiological scale, a pathogen is able to undergo natural selection within the host. In many instances where drugs are used, such as in the treatment of tuberculosis or shigellosis, the pathogen makes the intervention a part of its environment, so that resistance is acquired (Haila and Levins 1992; HWGNRD 1995). Pathogens may use a similar strategy in the external environment to achieve a selection advantage in artificially created reservoirs, which result from development and degradation of natural ecosystems. The greatest opportunities for disease can occur where there is least diversity and as such monistic versions of development can be associated with increased health risks. The ecology of individual diseases is also linked to human systems that maintain greater vulnerability of host and community. This is because general state of health and resistance is in part dependent on prevailing economic conditions that protect against pathogen contamination and which enhance nutritional well-being. Finally, in spite of similarities between systems in different places, it is important to consider the specific nature of different diseases and uniqueness of different places.

The Challenge of Integration: Reconciling the Use of Disparate Data Sources

Since this book is concerned with a range of interconnected factors, several areas of quantitative investigation are described. It is suggested that quantification of the variables targeted here provide both key results relating to proximate influences on incidence of cholera and dysentery, and a contribution towards understanding the role of other parts of a wider system proposed above. Cross-sectional associative analysis using aggregate values based on sub-areas of field sites is used to search for spatial association between rates of incidence of the diseases and the selected environmental and socio-demographic variables. The use of sub-administrative units of urban areas for micro-scale studies in Medical Geography has been appraised by Meade *et al.* (1979, 1983), Howe (1980), Giggs *et al.* (1980), and Learmonth (1986). Data was derived from health records, environmental field testing and structured interviewing using questionnaires. The temporal aspect of the analysis was achieved through repetition of data collection at the same locations for different periods of the year, and by asking questions relating to people's prior circumstances.

The strength of this approach in providing an indication of genuine association is dependent on both sample size and the area of the sub-locations. The larger the area and smaller the sample, the greater the generalisation that is being made on the nature of the phenomena within the boundaries. The ideal representation therefore becomes one in which disease incidence is measured as individual representative points and no spatial generalisation is made. In parts of the more technologically advanced countries health phenomena may now be represented at close to this scale using postcodes to identify a patient's place of residence to within at least $100m^2$. In the typical large scale epidemic circumstances of the rest of the world this is not possible and the spatial position of a disease case must be sought through aggregate sub-location of a city or district. In such instances, it is necessary to correlate spatial environmental information with a health area, rather than correlating individual health events within an environmental area. However, where the number of cases observed is very high, the inevitable loss of accuracy involved in this approach is rendered less significant.

A statistical limitation of aggregated data is caused by the modifiable areal unit effect (Oppenshaw 1977, 1984), where changes in the size of the areas or shifts in the boundaries inferring characteristics of individuals from data referring to a population, can create a completely different set of results. The phenomenon is also investigated by Waller and Turnbull (1993) and Morris and Munasinghe (1993). This and other aspects of the *ecological fallacy* determine that hypotheses can never be fully proven using spatial associative analysis, but rather that consistencies can be identified. The ability to do simply this, however, is a mark of the strength of the ecological approach that may outweigh its deficiency. This is because, in true Popperian tradition, the aim is to test whether new information is consistent with existing hypotheses rather than conclusively prove an association.

The debate on the relative merits of using ecological approaches or those based on individuals is well established. It has its origins in wider theoretical debates on spatiality and temporality that have marked the development of geography as a discipline concerned with both pattern and process. Within epidemiology there also remains a lack of conclusive judgement about its merits. For example, Kasl (1979) suggested that epidemiologists needed to develop guidelines for comparing ecological and individual level data as valid areas of causal inquiry. More recently Schwartz (1994, p819) responds to this in writing on 'the fallacy of the ecological fallacy' emphasising that, whilst 'ecological studies cannot usually be used as substitutes for individual correlational studies', they are 'necessary to examine structural, contextual, and sociological effects on human behaviour and disease development'.

There are limitations on the depth of analysis obtainable from areal measures of health and its contexts as individual chains of causation represent only a fraction of the reality and each component itself is the result of a complex genealogy or spatial history. For example, analysis of behaviour and people's perspectives on health and disease cannot be assessed remotely by observing large numbers of people as groups. To address this weakness, it is useful to collect information from individuals to provide more focused data on behaviour, as well as predisposing and micro-scale vulnerability to disease. However, it should be remembered here that there are also major limitations and confounding factors through making judgements about areas or groups based exclusively on personal accounts. For example, analysis at the level of individuals with no reference to the wider social and environmental context has its limitations since physical remoteness may be replaced by the distance of culture and class, misinterpretation of observed by observer, or vice versa.

To reduce the effect of 'social distance', participant observation is sometimes suggested. Johnston *et al.* (1986, p339) define this as enabling 'a sharing of activities, an understanding of meanings and actions and an appreciation of the logic and context of behaviour'. Potential difficulties with this are that if the observer's role as researcher is known, then the observed become influenced by the research itself and fail to produce unbiased representations. On the other hand it is morally questionable to hide one's true activities from the subjects. Also, representative generalisations are difficult to establish through 'participation', which may have only involved a few obliging households or communities. Alternatively, impartiality of the researcher may be lost through intensive involvement, leading to non-observing participation, the results of which need to be deconstructed and interpreted by third parties. Acknowledgement of how the researcher may constructively be part of the research process is viewed as action research by Carr and Kemmis (1986, p162) who refer to:

> A form of self reflective enquiry undertaken by participants in social situations in order to improve the rationality and justice of their own practices, the understanding of those practices, and the situation in which those practices are carried out.

However, though questions can concern the positionality of individuals, a potentially endless cycle of reflexivity can stifle the emergence of useful results.

The stance of the research described in this book was that by employing a multimethod approach, using both areal and individual representations, the weaknesses of one are compensated for by the use of the other, maximising the potential for accurate information. Hence, cross-sectional and spatio-temporal associative analyses at the scale of sub-areas of cities has been combined with point location information derived from individuals through interviewing. Though a qualitative approach is adopted in some instances, no claim of participant observation can be made. Protracted familiarity with the culture and context of the areas, through for example, employment within local structures and personal friendships, falls short of participation in the lives of the range of individuals being interviewed.[2] Theoretically the concept of participation in observational research may be flawed, since no individual can ever fully know the mind of the other, given any degree of cultural assimilation and involvement in their lives. Despite such limitations, the research uses wide ranging

---

[2] Between 1986 and 1989 I worked in the Conselho Executivo da Cidade da Beira (Beira City Executive Council) with a Mozambican Government contract. This was a period of limited external involvement in the city. Consequently foreigners, or 'cooperantes' working in Beira became relatively well integrated with their local situation, conversing entirely in the national language, Portuguese, and participating with the community in overcoming the everyday struggles of living in a city with almost no food or functioning services. This contrasts with the latter period of foreign involvement in Beira which is more characterised by 'expatriates' living in, and sometimes working from, the exclusive conditions of well guarded compounds, into which few local people are able to stray. The field work for this research maintained much of the same approach as the earlier period of employment, working from within local structures and with local staff.

information established from encounters with people affected by the issues concerned. This has been important in gaining an understanding of the behavioural interrelationships and structural contexts that influence incidence of the diseases in the locations studied.

Geographical Information Systems

The above discussion frequently refers to the challenge of integrating disparate data for research on health issues. Wider integration has become one of the major challenges for Geographical Information Systems in multi-dimensional and spatially based research projects (Martin 1991; Martin and Bracken 1993; Newby 1993). However, the principal dilemma of Geographical Information Systems is that, though they have helped stimulate the will to integrate geographical information, they are restricted in carrying this to full fruition by their own intrinsic limitations. For example, Geographical Information Systems have encouraged a resurgence of research reminiscent of Regional Geography, but they only address some aspects of what the Region was intended to mean. From Vidal de la Blache's (1845-1918) inclusion of possibilistic aspects of human relationships with the environment at the turn of the century, to Nigel Thrift's (1983) 'meeting place of human agency and social structure', the region in geography is well established as more complex than spatial geometry and quantified data. This was emphasised in regional studies of health, such as May's (1970) extensive work in East Africa, which included regional aspects of tradition and culture.

However, to throw out GIS because of these limitations is to 'tilt at windmills', for if its limitations are understood, its applications can be of great assistance to some aspects of health based research. An additional spin-off area of enquiry addressed by this research has been to consider useful applications for GIS in research on communicable disease in developing areas. This has become relevant since there is currently increasing interest in its potential development for health related research, disaster mitigation and urban planning throughout the Third World. To date there have been two main fronts involving GIS applications in health and disease research. One has typically involved the integration of remotely sensed information to assist in assessing macro scale environmental features and the effects of anthropogenic impacts, from which inference is made about disease vectors. Examples are the monitoring of tsetse and trypanosomiasis in Africa (Rogers and Randolph

1991; Rogers and Williams 1993; Epstein *et al.* 1993), and the remote sensing of harmful algal blooms (Epstein *et al* 1994, p20).

The other approach is more concerned with the spatial analysis capabilities of GIS, has been more developed for health issues of developed countries, and typically deals with postcoded disease data or decision support systems for locational purposes (Gatrell and Dunn *et al.* 1992; Gatrell 1993; Dunn and Woodhouse *et al.* 1995, Foley and Frost 1996). It is suggested here that both procedures have only been of indirect methodological use to the health issues of developing areas suffering from localised communicable disease. Firstly, the remote sensing approach has been too remote for dealing with the smaller scale environmental differences that are important as reservoirs for disease vectors, leaving many physiological factors influencing pathogens undetected. The second approach is limited by the fact that in most of the Third World there is less fixed demographic data, often no postcodes for locating disease cases, numbers of infected people are often too large to be isolated by individual co-ordinates, and events sometimes move too fast to be adequately recorded.

However, a third approach, which is currently gaining interest, and that has greater potential in these situations, is the use of GIS/GPS (Global Positioning Systems) combinations. Snow *et al.* (1993) use GPS's to map malaria cases on the coast of Kenya and le Sueur and Ngxongo et al. (1996) describe their use in investigating more thoroughly the epidemiology of Malaria in South Africa. Some further applications and more theoretical implications are demonstrated by the diarrhoeal disease research outlined in this book. GPS technology may be used to rapidly record the geographical locations of events and the stored information can be used interactively with a GIS. In effect, 'the GPS receiver becomes a digitising cursor and the earth is the digitiser's table' (Van Demark 1992, p5). Abler (1993, p132) suggested that a great attraction will be in the ability to 'create new maps interactively, in real time, amid the real phenomena the maps represent, while at the same time referring to and revising the background maps for the area contained in portable GIS's carried into the field'. In this manner GIS/GPS combinations can be applied to improving disease surveillance systems, particularly in emergencies such as those outlined in this book. A summary assessment of the worth of GIS and GPS as it has been experienced through carrying out this research is presented in Chapter 8.

Methods and Techniques

Comparing the Influence of Environment and Population Displacement on Distributions of Cholera and Bacillary Dysentery

The focus of the research on the different diseases of cholera and bacillary dysentery serves several purposes. In particular, it both helps answer specific questions concerning the individual natures of the two diseases, and serves as a method of comparative analysis. The two diseases are suitable for comparative analysis in that, whilst both are major diarrhoeal diseases, differences in pathogenesis suggests that patterns of incidence should vary. Comparison of the disease distributions with reference to environmental and demographic differentials can reveal more about probable associations than is possible by studying one disease on its own.

The hypothesis that incidence of cholera and bacillary dysentery are variably influenced by environmental factors relating to the ecology of their respective pathogens, is primarily based on the evidence that there are favourable environmental reservoirs for the cholera pathogen, *Vibrio cholerae*. The influence of favourable environmental reservoirs on incidence of cholera is tested through extensive data collection at multiple sites for the specific conditions of salinity and pH in the physical environment. In contrast, the pattern of incidence of bacillary dysentery was expected to differ to that of cholera, since there is no theoretical basis for it being influenced by these environmental reservoirs. Indeed, whereas large quantities of *Vibrios*, measurable in 10,000's, must be ingested to contract cholera, only small numbers of *Shigella dysenteriae* 1 are required to contract dysentery. Because of this *Shigella dysenteriae* 1 is believed to be the most communicable of bacterial diarrhoeas and better adapted to the human host than *Vibrio cholerae*. On the basis of this pathogenic difference it was therefore suspected that the spatial distributions of dysentery would be associated more closely with human environmental factors such as overcrowding and poor sanitation.

To date there has been a shortage of research on epidemics that draws on factors relating to the micro-ecology of diarrhoeal disease pathogens since much of the background information, presented in Chapter 1, was unknown until the 1980s. The testing of the hypothesis that the ecology of the disease pathogen and local environments influence the pattern of incidence of the disease is relevant to several scales of analysis. In sum, the foundations are established for inferring the relative importance of differing biological, environmental or social factors in patterns of incidence and nature of associating factors. On the basis of background information, it was also proposed that the spatio-temporal patterns of incidence from individual serotypes of these diseases could provide further indication of the interplay between endemic and epidemic areas of disease incidence. These are important avenues of enquiry, contributing to the debate on emergence and resurgence of diarrhoeal disease, and the development of preventative strategies.

The hypothesis that there is an association between population displacement, environmental change, and higher incidence of these diseases is based on the evidence provided by situations of forced displacement, refugee concentrations, and resultant epidemics. As outlined earlier, this has been identified for the case of refugee movements to camps in Africa (Shears and Lusty 1987), but remains to be determined for the case of rural-urban migration. There is also little indication of the extent to which forced and voluntary displacement processes affect health within urban areas of poor countries. Since many of the displaced people in Mozambique have been forcibly displaced to urban areas, it is hypothesised that this may be a key process behind their association with elevated incidence. The term environmental change is used here to cover both changes to the local environment favouring disease and changes in environmental experience and therefore further clarification of the role of each of these processes is required.

The health implications of environmental change through displacement is relevant to the hypothesis on the ecology of pathogens since resettling people may become exposed to new areas of endemic disease or contribute to creating the ecological conditions for a new endemic focus. In the broader sense, people recently relocated from another environmental zone can suffer more disease with exposure to their new environment, and the area of resettlement can undergo an environmental change as a result of their presence. Meanwhile, it also needs to be established to what extent socio-economic factors have made them more or less vulnerable to infection. The underlying theme becomes one of uncovering the extent to which health issues relate to a loss of local sustainable relationships between people and their environment. In addition to its intrinsic importance, the interrelationship between population displacement and health may therefore also be indicative of outcomes where people do not relocate but where there are health implications associated with disruption of local habitats. For example, global development processes are capable of increasing susceptibility through stimulating rapid environmental changes and/or a breakdown of societal well-being.

Selection of Field Sites

Three field sites, at Quelimane, Beira and Gorongosa, were selected for detailed study to allow investigation of the relationship between environment, health and displacement in three distinct environments, and with three contrasting experiences of displacement (Figure 3.2). The first site, Quelimane, formed the focus of earlier work (Collins 1993), in which preliminary evidence was found of the influence of physical environmental factors on the distribution of incidence of cholera. Quelimane was chosen for this earlier study because it had the highest rate of incidence during an epidemic between 1990 and 1991. In turn, as described in detail in Chapter 4, there were even greater epidemics of cholera and bacillary dysentery in subsequent years. Meanwhile, the city of Beira, 300 km to the south-west also had amongst the highest rate of incidence of cholera and dysentery in Mozambique from 1991-1994. Direct comparison between Quelimane and Beira is facilitated by the fact that both are estuarine, provincial capitals, and sub-divide into administrative wards for which data can be compiled.

Although the macro-scale environmental circumstances of the two cities have some similarities, variation in internal local environments were known to vary, providing an opportunity for comparison and therefore validation of associations. In addition, some major differences between the two are that Beira (pop 320,000) is a city with a faster developing economy and was approximately twice the size of Quelimane (pop 150,000).[3] Though each were severely affected by the war in Mozambique, Quelimane was more isolated than Beira, which remained accessible for most of the time via the Beira Corridor to Zimbabwe. Small quantities of road and rail traffic and an oil pipeline continued to operate along this corridor throughout.

A third site was selected that would provide significant macro-environmental contrasts, both with respect to the physical environment and

[3] By the early 1990s some parts of Beira developed rapidly, with extensive sprawling markets and the beginnings of major changes in policy were evident. At Quelimane infrastructural changes are less apparent as the city has failed to attract the same attention for development as Beira. Meanwhile Gorongosa had experienced only limited changes in conditions since the end of the war.

population characteristics. Gorongosa (pop 70,000) suited this requirement since it is a smaller rural and inland district capital situated in a different natural environmental zone at 300 metres altitude. For several years

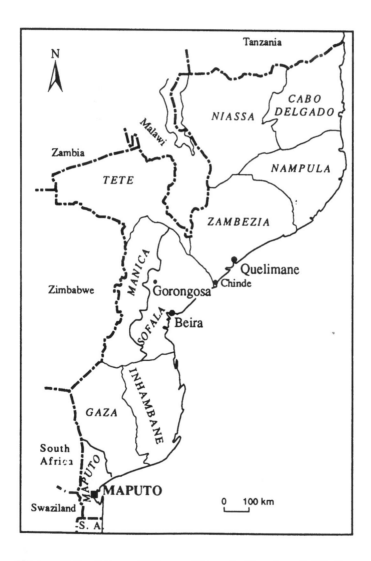

Figure 3.2   Map of Mozambique indicating field sites

Gorongosa was the focal point of the war in Mozambique, and it has also suffered recently from cholera and bacillary dysentery. Gorongosa was at many times completely cut off and over half its population were made up of people displaced by the war. A detailed background to these sites is presented in Chapter 4.

Sample Strategy

The health data used for this research represents all cases occurring within a defined time period, totalling over 10,000 individually recorded cases of cholera and dysentery. To a large extent the data represents the totality of cases from the beginning to the end of an epidemic wave in each city. In the case of Quelimane it has been possible to complete the observations for several epidemic waves of cholera by combining data derived from earlier work in 1991. Data for the 1992-1993 cholera epidemic in Beira are also complete. However, the data for dysentery in both cities were truncated since the early stages of these epidemics were not well recorded and the latter part was still going on at the time of completing the fieldwork. Despite missing data at the beginning and latter part of the epidemic a large quantity of continuous data was compiled comparable in magnitude to that collected for cholera. The cholera and dysentery data for Gorongosa were sections of the epidemics there.

Environmental tests were carried out at drinking water sites in nearly all of the administrative units (*bairros* or *unidades comunais*). On arrival at an administrative unit, general enquiries determined where water for consumption was obtained. This strategy was used because there were no existing maps of the water sources that people use in these areas, some of which changed from year to year. In some of the administrative units, all the water sites used for drinking were used in the analysis. In other locations, where there were too many sites to include them all, extra effort was made through local enquiry to select those with the heaviest usage. Where there were taps connected to the 'treated water supply' only a few examples were necessary since the main aim of the water sampling was to determine the nature of local environments. Although piped water in these areas reflected its local environment to the extent there were holes in the pipe, it generally reflects more the conditions of the source where the water is pumped. Further to this, at the time of carrying out this fieldwork, the piped water was only in operation intermittently. Consequently, most people were exposed to local ground water conditions for at least part, if not all, the time. There are a variety of types of well and this was taken into consideration in sampling sites for this study. In Quelimane they consisted of the following categories:

- Traditional wells, which usually consist of bare earth holes that are deepened regularly by hand.
- Shallow concrete lined wells many of which date back to colonial times. These vary between those which are open and those which are covered and have a hand pump on top, though not necessarily totally protected due to there often being cracks in the concrete.
- Bore holes sunk in more recent years by specific projects, although these have been restricted to only a few areas largely as a result of a lack of suitably thick fresh ground-water bodies. Some become inactive not long after installation due to silting up with the fine sand.

In Beira the wells consisted of the following categories:

- Traditional wells (similar to Quelimane).
- Shallow and open concrete wells. Many date from colonial times. Unlike in Quelimane, there are none with hand pumps.
- Oil drum and tyre wells. These are the most common and consist of makeshift improvisations used to prevent collapse.

In Gorongosa drinking water was collected from natural springs, the main river and some recently installed bore holes.

The method of selecting environmental sites by the distribution of water supply determined that more sites were analysed in some parts of the city than others. Areas with higher population typically had more sites analysed. This is because the initial enquiry procedure, in which local people were asked 'where is the drinking water?' produced a greater amount of focal areas from which to start the locating procedure. The strategy was deliberately spatial in its approach since a prime objective was to assess spatial associations with health statistics that are only accurately represented at sub-administrative level. Use of the cluster approach to sampling in this instance would have presented greater limitations since many areas would have been missed and much important comparative material would have been lost. Also, the emphasis of sampling more sites within one area would have meant including sites with only limited usage, whilst other sites around the city with heavy usage would remain under-represented. Potential bias in representing sub-areas with data generated from varying amounts of samples can be subsequently solved by not including sub-areas that turned out to have fewer than a minimum amount of sites. Soil samples were taken within a few meters of well sites.

The strategy of discovering environmental sites by use of local informants was facilitated by two hand-held Global Positioning Systems (GPS's) which were able to supply a co-ordinate for each location (accurate to 25 meters) after its selection. Their use in this way represents a distinctive feature of the survey design: remote selection of sites using existing maps in advance of the survey would have meant that less attention was given to the guidance offered from the local community. This survey demonstrates how the location of the sites can be accurately determined during the survey whilst benefiting from up-to-date and relevant information available amongst the local population. One effect has been that the sites have generally covered the most populated areas of Communal Units. Whilst the use of communal areas for associative analysis is problematical in that populations are unevenly distributed within sub-areas, those areas remain associated with the people registered as living within their boundaries. Therefore, though not morphologically precise, the choropleth maps generated from the sample remain adequately representative for comparison with the spatially registered health data. Use of sub-areas of Communal Units generated by the GIS techniques of 'buffering' distances around the sites and 'intersecting', in this context was found to add little to the visual representation and provided no new interpretation of the spatiality of the phenomena under observation.

A similar principle was employed for the selection of sites for interview. The starting point in this case was the environmental field site. Nearby clusters of housing were entered and a house picked out at random. This process was random to the extent that at first glance there are few distinguishing features between households within one group. The residents were approached and asked if they used the water of the site that had been tested. If the reply was negative then the house next door was used, until an occupant was found that used it. Though some of the questions concerned the whole household, one respondent was asked to answer the questions as an individual. Children under the age of about 14 were excluded from answering the questions due to fears about comprehension and reliability of answers from younger respondents. The location at which interviews took place were also given a co-ordinate using a GPS. The maps of the distributions of environmental and questionnaire sites were later generated from this information using a combination of base maps and co-ordinates transformed to UTM (Figures 3.3-3.6).

The sampling of field sites was given a seasonal dimension by carrying out the survey at two periods of the year. The first phase of sampling took place during the second half of the wet season (between early January and early April 1994) and the second phase during the first half of the dry season (between late April and late July 1994). For the second phase, most of the environmental sites that were used in the first phase were successfully relocated. In some instances a nearby substitute source was used. For comparative analysis only the repeat wells ended up being used and new respondents were randomly selected for interviewing. The carrying out of more questionnaire interviews during the second surveys served to approximately double the overall sample size, facilitate an assessment of consistency in survey results, and enabled a comparison of circumstances for two times of year. It also provided an opportunity for some more targeted, non-questionnaire, interviewing on themes that had emerged as important during initial analysis of the first survey.

Surveying Environment, Health and Population Displacement: Criteria, Variables, and Techniques

Since there is a limit to the number of variables that can be accurately quantified over a large area, only key factors suspected of influencing distributions of the diseases were isolated. The selected variables represent defining characteristics of the hypothesised elements in the environment-health-population displacement system relevant to the case of cholera and bacillary dysentery. The following describes and explains their use in the field studies.

Health data The research required large numbers of consecutive cases of cholera and bacillary dysentery, registered by place of residence and date of admittance, to enable the analysis of spatio-temporal patterns of incidence within the field sites. This was primarily carried out by use of hospital registry books. The age and sex of each case was also extracted from the same books to facilitate further epidemiological observations that could, for example, relate to patterns of endemicity. The quality of the information held in the hospital registry has improved in the last few years since new guidelines were issued by the Ministry of Health in Maputo in

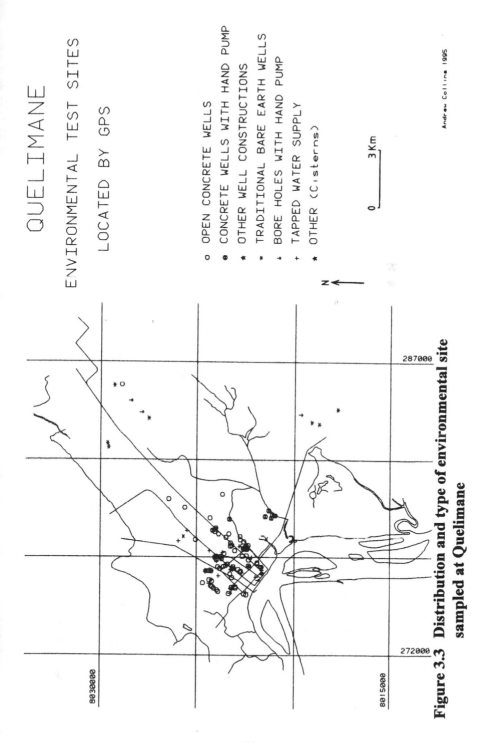

Figure 3.3 Distribution and type of environmental site sampled at Quelimane

73

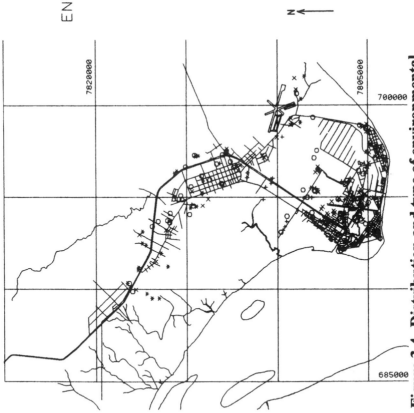

BEIRA

ENVIRONMENTAL TEST SITES

LOCATED BY GPS

o   OPEN CONCRETE WELLS

⊕   CONCRETE WELLS WITH HAND PUMP

×   OIL DRUM AND TYRE WELLS

*   TRADITIONAL BARE EARTH WELLS

↳   BORE HOLES WITH HAND PUMP

+   TAPPED WATER SUPPLY

*   OTHER (Cisterns)

N ←

0 _____ 3Km

Andrew Collins 1995

**Figure 3.4   Distribution and type of environmental
site sampled at Beira**

74

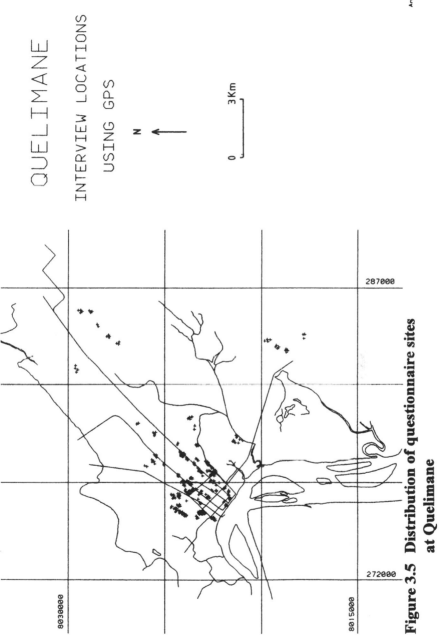

Figure 3.5 Distribution of questionnaire sites at Quelimane

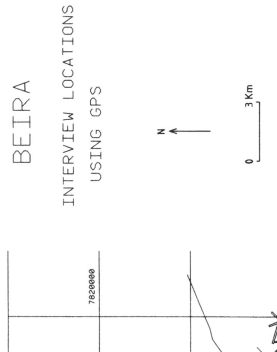

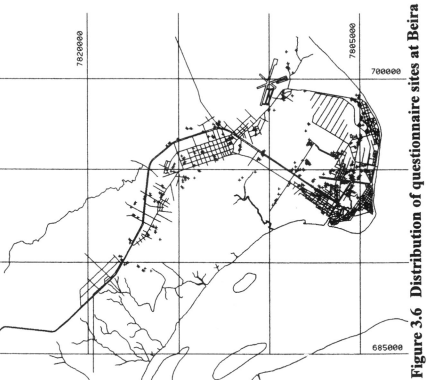

Figure 3.6 Distribution of questionnaire sites at Beira

the light of the increasing scale of the epidemics. In Quelimane, the quality of registration of cholera data also improved because the earlier study had emphasised the need to keep well kept books, and through the return of better trained staff from medical training in Cuba and former East Germany.

Although it is likely that some cases are not registered, since they do not make it to the hospital, there was little evidence available from hospital staff and health workers that this would have a significant affect on the distributions of the data. The likelihood of a distance-decay effect is minimised in Quelimane and Beira since health posts are located in both inner and outer areas. All cases of cholera and dysentery are dealt with by the main hospital, those that turn up at the health posts being referred on. This is a fairly rigorous procedure since part of the Government guidelines for control of these diseases was to have all cases treated in one location where isolated wards aim at preventing further transmission. However, in the more rural setting of Gorongosa, destruction of all health posts except for the central hospital during the war meant there was much greater possibility of cases from outer areas not being registered.

The identification of serotypes of cholera and dysentery relied on laboratory identification carried out at both Beira and Quelimane hospitals. Verification of the *Shigella* serotype was made by the Centro Epidemiologica, Ministério Da Saúde, Maputo. The laboratories aimed to monitor positive cases by culturing samples from one in every ten patients for the case of cholera. Verification of the dysentery serotype was made less frequently but produced consistent results throughout the epidemic, revealing that no other pathogen was responsible for the diarrhoea with blood symptoms. Conforming with common practice, the definition of an incident of the different diseases has been defined by the nature of the diarrhoea that the individual experienced during an epidemic period. For the case of cholera this is the classic 'rice-water stool', and in the case of dysentery 'bloody diarrhoea', symptoms distinct and familiar to the health staff registering the cases. The definition of a *case* conforms with the optimum described by Baqui *et al.* (1991) of the International Centre for Diarrhoeal Disease Research in Bangladesh, who recommend the occurrence of three or more loose stools or any number of loose stools containing blood, in comparative validation analyses.

Since the laboratories carrying out the microbiological tests maintained a register of positive identifications of cholera it was possible to cross-check the registrations made in the main registry books to confirm their reliability. The laboratory books were also able to supply the important information sought by this research on specific serotypes of cholera, since this was also established during the microbiological screening process. Whereas not every case of cholera is screened, the periods of different serotype prevalence at each site could be clearly distinguished since there was little mixing of the two.[4] All the extracted health records registering date of admittance, residence by sublocation, age and sex, were entered in chronological order into files classified by disease type and field site, in the database component of the MINITAB statistical package.

Physical environmental data Local physical environmental data was collected to facilitate an associative analysis with the pattern of incidence displayed by the two diseases. Using the selection technique described earlier, a total of 623 water samples and 165 soil samples were analysed. Water and soil analysis was carried out using portable Del Agua laboratories and the state-run provincial water-testing laboratories of Quelimane and Beira. Broader impressions were obtained through *in situ* observation of land use and vegetation, and by use of maps and air photography where these were available. To further facilitate an understanding of the role of background physical environmental influences and seasonality, daily rainfall data for the entire period of the epidemics for each site was compiled. This was taken from records kept at the airports of Beira and Quelimane, and from the NGO Redd Barna for Gorongosa.

Salinity has been indicated earlier as being influential on the survivability and toxigeneity of *Vibrio cholerae* in aquatic reservoirs and is one of the key environmental variables contributing to the hypothesis of an environmental influence on cholera. Comparable measures for salinity in and around the sites were established by recording the conductivity of the well water. This gives a quick and easy comparative measure for salt concentrations in water by measuring positive ion content (for a full discussion see Talsma *et al.* (1971), Wilson (1974), Mackereth *et al.* (1978), Chapman (1992), and Cairncross (1983)). The conductivity was measured at the field sites using a calibrated 'Palintest' conductivity meter.

---

[4] Serotype Ogawa has consistently been recorded in Quelimane and there was only one switch between Ogawa and Inaba and back to Ogawa for the case of Beira (this is discussed in detail in chapter 4). The Gorongosa serotypes were Inaba.

The level of pH forms the other key environmental variable implicated in influencing the viability of *Vibrio cholerae* in aquatic reservoirs. Water pH was determined at the field sites using a colour comparator and dissolvable tablets. The pH was measured in both water and soil samples since these can vary depending on the influence of rainwater, and because a better impression of the overall local environmental status can be obtained. Soil pH was measured using the Barium sulphate and Munsel colour chart standard technique on samples taken back to the laboratories.

Conforming with World Health Organization guidelines for assessment of the faecal pollution of drinking water (WHO 1983, 1985), and to assess levels of contamination in different areas, faecal coliforms were cultured and counted for all water sites. The presence of faecal coliforms in water means that pathogens related to the human intestines are also likely to be present, given the well-defined circumstances of epidemics such as these. However, a direct correlation between levels of faecal coliforms and prevalence of *Vibrio cholerae* has become questionable since the discovery that *Vibrios* may be autochthonous to the aquatic environment. There is still a lack of information on direct correlations with *Shigella dysenteriae*. However, a stronger correlation between dysentery and faecal coliforms than for cholera would be further evidence of the greater secondary transmissibility of dysentery through water, without the physiological constraints that apply to *Vibrio cholerae*. Faecal coliform tests were carried out using membrane filtration with apparatus sterilised in the field after each sample, incubation with lauryl sulphate nutrient at 44°C for 12-16 hours and a colony count.

Other micro-scale variables that were included were water turbidity as a supplementary water quality measure (WHO 1985, p4). Turbid water is more likely to harbour disease pathogens because it is constituted by suspended material, such as organic material, bacteria, algae, clay and minerals. However, despite its regular use in water quality surveys, it may be limited in identifying the worst sites for the same reasons as were outlined for faecal coliforms above. Turbidity values were determined by use of a transparent turbidity tube. Soil bulk density tests and a broad identification of soil type were carried out to facilitate a general assessment of compaction of ground surfaces. This was included in response to the suggestion from preliminary work that changes to the ground surface due to devegetation, flooding, and high population densities, may be associated with higher cholera incidence through resultant alkalinisation and salinisation of the local environment.

Soil bulk density was calculated by removing one vertical cylinder of earth of diameter 67 mm and height 98 mm and weighing after drying at a temperature of 105°C in a desiccator. The bulk density is derived by dividing the mass of the oven-dried soil by its field volume as described by Smith and Thomasson (1974, p42). Additional notes were made on factors such as the water odour, chlorine content for piped water (determined using a colour comparator and dissolvable tablets), and general condition of wells. This satisfied further requirements stipulated by the local authorities to whom a copy of all the water quality data for this research was submitted at the end of each phase of fieldwork. Chlorine content turned out to be consistently below the minimum (0.2mg/litre) required to eradicate pathogens from the piped water network (WHO 1985, p2).

The portable laboratories enabled a large part of the work to be done whilst visiting each sample site, minimising the risk of contamination that occurs when samples are collected and transported to other locations for analysis. The state laboratories were used primarily for sterilisation of equipment, battery recharging and for the soil analysis. In the case of Gorongosa, where there is no laboratory, the kits were recharged using the guest house generator and sufficient material transported to the area to avoid the need for the main resterilisation procedures.[5]

Further details on use of water supply, sanitation and local environment were established through sub-sections of the questionnaire interviewing that accompanied the environmental analyses.

Questionnaire interviewing The principal criterion of the questionnaire interviewing was to provide enough information to be able to test the hypothesis that there is an association between population displacement and higher incidence of cholera and dysentery through changes in susceptibility and/or environmental change (the questionnaire can be consulted via the author). The main comparisons that were sought through the questionnaires were between the living circumstances of groups of voluntary and forced migrants and longer term residents, and between living circumstances before and after resettlement. The aim was to establish the role of population displacement in increasing vulnerability to disease, and indirectly to assess the extent of increases in disease incidence caused by local environmental changes. An answer to the latter question

---

[5] A maximum of 48 cultures could be carried out in one period using pre-sterilised petri-dishes. Soil samples were analysed at the Beira laboratory.

can partly be gained based on the rationale that health impacts resulting from changes to the local environment would also affect the health of less mobile people in the same area. On the other hand, health outcomes resulting from the changed circumstances of being displaced would not apply to the non-displaced people.[6]

Other sections of the questionnaire were designed to indicate the possible variations in circumstances that contribute to increasing exposure to disease hazards and /or changes in susceptibility to disease through socio-economic and behavioural factors. In particular, questions centred around water supply, sanitation, fuel and crops, since these are potentially interrelated with health and diarrhoeal disease. For example, better water supply and sanitation facilities protects against exposure to pathogens; availability of fuel enables food to be cooked and water boiled to kill pathogens; and ownership of land can improve disease resistance through improved nutrition. Additionally, variation in these aspects of primary subsistence serves as an indication of more general socio-economic and livelihood well-being of households, reinforced by questions on economic activities, and the condition of the house and immediate neighbourhood. Comparative health data were also sought from the questionnaires by asking whether the respondent had suffered from cholera and/or from bloody diarrhoea within the last three years. Additional questions concerned the type and source of remedy used, extent of community interaction and co-operation in health issues, and perception of the causes and means to reducing incidence of cholera and dysentery (including what the local authorities and the government could do). Further indications of the overall circumstances at the field sites were sought through questions concerning changes in the availability of drinking water and fuel and whether respondents thought they were suffering more illness than previously.

It must be noted that there is a potential limitation on the use of questionnaires for retrospective study of disease incidence through loss of accurate recall of individuals. One landmark study by Forsberg and Van Ginneken *et al.* (1993) compared data from cross-sectional household surveys of diarrhoea incidence with the same locations as large scale

---

[6] The use of a 10 year limit for asking questions about previous circumstances was employed since it was considered that beyond this period it would not be likely that questions of immunity, susceptibility, adaptation and integration would be very relevant. Further explanation of the use of time periods in classifying residents as 'recently settled' or 'established' appears in Chapter 5.

surveys and within a narrow time margin. They found that the differences were too large to be accounted for by true variation in the variable being studied and suggested that validity problems could be due to response and recall errors. They also recognised that the programme had a 'positive' effect on the behaviour of health workers and target groups in the community and recommended better training of surveyors. A further key study on the reliability of health interview surveys has been carried out by Fabricant and Harpham (1993) using reinterviews. The results show that non-sampling errors were much greater than errors due to sampling, with certain types of question subject to greater error than others. Whilst much attention is typically paid to sampling errors, and they are relatively well understood, arguably less attention has been paid to this greater source of error.

Some of these weaknesses in the questionnaire approach have been reduced in this research. Firstly, the definition of a case was defined as someone who reported having had their condition confirmed at the health clinic or hospital, rather than simply having had diarrhoea. This helped to eliminate those cases of less severe diarrhoea caused by other pathogens and meant that recall errors were less likely. Recall was also assisted by the fact that knowledge of death through cholera or dysentery when not treated was good, such that most people would seek help or be carried to clinics where their condition could be confirmed.

The questionnaire was translated from original English drafts into Portuguese and the syntax further examined by one of the research assistants provided by Centro de Higiene Ambiental e Exames Medicos (CHAEM) in Beira, whose other employment included teaching English at a local night school. Further consultation on the content of the questionnaires and small alterations were made on the advice of an employee of the government planning office who was native to the region, spoke all the dialects, and had previous experience of questionnaire surveys in that city. The same employee worked as a research assistant for the interviewing in both Beira and Gorongosa where similar dialects are used. A local interviewer with previous training and experience of health questionnaire surveys was also provided by the Direcção da Saúde da Cidade in Quelimane. All communication for the implementation of the field work in Mozambique was carried out in Portuguese. Most interviews were also carried out in Portuguese since this is widely spoken by all sectors of urban Mozambique, and most rural areas.[7] However, ability to speak Portuguese was not a factor in the selection of respondents and there were some instances where the local interviewers had to communicate in Mandau (Beira), Masena (Beira), Chuabo (Quelimane), and Chirgorongodzi (Gorongosa).

Interviews typically took place with three people present, interviewee, interviewer and researcher, the structured part of the interview being administered by the local assistant, introduced above, who spent time in prior consultation on how to administer this questionnaire successfully. By having an assistant to administer the questionnaire there was more opportunity for the 'researcher' (myself) to simultaneously make extra notes and observations whilst present at each interview, supplementary to the information recorded on the standardised questionnaire.

Demographic data Data on the population of each sub-area was acquired from local government departments, such as the Direcção de Saúde de Quelimane, the Direcção de Saúde da Beira, and the Conselho Executivo da Cidade da Beira. Those for Quelimane had been compiled by the *chefe* of each Bairro within the last few years. In Beira, there had not been a count since the 1980s and a projection of the data had been used to provide the 1994 figures. The Gorongosa figures were believed to be the most accurate since there had been recent and regular assessment of numbers, by the local administration and the NGO 'Food For The Hungry', for distributing aid. It is accepted that there is likely to be errors in the population totals, particularly in the case of Beira. However, the figures were considered adequate for comparing rates of incidence between sub-locations.

Data Analysis

Mapping the Problem

The Geographical Information System (GIS) 'ARC INFO' was used both to create the maps that have been used for this research, and as a database

---

[7] Following independence in 1975 one of the Government's key campaigns was literacy. Portuguese was officially maintained as the national language as a means to creating national unity between the 12 major language groups.

of original, transformed and statistically-derived data. The map compilation stage was particularly important since, unlike in most more developed parts of the world, obtaining existing good maps at a suitable scale with the desired information was only partly successful. Though some old plans were acquired, there were none available for Quelimane or Beira with co-ordinates visible, making it initially difficult to work with geo-referenced data. The following procedure using ARC INFO functions resolved this shortcoming and demonstrates how GIS/GPS combinations can be applied to problems of this type in parts of the world lacking up-to-date and detailed cartographic coverage. This could be particularly useful for dealing with disaster situations in remote areas where GPS point analysis is required and good maps are scarce.

The best of the existing plans of the three areas were selected and separate layers or *coverages* of information digitised, such as administrative boundaries, roads and rivers. Since no grid or co-ordinates could be taken from the plans, an artificial grid was created. Whilst in the field the GPS was used to give co-ordinates to several key features represented on the map, such as major road intersections. These locations were digitised as *ticks* or control points on the ARC INFO coverages. The tick positions were updated in the ARC INFO TABLES mode with the UTM values derived from the GPS geographic co-ordinate values. 'TRANSFORM' commands were then used to project the old maps and plans into a real world co-ordinate system suitable for use with the GPS generated data, subsequently used for indicating the position of sample sites. In the case of Gorongosa, this procedure also facilitated the drawing of part of the map itself using the GPS to locate principal physical features whilst trekking the area.

Cross-sectional Spatial Analysis

Rates of cholera and dysentery for each sub-zone were calculated. The density of population for each sub-area was taken into account using areas measured by ARC INFO. Differences in the rate of incidence of the two diseases were compared by subtracting one from the other for each sub-area and then mapping the results. Further statistical investigation of the similarities between the two disease distributions at the different field sites was established using correlation coefficients, an index of dissimilarity based on the Lorenz curve, and the chi-square statistic. Differences between standardised residuals, calculated separately from observed and expected rates of incidence of each disease, were mapped. Where there was significant correlation between the two diseases, regression analysis was used and the residuals mapped. These were also compared with the spatial distribution of environmental variables. Where at least seven field sites were tested within one area an averaged value for the environmental variable was calculated.[8] Correlation coefficients and significance values were determined for associations between rates of cholera, dysentery, population density, and all the environmental parameters. In the case of a significant initial correlation, residuals from regression analyses were investigated and mapped to reveal possible secondary associations.

Spatio-temporal Analysis

The epidemic curves for the two diseases were plotted and correlated with monthly precipitation rates for Quelimane and Beira and some sporadic rain data for Gorongosa. To clarify the role of seasonal dimensions to water contamination, levels of faecal coliform contamination in the water supply were compared for two periods of the year. Further environmental influences on the spatial diffusion and persistence of the diseases were analysed using graph plots to assess the degree of spread from the sub-areas that represented the main core of the epidemic. Analysis of change in environmental parameters for the well sites was made by correlating the repeat data for the two survey phases. A correlation matrix for disease rates, population density and the environmental variables was determined so that phases 1 and 2, the two seasonal periods, were treated separately. This was to see if there was indication of stronger association during different periods of the year.

A qualitative approach was also used to analyse changes in infrastructure that relate to health, such as housing, water supply and sanitation, based on key information gathered in the field sites and existing documentary material. The implications for health of structural adjustment were considered through local discussion and observation, focussing for example on its behavioural consequences as well as its influence on disease hazards in the environment and human vulnerability.

---

[8] Some areas with less than seven samples were omitted from this part of the analysis, due to the possibility of too few sites providing spurious representation of the sub-area's physical environment. The minimum number of seven samples required for inclusion of a sub-area was used for practical reasons, since below this level few sub-areas needed to be excluded.

Despite achieving wide ranging primary and secondary data for this research, some limitations are recognised. For example, in carrying out spatio-temporal analysis water quality was only sampled at two times of year. Ideally and with more extensive resources this would have been carried out on a continuous basis. Although 748 successful interviews were achieved, the survey could also have been improved by interviewing on the magnitude of the health data, which consisted of 10,000 cases of cholera and dysentery. It could be argued that there is a weakness in the research strategy in that those interviewed are based on a different population to the cases registered in hospital registries. It would have not been possible to try to locate names registered in hospital admissions books, since only the *bairro* within which they lived was accurately recorded. It should also be pointed out here that there was no overall census data, and that the region has been subject to dramatic changes in recent years. Ultimately practical constraints on the quantity of data achieved can lead to inference in research analysis. Of particular note is the well-established limitation of using group analysis to infer about individuals and the limitation of using individual analyses to infer about the group. Nonetheless, it is the opinion of the author that this research represented one of the most extensive and cost-effective urban surveys carried out in central Mozambique in recent decades.

4 The Disease Environment of Beira, Quelimane and Gorongosa as Background to Incidence of Cholera and Bacillary Dysentery

This chapter describes the field sites with respect to environmental, demographic and contextual characteristics that have been suggested as influencing the incidence of cholera and dysentery in the previous chapters. Elements proposed as proximate determinants of disease in the systems approach outlined in Chapter 3 are also identified. This provides a location specific background in advance of more detailed analyses of spatial associations and interconnectivity in subsequent chapters. First, a macro-scale analysis of incidence of the two diseases is presented. This is followed by an account of background geophysiology, environmental changes and seasonality at the sites. Next, characteristics of the population and recent mobility are described. The latter part of the chapter introduces use of land and water and background infrastructural features.

Variability of Cholera and Bacillary Dysentery in the Research Area

Cholera associated with the contemporary pandemics affecting Africa arrived in Mozambique for the first time in July 1973 at the capital Maputo. By 1974 it had spread to 5 other provinces, including Sofala and Zambézia, and 753 cases with 90 deaths had been reported (Aragon and Barreto et al. 1994). An approximation of subsequent annual incidence is provided by the epidemiological department of the Ministry of Health (Figure 4.1). During the period between 1973 and 1993 there were only 6 years when cases of cholera were not registered (Barreto 1994). The first major epidemic is recorded as occurring in about 1983 with a focus on the south of the country. One reference to this states that there were in excess of 10,000 cases with 447 notified deaths (Cliff and Noormahomed 1988). The broad explanation for the epidemic was that the war in Mozambique had created ideal conditions for the spread of infectious diseases, with an increase in crowding, decreased access to water, and malnutrition (Cliff and Noormahomed 1988, p721).

A study by Rutherford and Mahanjane (1985) amongst displaced people in Gaza and Inhambane Provinces in 1983 found that on average mortality rates were 96 per 1000 per year and morbidity 283 illnesses per 1,000 per month. Whilst malnutrition was the highest cause of death (35 per cent) followed by diarrhoea (27 per cent), the most common morbidity diagnosis was diarrhoea (44 per cent). Detailed information at provincial level for the centre and north of the country during this period is not available though incidence is understood to have decreased nationally during the period 1985-1989 (Figure 4.1). Consistent with this assertion, Cutts (1988) makes no reference to cholera during a survey of target disease incidence rates in the City of Quelimane in 1986. However, incidence of diarrhoea from other causes remained high with an average 115 cases per 1,000 people per year and average mortality rate of 4.2 per 1,000.

The more recent wave of major epidemics, which began in 1989, coincided with a global surge in incidence of cholera during which the fastest spread and rates of increase were found amongst African countries. By the end of 1992, Mozambique had the highest number of cases and highest rate of incidence on the continent (WHO 1993a), taking second place ,to neighbouring Malawi in 1993 (WHO 1994b). During 1990 and 1991 Zambézia was by far the most affected province with more than 3,000 reported cases. Cholera subsided throughout the country between July 1991 and November 1991 before a new epidemic took off and lasted through to May 1993. During this period incidence was much higher in all provinces than during 1991 except in the cases of Nampula and Cabo Delgado, which are in the far north of the country (Figure 4.2). The drought of 1992 coincided with the period of highest incidence and this has been implicated as an associating factor due to the reduction in availability of clean water and through increased vulnerability caused by disruption of the food supply (Aragon and Chambule *et al.* 1993; Aragon and Barreto *et al.* 1994).   Cholera was considered as having waned or disappeared in most areas by mid 1993, attention instead being focused on the dysentery epidemic which by then was widespread and severe. However, new surges

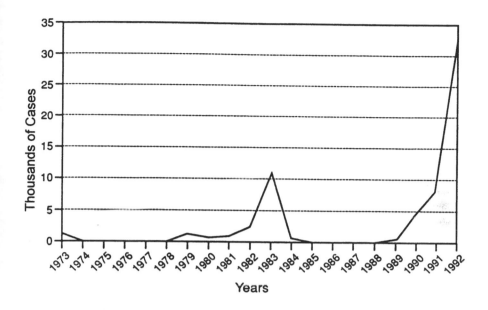

Figure 4.1   Reported cases of cholera in Mozambique for the period 1973-1992

Source: Gabinete de Epidemiologia, Ministério da Saúde, 1993, p.25

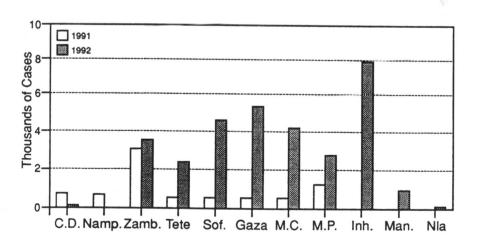

Figure 4.2   Cases of cholera in Mozambique by province for 1991 and 1992

Source: Gabinete de Epidemiologia, Ministério da Saúde, 1993, p.25

of cholera occurred in the north of Nampula Province and neighbouring south of Cabo Delgado Province which had been previously less affected. The first cases were registered in July 1993 and about 8,000 people were reported to have been treated by November 1993 (MSF 1993a, 1993b). This was brought under control by the end of the year and confirmed reports of cholera in Mozambique since this period have been minor. However, there has been plenty of conflicting data.[1] Potential errors have been reduced in the health data used for the more detailed analyses presented in this book by only using data collected directly from locally maintained records in the field.

Dysentery, otherwise referred to as bloody diarrhoea, spread into Mozambique from Malawi during the second half of 1992. It had been reported as entering the Central region of Malawi from Zambia at the beginning of 1992 and had taken hold amongst the Mozambican refugees in the south by June (Paquet 1992). Its origins to the north and interior of Africa meant that *Shigella dysenteriae* 1 was suspected before any laboratory confirmation being made, since this pathogen was known to have been causing epidemics there since 1979 (WHO 1988; Ries and Wells *et al.* 1994). By May 1993 estimates of 10,000 cases and 100 deaths for Mozambique were being made by the Ministry of Health and the situation was declared an absolute epidemic and out of control (Tempo 1993). A total of 47,483 cases and 199 deaths were later reported for the entire year (Aragón and Barreto 1995), although many cases are suspected as having remained unrecorded. The dysentery epidemic was continuing to occur at the time of editing this publication. Accurate country-wide data for the earlier part of the epidemic is not complete due to the rapidity of spread, difficulty in diagnosing cases of a 'new illness', and because initially, unlike cholera, it was not classified as a WHO recorded disease. At local level good information was available for the selected field sites

---

[1] Figures presented in the *Weekly Epidemiological Review* (1994) of the World Health Organization, Geneva appear to be in error. They report receiving notification of 4,551 cases of cholera in Mozambique during the period 11th to 17th February 1994 (p.52) and include Beira and Quelimane as infected areas (p.49). The research described in this book was not able to find evidence of cases during that period despite visits to hospitals, health posts and local government offices in the area under question. MSF (1994a) also report no cases for this period. However, up to 400 new cases occurred in Beira during September and October 1994 (MSF 1994b). There may be several explanations for large scale errors such as these. Reporting by WHO might be subject to a lengthy time lag in getting information from the field to Geneva and therefore it relates to some other period, the reported cases were not cholera but dysentery, or some other administrative error has occurred.

through reference to the hospital and health post registry books, which improved in quality following a decree by the Ministry of Health to start registering cases with as much rigour as had been done for cholera.

Despite dramatic increases in incidence of diarrhoeal disease in Mozambique during the 1990s the overall death rate has been decreasing. This is displayed by the Ministry of Health data presented as Figure 4.3, and may reflect the intensification of Government and NGO emergency assistance programmes which promote Oral Rehydration Therapy, antibiotics for severe cases, and provide isolated diarrhoea wards at hospitals. However, it should be noted here that since death rates are calculated as the percentage of the overall number of affected people, higher morbidity in recent years has meant increases in actual numbers of deaths. These figures demonstrate that, although curative medicine has been partly successful in treating cases, the main challenge to combating diarrhoeal disease remains one of preventative health care aimed at reducing initial morbidity.

Though the countrywide pattern of incidence of the diseases cannot be

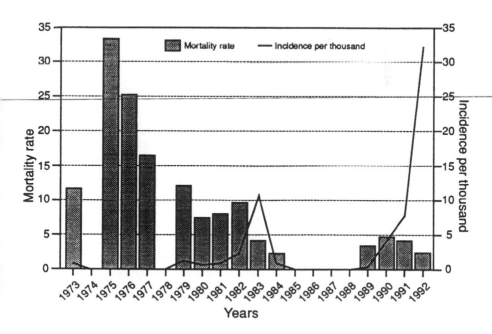

Figure 4.3   Annual incidence and death rate from cholera in Mozambique for the period 1973-1992

Source: Gabinete de Epidemiologia, Ministério da Saúde, 1993, p.29

explained by singular causes some initial broad associations can be suggested. For the case of cholera, Mozambique's macro-scale geographical features are characteristics that have been associated with endemic areas in the past. These include its low elevation and estuarine cities, high temperatures and humidity, heavy seasonal rainfall, and increased concentration of population because of war (Adesina 1975; Merson 1980; Miller *et al.* 1982, 1985; Learmonth 1988; WHO Features 1990; WHO Technical Report 1991). This is also borne out to some extent by the higher incidence that has generally been reported in coastal regions and cities within the sedimentary basin that occupies about 31 per cent of Mozambique.

Using the finer resolution of sub-provincial areas the distribution of high and low incidence continues to present a diverse pattern. The anomalies of an uneven distribution of cases at sub-provincial level were pointed out by health workers at the Provincial Directorate of Health for Zambézia in 1991 where the main cholera epidemic that year was occurring. Having compiled estimates of known cases by district, no clear explanation was apparent for the pattern of incidence. During that period all parts of the Province were considered to be in a state of crisis. As such, areas of both low and high incidence were suffering disruption by war and malnutrition. The universality of poverty in Zambézia also suggested that additional place specific factors were influential on the pattern of incidence. A lack of accurate quantitative data during this period, such as demographic figures for the individual districts which would enable the calculation of rates of incidence, limited any more detailed an analysis. However this has been possible for the major urban areas used in this book.

Some environmental contrasts between sub-areas of the provincial capital of Zambézia, Quelimane have already been identified (Collins 1993). One indication from this preliminary work was that there is a physical environmental explanation to the distribution of incidence of cholera defined in terms of higher salinity and alkalinity in some parts of the city. However, further unanswered questions related to the role of population displacement which was also a feature of the areas of higher incidence. Local health workers and members of the public informally contended that displaced people were associated with high incidence of the disease. Two years later displacement was reported in the National Press as being a factor in the intensification of disease in general (Mohomed 1993). This was suggested primarily for the case of Malaria but a similar association was implied for other diseases. The explanation was that many people who previously lived in non-infected areas had moved to areas where there was already a manifestation of the disease but that this intensified due to their presence. However, details of the mechanisms that might be involved had not been investigated. Further to this, the uncontrolled growth of urban populations caused by displacement has, in generalised terms, been mentioned as a factor behind the recent increase in incidence of cholera by Aragon and Barreto *et al.* (1994).

The case of bacillary dysentery presents an added challenge to understanding varied causes of diarrhoeal disease within Mozambique. The epidemic spread from the centre of the Continent and via the Malawian refugee camps. Though it is not likely to have been the only route, the progression of reports of outbreaks within Mozambique, which started around northern Tete Province (MSF 1992a, 1992b), suggest a link with the movement of refugees to and from the Malawi camps. At the outset of investigations, there is therefore some evidence suggesting a demographic explanation for the spread of dysentery, in contrast to the environmental explanation advanced for the cholera epidemic. The rapidity of the spread of dysentery meant that it often broke out in areas where cholera was just being brought under control, such as in the provincial capitals of Quelimane and Beira at the end of 1992. Meanwhile, local personnel running the wards at health centres noted that dysentery seemed to affect a wider range of people than cholera did, citing the fact that the more materially 'well-off' were also being affected. The persistence of dysentery, and the apparently different pattern of infection to cholera reinforced the need to investigate associating factors of diarrhoeal disease with respect to the individual pathogens responsible.

Recent Morbidity and Mortality in Quelimane, Beira and Gorongosa

During the 1990-1991 wave of cholera in Mozambique, Zambézia Province was the worst affected. The District of which Quelimane is a part had the highest rate of incidence out of all the districts in the Province, calculated as 53 cases per 10,000 by the Dirrecção Provincial de Saúde da Zambézia (Delgado and Azevedo *et al.* 1992). This compares with about 6 per 10,000 for the country as a whole and 15 per 10,000 for Zambézia Province. The first diagnosed case in this epidemic occurred in Unidade Communal Chirangano on the 17th of July 1990 (Figure 4.4). The patient had been host for one week to a relative from Beira who had been suffering

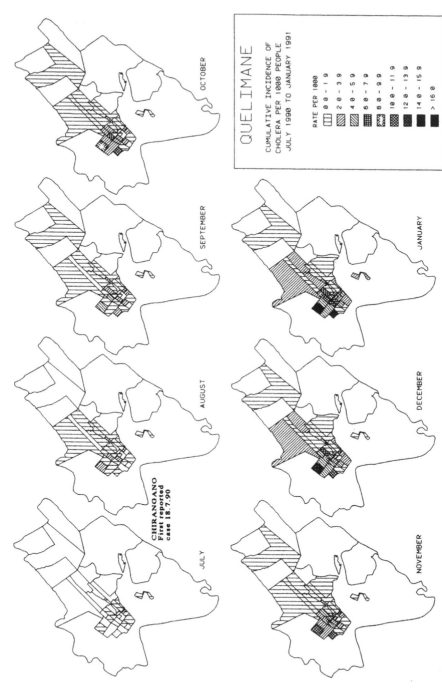

Figure 4.4 First reported case and cumulative incidence of cholera at Quelimane, 1990

from diarrhoea. The main spread of the epidemic throughout Zambézia appears to have occurred after its becoming established in Quelimane. However, some cases were reported earlier in the southern District of Chinde (Figure 3.2), in the Zambezi river delta, as early as February 1990 (Delgado and Azevedo *et al.* 1992, p5).

The first diagnosed case of cholera in Beira during the 1990-1991 epidemic occurred at the earlier date of 9th June. The origin of this infection remains unclear, though the patient was resident in a large concrete building in the inner part of the city (Cunguara 1991). A possible link with Tete Province was made because a visiting sick relative had come from there (Cunguara 1991, p23). However, the diagnosed case had been ill before the visit from Tete and no proof is available that the cholera came from that region. In general, there is no clear evidence that the 1990-1991 epidemic originated outside the country and it is therefore reasonable to suggest that it could have represented resurgence of the earlier epidemics of the 1980s.

In Sofala, the disease started in Beira before spreading into other districts, as with earlier epidemics. The province was the second most affected in 1974 with 259 cases. In 1979 a further 64 cases were registered and in 1980-1981 there was an epidemic with 1,161 registered cases and 114 deaths (Cunguara 1991, p22). The data for the period of 1981-1982 is reported by Cunguara (1991) to have revealed that incidence of cholera spread from Beira to the Districts of Dondo, Nhamatanda, Buzi, Caia and Marromeu. These are all low lying districts with population concentrations at or near to large rivers, such as the Pungwe, Buzi and Zambezi. The central and generally upland District of Gorongosa is not thought to have been affected at that stage. Given these circumstances of low lying riverine and estuarine environments an overall physical environmental association is also feasible for this epidemic.

No detailed data is available for the period 1984-1986 in Beira.[2] However the City Health Department acknowledge that there were

---

[2] The period 1984-1986 was a particularly difficult time in Beira's history which lacks statistics on health and well-being in general. During this period it was one of the few disaster affected regions of the world with almost no aid or media coverage. The essential link to Zimbabwe was cut off for much of the time and local residents refer to famine on the streets. There may have been many unregistered cases of cholera since the central hospital was functioning at only a minimum level with no electricity or regular water supply. Some foreign assistance was received via a few Soviet medics and international *cooperantes* who assisted Government departments but often with limited backup.

substantial quantities of cases. One of the few reports on disease incidence shows that there were an estimated 437 notifications of diarrhoea per 1,000 people amongst the under 5 age group in Beira as opposed to 132 per 1,000 in Quelimane (Cutts 1988, p236).

The 1992 epidemic The 1992 epidemic was the biggest in a 20 year history of the seventh pandemic El Tor cholera in Mozambique. Figures vary in different accounts but generally conservative estimates indicate that there were nationally around 32,000 cases and 780 deaths within the year (Aragon and Chambule *et al.* 1993; WHO 1993a). This represented the highest annual total in the history of cholera in Mozambique, three times higher than in 1991 and 8 times higher than in 1990. The previous highest had been in 1983 with 10,745 cases and 447 deaths (Aragon and Chambule *et al.* 1993, p.15). The dramatic rise in the figures is suggested by Aragon and Chambule *et al.* (1993) as being partly due to changes in the way that positive cases were included. For some areas only clinically proven cases were previously counted, whereas more recently all cases of severe diarrhoea in an area supporting some positive tests for cholera are included. This source of error would suggest that earlier figures were under-estimates and therefore that the real contrasts with the 1992 figures should be less pronounced. However it is unlikely that this would affect the overall trend of increasing numbers of cases with the latter epidemic, which is known to have also increased in other parts of the continent.

A distinguishing feature in 1992 was that three new provinces became affected since the 1990-1991 epidemic, and that one of these, Inhambane, had the highest number of cases (Figure 4.2). Increases were most dramatic in Provinces that had fewer cases during the previous year, except in Cabo Delgado and Nampula where there were decreases on an already lower rate of incidence. In Zambézia, the focus of the biggest epidemic during 1991, there was a marginal increase in cases, whereas in Sofala the number of cases increased well beyond that of the previous year to be more than Zambézia. This pattern at the outset suggests that cholera in 1992 could have been related to a new epidemic. It was separated from the previous one by three months of zero incidence during August, September and October of 1991 and displayed a different pattern of incidence.

Additional features of the 1992 epidemic were that it was also more widespread at sub-provincial level, breaking out in districts previously unaffected. This included the District of Gorongosa in the centre of Sofala Province which by the latter part of 1992 had 'at least 600 cases' and '165 deaths' (MSF Dec 1992, p10).[3] The Gorongosa epidemic was occurring at the same time as the arrival in and around the town of people from other parts of the district occupied by RENAMO. By far the largest surge in arrivals was the estimated 12,000 newcomers in October 1992 (MSF 1992a). This followed the signing of the National Peace Accord and temporary lifting of restrictions on population movements by local RENAMO commanders. Apart from the demographic figures presented to MSF by local representatives working for the Government, no more detailed information on an association of displaced people with disease incidence was readily available at this stage. The 1992 drought also seriously affected the district before the start of the epidemic. The famine caused by this was a major reason for population movements to government areas, where there was more aid at that time. Reports by MSF (1992a, p6, 1992b, p10) record that 561 children were receiving emergency feeding for advanced malnutrition at their base next to the health post. Also, summary statistics provided by the Nucleo Estatistica Provincial (unpublished) show that malnutrition was highest in Gorongosa District during 1992, with 45 per cent of children being affected compared to 14.5 per cent for the Province as a whole.

A further change occurred in Gorongosa as the rivers from which people drink moved into flood with the coming of the rains, causing water quality to visibly deteriorate. In response to this Agua Rural, the state owned rural water supply company, and MSF report initiating plans for construction of 3 new bore holes with hand pumps (MSF 1992a, p3). The case of the 1992 Gorongosa epidemic demonstrates a complex of politico-demographic and environmental factors that, at a superficial level of enquiry, presents difficulties in establishing the main cause of the disease. However, there is no suggestion of resurgence from an earlier endemic state as has been suggested elsewhere.

The dysentery epidemic arrived in Gorongosa as the cholera epidemic waned. Surprisingly this information does not appear in MSF reports which only sporadically mention cases of serious diarrhoea after June 1993 (MSF 1993c), and specifically dysentery in January and March of 1994 (MSF 1994c; MSF 1994d). During earlier field work in Gorongosa District

---

[3]No exact figures are available although, during a period when accurate registration took place between 20th November 1992 and 22nd December 1992, this research confirmed that in excess of 200 cases were recorded in the health centre registry. Official data for this district indicate much lower figures.

in April 1993, the Director of the health post said that they had treated 35 cases in December and 28 in January and that there had been further cases since then. However, key informants, such as the local Government representative for religious affairs and two local senior citizens, said that actual cases of bloody diarrhoea appeared substantially higher. It was public knowledge that even the Government administrator was suffering from bloody diarrhoea. A visit into the RENAMO areas of the district 50 km to the north-east, still isolated from the rest of the country during that period, confirmed that the dysentery epidemic was widespread in those areas too. People in advanced stages of dehydration and known to be passing blood in their stools could be seen staggering around the site where the interviews were being carried out with the RENAMO administrator and director of health on 5th May 1993 at Vunduzi, near to the base of Mt. Gorongosa. Unfortunately, numbers of cases and other demographic information were withheld, despite a formal request for medicines to treat the dysentery in that area. By the end of July 1993, the Gabinete de Epidemiologia of the Direcção de Saúde in Maputo indicated 425 cases of dysentery for government held parts of Gorongosa (unpublished data).

During the period after December 1992 population movements decreased substantially in comparison with the previous quarter year. Movement of population around the district at this time subsided because people had become 'tied' to cultivation and the forthcoming harvest that ended in late July. Return movements of refugees to this area from neighbouring countries were also minimal since people were waiting to see if the Peace Accord would hold before committing themselves to resettlement. On the face of it there therefore appears no strong background evidence that population movements were a major factor in the dysentery epidemic in Gorongosa.

Pathogenesis of Cholera and Bacillary Dysentery, and its Significance

Spatio-temporal variations in serotypes of pathogens causing acute diarrhoea provides a further basis for identifying likely influences on incidence of cholera and dysentery. This sub-section introduces the nature of the bacilli concerned, and suggests these are associated with different areas.

The seventh pandemic of El Tor cholera began in the Celebes Islands in 1961, spread through Asia in the 1960s, and to the Middle East by 1970 (Figure 4.5). In August 1970, the first cases in Africa this century were identified in Guinea (Glass and Claeson *et al.* 1991). The same El Tor cholera spread to 30 of the continent's 46 countries increasing and decreasing with numerous epidemic foci. By 1990 the affected countries of Africa accounted for 90 per cent of the world's cholera cases. Since the El Tor biotype was identified the epidemic in Mozambique has correctly been associated with the wider African epidemic from the outset. However, little attention to date had been paid to the varying serotypes of El Tor. Whilst this is an important aspect of much laboratory work, epidemiological and other field studies referring to incidence of cholera often fail to pay attention to its possible significance in explaining disease distributions. It is particularly relevant now that there is an increased understanding of the role of aquatic reservoirs, dynamic ecologies, and possible evolution of new pathogens through selection advantages in changing environments (Chapter 1).

In Quelimane, serotype Ogawa was identified throughout the epidemics of 1990-1991 (Collins 1993, p325) and 1991-1993. However, in

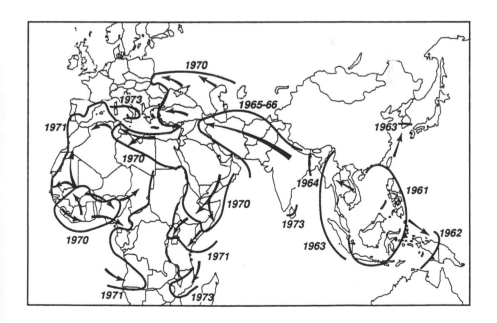

**Figure 4.5   Expansion of the seventh pandemic of El Tor cholera
                between 1961 and 1991**

Source: WHO, 1992a, p.210

Beira, whilst serotype Ogawa was identified for the first epidemic (Cunguara 1991, p23) Inaba was identified for most of the second. A small amount of Ogawa cases reappeared in Beira during the fading months of the second epidemic. Information for Gorongosa has relied on the results of a few specimens that were sent to Beira for analysis. These were reported by the health workers in Gorongosa to have produced the same results as for Beira at that time, indicating that they were also serotype Inaba. Interestingly, a recent study carried out by Folgosa and Valdivia *et al.* (1994) for Maputo city and Province between June 1991 and June 1992 reveals a pattern of serotype prevalence similar to that of Beira city and its surrounding province. For Maputo, serotype Inaba accounted for 89.9 per cent of 952 positive samples taken and serotype Ogawa for the remaining 10.1 per cent. The Ogawa cases were mainly in the city and occurred at the beginning and end of the main epidemic period.

The differing serotypes suggest two separate epidemic events for the early 1990s. Thus whilst Ogawa had become locally persistent and strong in Quelimane, it lost its advantage to the Inaba strain in other parts of the country. The more virulent Inaba strain was also able to take hold in new locations that had previously avoided the Ogawa epidemic. The pattern of much higher incidence of cholera in Quelimane in 1990-1991, and much higher incidence in Beira in 1991-1993 also supports this hypothesis of resurgent and new disease epidemics. Meanwhile, given that El Tor cholera provides insignificant immunity to subsequent infection from a different serotype (Clemens and Sack *et al.* 1990; Sepulveda and Gomez-Dantes *et al.* 1992), it is reasonable to suspect variation in background environmental factors as determining the differing distributions of the serotypes. Thus Ogawa seems to have been better adapted to Quelimane, whilst Inaba may have found a particularly suitable niche in Beira during the latter epidemic.

Observation of the distribution of diarrhoeal disease attributable to *Shigella dysenteriae* 1 provides a further clue. Since this epidemic first arrived in 1992, and there is also no evidence of pre-existing immunity, it could be suspected of behaving in a more similar fashion to the latter widespread Inaba serotype of cholera than to the earlier and more localised Ogawa serotype. More detailed results achieved through closer analysis in the field sites described here examine the validity of this assertion.

Physical Background and Geoecology of Disease at the Field Sites

As noted in Chapter 3, Quelimane and Beira are both provincial capitals on the central section of the Mozambican coastal plain. Quelimane is a sea port on the north bank of the River Cua Cua (formerly Rio dos Bons Sinais) in Zambézia Province and is about 300 km north-east of the port of Beira, which is situated at the mouth of the Pungwe river in Sofala Province. Some of the macro-environmental circumstances of the two cities are similar. However, regarding localised environmental factors of importance to an analysis of diarrhoeal diseases there are significant differences between and within these sites. Vila de Gorongosa is a smaller district capital situated 160 km north-west of Beira in the central upland zone of the country. The macro-scale physical environment at Gorongosa is significantly different to the other two sites because it is smaller, inland, 300 metres above sea-level, and has a different underlying geology.

Habitat Differentials and Preliminary Evidence of Environmental Reservoirs for Disease

As part of the sedimentary basin that occupies about 31 per cent of Mozambique, the zone within which Quelimane and Beira are situated is composed of sands with fine sands at the surface, micas and layers of clay. The immediate area in and around Quelimane is characterised by prolonged sand dune ridges, known locally as *morundas*, shallow depressions between them and coastal plains, some areas of which are covered by mangroves (Figure 4.6). The estimated heights of the sand dunes are between 5 and 10 meters above sea-level and they vary in dimension up to sizes of about 500 meters by 2,000 meters. The low areas between the dunes are poorly drained, sandy but with a certain amount of organic and clay material, and are permanently flooded for the wet part of the year. The layers of clay or high clay content in the sand are relevant factors to note in the context of water borne disease as seepage may be prevented or restricted, causing stagnation of groundwater that might otherwise be undergoing a continuous process of filtration.

The coastal plain consists of some grasslands and a drainage network of streams some of which are permanently in flood. These areas are characteristically very saline. Mangrove areas beside river inlets and small lakes, which flood at high tide, are also high in salinity and clay content.

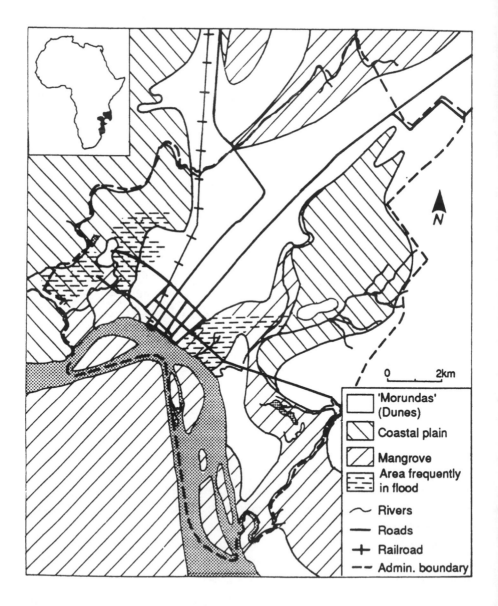

Figure 4.6   Main physical features of Quelimane

The drainage system consists of a large number of rivers and streams on which the salinizing influence of the ocean is known to remain up to a distance of 30 km inland in some cases. The presence of fresh water in the area remains largely restricted to shallow lens-shaped water bodies with a limited regional extension. However, no detailed information on the location of this water is known, the only recent hydrogeological survey for Quelimane concluding that:

> Their extent does not obey the laws for a situation of hydraulic equilibrium due to the presence of clayey layers that hamper the groundwater flow, the variation of the groundwater level during the seasons, the tidal effect and occurrence of recent floods. (Direcção Nacional de Aguas 1991 p2 author's translation)

The composition of the natural environment at Beira is similar to that of Quelimane in that large areas are flat swampland but it is generally characterised by a coarser sand. Part of the city directly borders onto the sea and has continuously suffered from coastal erosion. The critical drainage level is 7.5 metres, representing the level of the highest tide above which rainwater does not have any outlet to the sea. Permeability is poor due to the high clay content and rainwater sometimes stays for weeks on or close to the surface. Saline inundation is greatest in the low lying parts of the south of the city where flooding occurs along the drainage canals. The dune areas, and areas above 7.5 metres include some of the down town areas and a narrow coastal strip. Larger areas occur further inland at Manga and Inhamizúa and in hindsight it might be argued that this would have been a more suitable site for the development of the main habitational part of the city, rather than the water logged areas near the sea port. There are mangrove areas on the coast to the north, along the banks of the Pungwe River and some small surviving areas on the stream like River Chiveve in the centre of the city, which is practically blocked off at its exit to the Pungwe river.

Both cities typify environmental conditions that assist water-borne diseases since flooding is frequent. However, a more detailed analysis of the environmental conditions has been necessary to assess the possible role of aquatic reservoirs in maintaining endemic disease such as cholera since specific geochemical parameters vary from place to place, such as in the balance of saline and fresh water inundation. In Quelimane saline intrusions permeate large areas in and around the city, whereas in Beira they are more restricted. Instead, flooding in Beira is often caused by rainwater. Given that it has recently been shown that *Vibrio cholerae* is able to survive, be dormant, and establish toxigeneity in more saline and less acidic conditions it might be suspected that the physical conditions at Quelimane present more favourable circumstances for endemic cholera. However, analysis at this larger scale of comparison presents only a very generalised impression and requires examination at a more localised scale.

By way of environmental contrast the area in and around Vila de Gorongosa is very well drained with coarse *terra rosa* sands, perennial rivers and a dendritic pattern of intermittent streams (Figure 4.7). The area within which the district capital, Vila de Gorongosa is situated is a raised watershed about 300 meters in altitude and, apart from the Mt. Gorongosa range to the north, represents the higher part of the district. The Mt. Gorongosa range is about 30 km by 20 km, up to 1,863 metres in altitude and starts at about 20 km from the town. The natural biome of the region within which the town is situated is tropical dry forest. There are no areas of ponded up or slow moving water and therefore an aquatic reservoir for *Vibrio cholerae* is not suspected.

Recent and Localised Environmental Changes

Major negative environmental changes associated with human activity have not occurred in Mozambique to the extent they have in many other African countries. However, the view that Mozambique's natural environment may have escaped being degraded is rapidly changing. Large scale foreign owned logging operations are underway in several areas of the interior, such as in Gorongosa District, there are plans for intensive agriculture in the north, mining schemes, and the fish stocks previously reduced by Soviet trawlers are now exploited by Japanese industry. The impact of the accelerated development activity has barely been investigated. As recently as the early 1990s, O'Keefe and Kirkby *et al.* (1991) wrote a review of potential environmental problems suggesting that none of those outlined by Timberlake (1985) as characterising the crisis in Africa were significantly present at a national level. However, they concluded that some issues were locally relevant and in particular referred to the implications of high population concentrations resulting from the conflict, in the coastal zone, around major cities and along transport corridors.

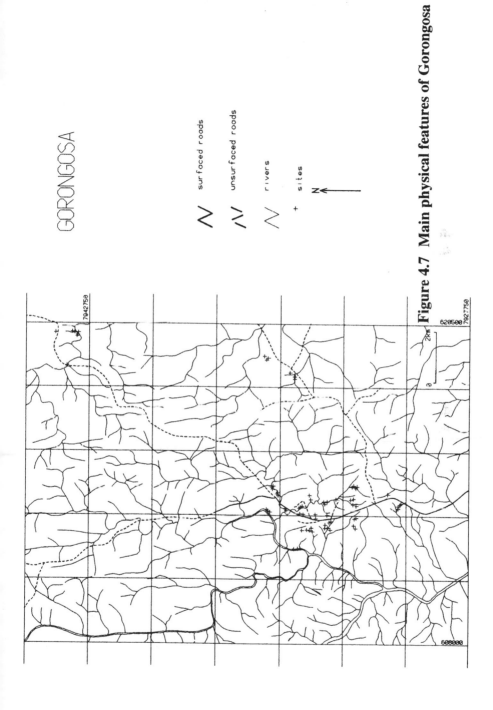

GORONGOSA

surfaced roads

unsurfaced roads

rivers

sites

N

Figure 4.7 Main physical features of Gorongosa

Some of Timberlake's environmental changes listed by O'Keefe and Kirby *et al.* (p308) are particularly relevant to health issues in the field sites investigated in this research. For example, resource overuse, fuelwood scarcity, soil degradation, and reduction in water availability and quality are processes that can both affect the overall balance of human well-being, and contribute to altering specific ecologies of disease pathogens. In the littoral zone within which Quelimane and Beira lie, it is reasonable to suspect that processes of devegetation that reduce soil acidity, or compacting of exposed soils that alter the fresh water balance of the aquifer are particularly relevant. An accumulation of salts builds up at the ground surface where there is regular flooding of exposed areas followed by evaporation. Salt concentrations measured at above 4 mS^{-1} (milliSiemens) in conductivity starts to destroy remaining non-salt tolerant vegetation (Thompson and Mannion *et al.* 1986). This process can be applicable to both flooding caused by sea-water and that caused by freshwater since the origin of the salt may be the soil itself. Reduced productivity of crops through environmental change increases susceptibility to disease through malnourishment, and fuelwood shortages can mean greater consumption of insufficiently cooked food and unboiled contaminated water. Even at times when a population receives food aid, such as in these field areas, it is often the small amounts of supplementary produce grown locally that provide the necessary vitamins and minerals for a healthy diet.

Urbanisation has also caused a variety of environmental changes in the field sites. In the cases of Quelimane and Beira, there is a distinction between changes that have occurred in the 'cement' city and those in the areas of 'spontaneous settlement',[4] classified as indigenous zones in colonial times. The 'cement' zones of the ex-colonial cities, are formally planned areas that include corrugated metal and timber buildings from the early part of this century, concrete residences, and more modern blocks of flats and offices. In the case of Beira in particular these are largely areas that have been artificially raised in elevation by sand infilling. However, much of the process of raising the level of the land remained uncompleted.

---

4 The term 'areas of spontaneous settlement' is often used in local planning offices in Mozambique to describe zones which have not been planned on the basis of a detailed urban structure plan and where the majority of occupants do not hold official documents for their occupancy. These predominantly consist of zones adjacent to what was considered the European city in colonial times. However, the term is recognised as controversial in that it fails to recognise unspontaneous mechanisms that operate at neighbourhood level.

The urban infrastructure of roads, sewers, drainage channels, treated water and electricity follows the same incomplete pattern and largely bypasses the former indigenous areas. These are situated on lower ground and are prone to flooding.

Beira is the city in Mozambique requiring the most artificial landfill and protection against the natural environment making it particularly dependent on maintenance. For example, groynes around the coast, a defensive sea wall along the estuary front and a 2 km long stretch of casuarinum trees, originally covering 100,000 m^2 to stabilise the sand and protect against the sea, all require maintenance. Drainage ditches originally designed to let fresh water out without sea water taking its place and used to reclaim areas for cultivation and grazing do not function. As such, environmental changes in the core of Beira have been largely linked to engineering initiatives taken during its colonial history, which no longer serve their intended function. Meanwhile the population has continued to grow rapidly so that increasing numbers of people are being exposed to these failing features of the city. In *bairros* near the concrete core of the city, pressures on the environment have come about more as a result of population increase, high density housing, depletion of vegetation, and flooding. The quality of the environment improves in the outer northern suburbs that benefit from being less congested, well vegetated with mango and palm trees and situated at a slightly higher elevation.

The contrasts between the concrete city and adjacent *bairros* is also pronounced in Quelimane, though in this case there is much greater homogeneity in housing type. Typically, most non-concrete housing is neatly constructed out of the products of the coconut palm. Main timbers are made from the trunk and the palm leaves are woven together to form the walls and roof. Alternatively, baked mud or reeds are used for the walls. In Beira, the equivalent housing is more often wattle, reed, tin, mud or made from cast-off products from the concrete city creating an appearance more reminiscent of a shanty town.

Vila de Gorongosa is made up of mud huts with grass roofs save for a few concrete buildings alongside the main roads. The main environmental impact of the town's population increase has been through removal of the vegetation cover for housing and fuel. This was particularly thorough in and around the town during the conflict when the residents lived under near siege conditions. Rills and gullies caused by soil erosion became widespread and the soil quality deteriorated due to its over exploitation. The density of housing is not as extreme as can be found in the larger cities but is far more than what occupants experienced before the conflict. Where people have now resettled away from the town their preferred distance between houses is typically in excess of 200 metres whereas in central Vila de Gorongosa they have been as little as 10 meters apart. Whilst the physical environment at Gorongosa looks less likely to be one where disease pathogens such as *Vibrio cholerae* could survive in the natural environment, it has represented a concentration of human poverty where susceptibility to disease is likely to be high.

Seasonality

The focal areas described here are situated within a sub-equatorial zone the southern limit of which extends to just south of Beira. The climate is therefore divided between a humid tropical wet season and dry warm winters with variations from place to place being mainly a function of elevation and fluctuations in air flow above the Mozambique Channel. There are typically much drier conditions at Gorongosa since it is over 100 km inland and 300 metres above sea level. At Quelimane the maximum monthly temperature varies between 27°C and 33°C, and the minimum, between 16°C and 24°C. (Direcção Nacional de Aguas 1991). At Beira, the average temperature of the hottest month, January, is reported as being 28°C and average of the coolest month, July, as 21°C (Serviço Provincial de Estatística 1993). The greater part of the rainfall comes in torrential storms and the average per annum has been reported as 1428 mm at Quelimane (DNA 1991) and 1551mm at Beira (SPE 1993). Reliable climatical data for Gorongosa was not available over a sufficient time period to calculate comparable data. However, figures from the aid agency, 'Redd Barna', who maintained data for the drier than normal period of 1993-1994, show that January was the wettest month with about 300 mm of rain and that the months between May and November had almost no rain. This is considerably less than at Beira or Quelimane.

A seasonal pattern to human activity is also to some extent apparent in these places through the timing of the two main harvests. Whilst some crops, such as cassava, are grown throughout most of the year, rice is sown at the beginning of the rains and harvested after it dries. Sweet potatoes often take its place and are harvested just in advance of the main rains. The coming and going of the main rains is therefore associated with an increase in movement of people travelling to and from their fields. Whereas these are sometimes near to the house, many people in the urban areas have to travel backwards and forwards to outlying areas. During a disease epidemic this increased mobility enhances secondary transmission from area to area and could be a further explanatory factor in explaining seasonal patterns of incidence. In Gorongosa the two main crops, maize and sorghum are grown simultaneously with a main harvest in July. Vulnerability through reduced nourishment also takes on a seasonal dimension should a harvest fail and aid is not forthcoming or nutritionally insufficient.

Land and Water Use

The main populated areas of Quelimane are on the *morundas* (sand dune ridges), habitation in other areas of the city being restricted to small temporary fishing settlements. Save for some informal and formal sector employment in the city centre, some small scale livestock production, and fishing, most local economic activity is agricultural. The cultivation of palm groves, cassava and maize is restricted to the *morundas* whilst rice and sweet potato are rotated on the lower areas between them, known locally as *entredunas*. Much of these more acidic and less saline areas are therefore not used for population settlement.

Some of the main parts of Quelimane are served by piped surface water from the river Licuari 50 km away. However, this supply was limited to certain times of day only, poorly filtered and chlorinated, and at times of drought ceased to function. Consequently the major supply of water was from the wells, and it is there that one might suspect to locate the most significant contamination linked to diarrhoeal disease epidemics. The remnants of an urban sanitation system, established in colonial times, supports some of the concrete areas of the city. However, the vast majority of people in both the concrete and other zones of the city only have access to rudimentary latrines. The presence of exposed faeces in and around the city was evidence that many people do not possess or use even the rudiments of a sanitation facility. Health care is centred on the provincial hospital in the concrete city bordering the river and this has been a focus of aid and assistance from NGO's in recent years. The municipal area of Quelimane is divided into 5 *bairros* representing major zones that subdivide down to a total of 39 smaller *unidades comunais* (communal areas) which are displayed in Figure 4.8.

Beira grew to be a considerably larger urban centre than Quelimane with historically significant functions as an international port, industrial

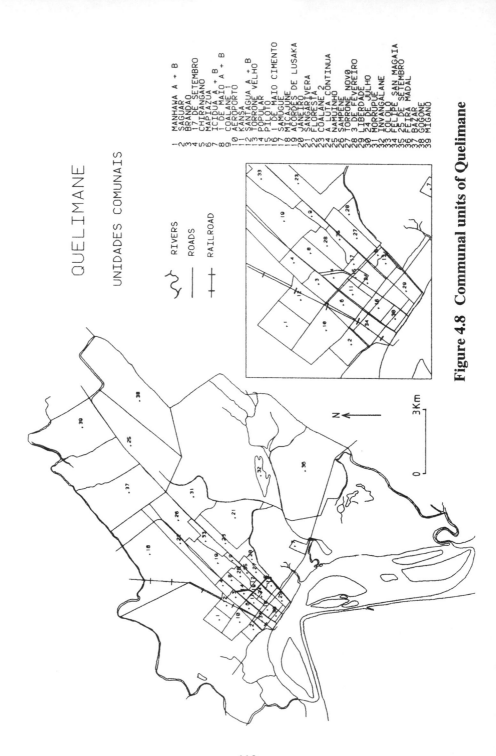

Figure 4.8 Communal units of Quelimane

QUELIMANE

UNIDADES COMUNAIS

RIVERS
ROADS
RAILROAD

1 — MANHAWA A + B
2 — SAGUAR
3 — BRANDAO
4 — 17 DE SETEMBRO
5 — CHIRANGANO
6 — MAPIAZUA
7 — ICIDUA
8 — CODE MAIO A + B
9 — CODE MAIO A + B
10 — AEROPORTO
11 — KANTA
12 — SANTAGUA A + B
13 — TORRONE VELHO
14 — POPULAR
15 — PILOTO
16 — 1 DE MAIO CIMENTO
17 — SAMGUE
18 — MICAUNE
19 — ACOPDES DE LUSAKA
20 — JANEIRO
21 — SANARVERA
22 — FLORESTA
23 — COALANE 2
24 — A LUTA CONTINUA
25 — NAMILINHO
26 — SAMPONE
27 — TORRONE NOVO
28 — 3 DE FEVEREIRO
29 — LIBEDADE
30 — 24 DE JULHO
31 — MORRUPULHO
32 — INVANGALANE
33 — COLONE
34 — POPULAR
35 — FELIPE SAN MAGAIA
36 — 25 DE SETEMBRO
37 — FEIRA MADAL
38 — BAZAR
39 — GOGONE
   — MIGANO

0   3Km

N

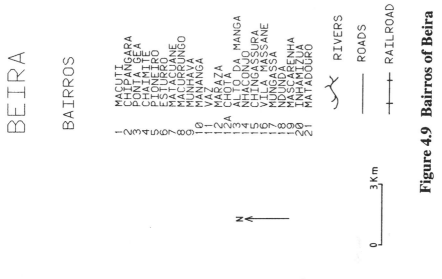

BEIRA

BAIRROS

1 — MACUTI
2 — CHIPANGARA
3 — PONTA GEA
4 — CHAIMITE
5 — PIONEIRO
6 — ESTURRO
7 — MATACUANE
8 — MACURRUNGO
9 — MUNHAVA
10 — MANANGA
11 — VAZ
12 — MARAZA
12A — CHOTA
13 — ALTO DA MANGA
14 — NHACONJO
15 — CHINGASSURA
16 — VILA MASSANE
17 — MUNGASSA
18 — NDUNDA
19 — MASCARENHA
20 — INHAMIZUA
21 — MATADOURO

〜 RIVERS

—— ROADS

+—+ RAILROAD

N ←——

0 |——| 3 Km

Figure 4.9 Bairros of Beira

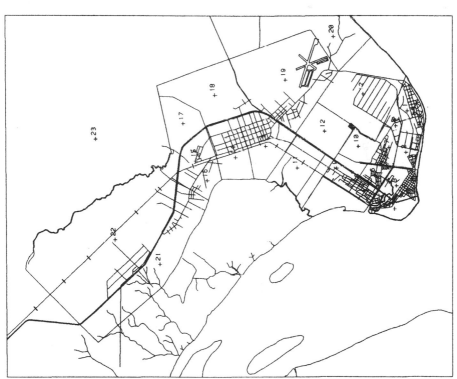

111

centre and tourist attraction. The municipality, which is divided into 22 *bairros* (Figure 4.9) and numerous smaller communal units has wide ranging land uses and is environmentally varied. The central business district, port, industrial estate and railway yards constitute much of the south west sector of the city around Bairro Chaimite. The main residential areas, previously inhabited by the Portuguese, hug the sea coast line to the east, centre on the Bairros of Esturro and Matacuane, and sporadically occupy outer *bairros* at Alto da Manga and Nhaconjo. Blocks of flats are interspersed in and around the central business district and spread out along the main roads from the centre (Pioneiros), most other inhabited land being made up of 'spontaneous settlement'.

In the less densely housed zones, typically away from the urban core, houses are surrounded by small scale cultivation associated with humid savannah, typically rice, sugar cane, maize and cassava. Larger tracts of land between the urban core and outer suburbs, too low lying for habitation, are used almost exclusively for rice cultivation. The outer zones of the municipality are made up of small farms formerly owned by private Portuguese land-owners, which produce vegetables, fruit, ducks, chickens and goats. A few maintain their original owners but most became nationalised when the owner left the country after Independence or died, or were bequeathed to the *empregado* (servant) who remained on the site. New and old areas continue to be sold off by the city council in its quest to generate more funds, a result of pressures caused by the latest austerity programs. Nearly all officially set out plots of land within the municipality have been occupied in the last few years, only leaving room for expansion in the outer zones of Inhamízua 18 km from the centre, or in former rice growing areas, liable to regular flooding and for which a fee must be paid.

Water is piped into Beira from a pumping station at Mutua, by the river Pungwe nearly 50 km from the city. The water rarely meets WHO guidelines for chlorine content and at best is only connected for short periods in the morning and evening. The supply was completely inoperable for periods of up to six months during the late 1980s due to sabotage of the electricity supply which is needed to operate the main pumps. The supply resumed with the installation of a generator powered by aircraft fuel in 1989. However, data released by Aguas da Beira (1993) show that there was a steady reduction in output between 1990 and 1993 (Figure 4.10). During the later part of 1992 the supply was halted altogether because of the drought. There is currently a large scale project underway to update the piped water supply to the city, though the distribution of localised improvements associated with this scheme remains unclear. As in Quelimane, the well water supply has been vital for Beira residents, since there are no bore holes and NGO involvement in assisting this sector has been minimal.

Beira has the worst reputation in Mozambique for its sanitation difficulties. The concrete city is served by the original sewage system installed during colonial times, but this is operated by pumping stations that often cease to function and, when working, effluent is discharged into the estuary to the north of the port area. Residential areas away from the central area and coastal strip operated in the past through a system of septic tanks and the areas of 'spontaneous settlement' were not covered. Makeshift latrines or use of no facility at all has therefore been widespread. Health care is centred on the Hospital Central da Beira and five health centres, serious cases of illness being referred to the bigger institution.

One of Gorongosa's greatest assets has been the presence of natural springs. However, these are sometimes considerable distances from where

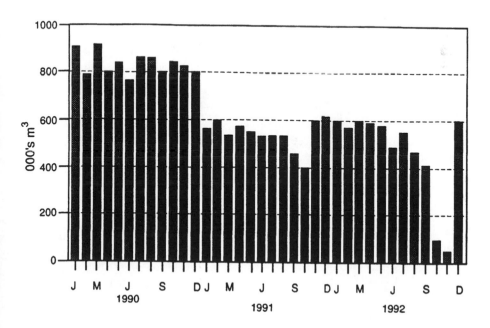

Figure 4.10 Output of piped water supply to Beira, 1990-1992
Source: Comissão Provincial do Plano de Sofala, 1992 p.35

people live and often do not provide water fast enough to meet the demand. Consequently people also use other sources, such as the main river, two old open wells (almost dried up since the 1992 drought), and some recently installed bore holes, which have mainly been successful. Vila de Gorongosa is an urban area in that it houses over fifty thousand people, but in other respects it functions as a rural settlement. There is no electricity supply or formal drainage system and domestic animals roam freely amongst the huts. The remains of the old surfaced road which links it to the main Beira Corridor less than 100 km to the south ends nearby after which there are only unsurfaced roads, some of which were beginning to be de-mined at the time of carrying out this research. One of the few buildings dating from the Portuguese era is a small district hospital which most victims of serious disease try to reach.

Population Differentials and the Role of Displacement as a Cause of Disease in the Field Sites

As outlined in Chapter 1, the spread of a communicable disease occurs against a background of terrain factors which guide its direction and magnitude. But the terrain is made up of local environments and people, the relative influence of which is dependent in part on the nature of the pathogen causing the disease. So far this chapter has introduced three different urban areas with respect to disease incidence, pathogenicity and characteristics of the physical terrain. The next subsection provides a background to demographic aspects of the terrain environment and describes how changes, caused by population displacement, may influence incidence of cholera and dysentery in these areas.

Demographic Profiles

The demographic background to central Mozambique has been shaped by events beyond the control of most of its inhabitants. Colonialism, revolution, rural destabilisation, and post conflict economic adjustment have contributed to altering the relationship between local communities and their habitat.

In the colonial era the distribution of the population was influenced by the growth of urban areas around ports, the marketing of exploitable resources in the more fertile areas, and the establishment of lines of communication with the interior. The main urban areas, such as Maputo, Beira, Quelimane and Nacala were established as sea-ports with smaller towns, such as Tete and Chimoio situated on major transport routes in the interior. The urban areas swelled as demand for a locally resident work force grew.

During the early phases of the post-colonial era in the second part of the 1970s, it became Government policy to try to discourage further urbanisation and the theme 'Vamos voltar para os distritos' (Let us return to the districts) was promoted on the radio and advertising hoardings. This theme was still apparent around urban areas as recently as 1987. During some of its more radical moments, and in keeping with this policy, the Government used its *Operação Produção* (Operation Production) campaign to remove some sectors of the urban community to live in communal villages in rural areas. For example, prostitutes, of which there had been many in the main cities during the late colonial period, were taken from Maputo and resettled in remote communal villages in Niassa Province 3000 km to the north. However, many communal villages, such as 'Aldeia Fidel Castro' in the south of the country and 'Aldeia Josina Machel' in Sofala Province were not forced, instead attracting the popular support of a population recently liberated from imperial servitude. The case of 'Cooperativa Heróis Moçambicanos' is described in some detail by (Lappe and Varela 1980).

The war eventually halted any further notion there may have been for advancing ruralisation since most areas of Mozambique became too dangerous for regular activities. The population restricted themselves to only making essential journeys and population pressure zones developed in the relatively safer areas. Only vague approximations for the amount of people physically displaced as a result of the conflict can be made. Primarily using data from the Departamento de Prevenção e Combate às Calamidades Naturais, Green (1992) has estimated that over half the country's population were displaced in one way or another. This comprised more than 1.5 million international refugees and 6 million internally displaced. Further demographic impacts resulted from extreme climatic events, such as the drought of 1992 which gravely affected the whole country, and about 0.5 million people in Sofala Province alone (Serviço Provincial De Estatística 1993, p15). Further displacements result from flooding, such as those that have affected large areas of Sofala and Zambézia Provinces during the first part of 1997 (MSF 1997).

Following the formal ending of the conflict in October 1992, return movements to former locations of residence have been irregular. The pattern of return of the internally displaced stopped and started as a result of the timing of harvests and changes in actual and perceived security. A large part of the return process for refugees in neighbouring countries was additionally subject to the timing of organisational assistance programmes, which were slow in being implemented. Though many Mozambicans had already made their own way home, the large numbers included in the UNHCR repatriations were only occurring by July 1993 (UNOHAC, 1993). By June 1995 UNHCR completed the largest programme of repatriation undertaken in Africa (MSF 1995). However, return movements of internally displaced people residing in urban areas has been much more limited.

For example, amongst 132 people displaced by war identified from a cluster sample used by the Commisão do Plano for Bairro Munhava, Beira (Figure 4.9) in January 1994 (unpublished data), 64 per cent said they wanted to return but only 16.5 per cent of these confirmed that they were ready to do so. Thirty three per cent of those interviewed said that they did not want to return and an unclear response was offered by a further 3 per cent. There is no evidence that the rate of urbanisation in Mozambique has significantly slowed due to return migration of forcibly displaced people. This is because birth rates remain high and mask any significant changes in population caused by those gradually resettling in the rural areas. Consequently, the sub-locations in Quelimane and Beira that have been associated with high numbers of displaced people have maintained a populous and congested appearance. This will be able to be verified more precisely with the publication of the 1997 national census, the first of its type since 1980.

In Gorongosa, where some sub-locations had been set up exclusively for displaced people, named individually according to the origin of displacement, evidence of emptying out was becoming more apparent by early 1994. Since the tradition in the Gorongosa area is to break up your hut before departure to prevent evil spirits using it, the hut debris that remains in these locations provides an indication of zones from which there has been an exodus.

The age and sex structure for the research area is broadly typical of low-income areas of the Third World, with a large percentage of people in the younger age quartile, and a very small percentage in the upper age quartile. Figure 4.11 displays the situation for the Province of Sofala. An extra feature is the indent in an otherwise regular bell shaped pyramid caused by the relatively lower numbers of young men. This is understood to be attributable to death or absence during conflict, avoidance of registration through fear of conscription, and relocation for educational or employment purposes. The latter of these included moves to Maputo, neighbouring countries (in particular to South Africa), and to other parts of the world such as Cuba and the former East Germany a few years back. It is not clear to what extent these factors have affected the overall higher number of women in the province since the higher numbers are also found in the 0-14 years age group. A probable, though generalised explanation, is that larger numbers of female children reflect a genetic survival advantage over males, and that this is exaggerated because of very high infant and under 5 mortality rates. UNICEF (1991) recorded 173 deaths per 1,000 live births for infants under one year of age and 297 deaths for infants under 5

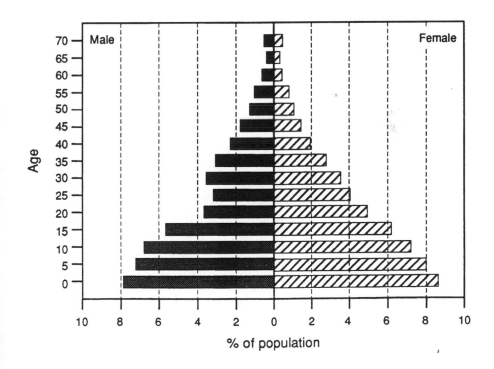

Figure 4.11 Population pyramid for the Province of Sofala
Source: Comissão Provincial do Plano de Sofala, 1992, p.35

years, the highest in the world for that year. The reversal of the trend, with higher numbers of males than females in the 35-75 years group is due to the lower quality of life that women still experience in most parts of the Third World.

The Role of Population Displacement in Diffusion of Cholera and Dysentery

Recent mobility and population displacement is hypothesised by this research as being part of the background terrain against which the pattern of disease incidence is determined. It is well established that diffusion of communicable diseases occurs through secondary transmission since pathogens are transported by people from place to place. For example, transporting of pathogens from one area to another with a highly mobile population has resulted in cholera and dysentery affecting all provinces of Mozambique. However, rather than explaining the pattern of incidence, this simply confirms communicability of diarrhoeal disease and the potential for all areas to be part of a major epidemic. Less is known about the association of incidence of disease with recently mobile people in their new place of residence. The recent background information on cholera and dysentery and preliminary research indicated that in Mozambique an association with displacement may operate in a variety of ways. Increased mobility may be associated with poor health through exposure of migrants to new disease ecologies, the impact of migrants on existing ecologies and, altered resistance to disease. A further category can be considered as including both changes in biological and socio-economic resistance.

High incidence of cholera and dysentery within the region provides some initial suggestion of an association with population displacement, as in cases of cholera in the external refugee camps of Malawi in 1987 (Moren *et al* 1991a, 1991b; Hatch and Waldman 1994), and of variable combinations of cholera and dysentery in Malawi, Zimbabwe and Swaziland in 1992 (Aragon and Chambule *et al.* 1993, p16; Paquet 1992, Personal communications; WHO Geneva 1993b; Zimbabwean government employee in Manicaland 1992). However, with respect to the internally displaced, the association requires a closer analysis since movements have been more complex and patterns of incidence unaccountably irregular. Movements have been in many different directions and for varied reasons. There are non-forced movements which would have taken place with or without a war, such as marriages and rural-urban push and pull influences.

Forced movements have been both due to direct uprooting by war, and other movements indirectly caused by the war, such as drought induced displacements that would be avoidable with the operation of the wider ranging coping mechanisms of peacetime.

A large part of the population of all three sites was made up of people who had been forcibly displaced or had voluntarily relocated at some period. One outcome of displacement may be the development of coping mechanisms that buffer against negative health impacts. Alternatively, a long term background of displacement of livelihoods could represent a cumulative negative influence on well-being and health. Whichever is more significant, longer time periods spent in the same place causes differentiation between 'non-displaced' and 'displaced' people to be less evident. This is particularly likely to be the case in areas undergoing major processes of change, such as urbanisation affecting all inhabitants. However, by far the biggest and most rapid displacements of population occurred in the 1980s as a result of the recent war. It is the health implications of these that have been of immediate importance since they preceded the countries' biggest disease epidemics on record.

Some of the post-conflict movements are also of interest here. The 1992 epidemic of cholera was well established before the signing of the Peace Accord in October 1992 but increased substantially in the following two months. One possible explanation for this increase, in addition to environmental seasonality, is that population movements intensified. In the provinces of Sofala and Manica thousands of malnourished, and often diseased, people left RENAMO areas for the area around the Beira Corridor to gain better access to food aid. At this period, the exodus from these remoter areas was greater than the movement of people returning to their home areas. It meant a spreading out of the poorest and most susceptible people in the country previously closeted behind RENAMO lines. It is however unclear whether this pattern applied to all other parts of the country. Whilst some commentators (Hoile 1989) have claimed that conditions were better behind RENAMO lines, the author's own interviews with former civilian captives who escaped indicated that there were areas with a lack of subsistence, forced labour and death amongst an incarcerated population.

Whereas the association between refugee concentrations and epidemics of cholera and dysentery is already very clear for several locations in Africa, a similar association with internally displaced people in pre-existing urban areas has not been obvious. Health records do not provide information that enables differentiation between migrant and non-migrant populations or reasons for migration. Though some sub-locations of the field sites used in this research are known to be zones into which large amounts of displaced people resettled, no existing work has investigated the relative disease burden of displaced to host populations. A complex mix of displaced people and long-term residents potentially confounds an oversimplified account of disease association in these areas.

In Quelimane, the areas in and around Manhawa were the main zones allocated to displaced people during the 1980s. However, this zone was not uninhabited before their arrival and expansion from within the city has meant that local people have also had to settle there. Other displaced people benefited from the hospitality of existing relatives in the urban area and are therefore more dispersed. The area in and around Manhawa supports the poorest living conditions in Quelimane and this is one reason why displaced people ended up settling there. Unlike most of the rest of Quelimane, this area has almost no vegetation other than some clumps of sugar cane. An older resident of the area claimed the zone had previously been better vegetated and this can be confirmed through consultation of arial photographs kept by the Direcção Provincial de Planeamento Físico. An explanation for the significantly higher rate of incidence of cholera in that part of the city, provided by the epidemiological unit of the Dirrecção de Saúde da Zambézia, was the following:

> The greater part of the population is made up of refugees and the living conditions are not good, the level of education is low and in most cases it does not exist; environmental hygiene is very bad. (Delgado and Azevedo *et al.* 1992, p9. Author's translation)

The same report refers to the lack of piped treated water, open air defecation, a high water table and transmission through the increased activities of buying and selling food in an unsanitary environment. Recommendations included increasing clinical tests for cases, intensification of preventative action with respect to water, latrines and food, and support of the government programme 'Luta Contra a Cólera' (Struggle against Cholera) which is based on WHO guidelines.

Population Displacement or Unsustainable Places?

A background to how displaced people may be predisposed to higher infection from communicable disease has been presented in Chapter 2 and serves as a theme for quantitative investigation throughout this book. However, even a cursory review of the environmental circumstances in which displaced people found themselves in the sites described here suggests the likelihood of an association.

At all three sites during the years of conflict there was limited space within which to resettle. Many *bairros* already had a high population density and those that did not were occupied by intensely cultivated plots, the military, or represented areas on the periphery of the city that were too prone to 'bandit' attack to provide adequate security. Displaced people without pre-existing family affiliations in the city were more likely to inhabit environmentally marginal areas, unfavoured by the long term residents, but safe from attack. There is therefore an unclear cycle of causation between high densities of recently settled people and the condition of their local environment. For example, it was suggested in earlier reports that the presence of large numbers of displaced people in the area in and around Manhawa in Quelimane assisted the local environment in becoming devegetated and degraded (Collins 1991, 1992; Chambule and Azevedo 1994). However, this area may have already been susceptible to environmental degradation in that it was situated at the edge of flooded areas, considered marginal, and normally avoided for habitation. As such it was the unsustainability of the place of resettlement rather than the impact of the newcomers that was the underlying factor in determining the nature of the environment-disease interaction.

The nature of the place of resettlement is also related to infrastructural factors, especially in the 'cement' parts of the cities where displaced people have resettled in a variety of locations. In Beira this has included along drainage canals, in the remains of the Grand Hotel, in the basements of apartment blocks, and under the floors of stilted houses. There is often no provision for sanitation, and deficiencies in the water supply, but it remains unclear whether this was significantly worse than for longer term residents. Since these areas are characterised by a built environment, less influence from natural environmental reservoirs for disease pathogens is suspected. However, with low levels of hygiene and little opportunity to cultivate food to supplement their diet, these areas have represented zones which are often unsustainable for maintaining adequate defences against disease infection. In Gorongosa the unsustainability of resettlement locations for displaced and host populations related primarily to constraints brought about by restricted movement. The immediate vicinity of the town became increasingly unsustainable due to intense cultivation and harvesting of fuelwood which caused land degradation. However, because the pre-existing environment was different to that of the coastal area, the resultant ecological implications for disease and health can not be assumed to be the same. For example, there is likely to be fewer microcosms of saline water, a different pH and the process of environmental change is likely to be different for upland areas.

This chapter has provided a background to local factors which are relevant to the assessment of environment, health and population displacement based on three key sites in central Mozambique, as well as hinting at wider contextual factors which need to be taken into account. In the next chapter, detailed associations between environmental circumstances and the incidence of cholera and dysentery are investigated. Chapter 6 will review more detailed evidence for and anomolies in an association between migration and population displacement and increased incidence. Structural adjustment and changing aspects of community behaviour are considered in Chapter 7.

5 Environmental Influences on the Distributions of Incidence of Cholera and Bacillary Dysentery in Quelimane, Beira and Gorongosa

This chapter presents the results of the environmental associative analysis carried out in the three field sites between October 1993 and July 1994. The key findings are that in Quelimane there is a variable spatial pattern of cholera and dysentery consistent with there being a favourable physical environmental reservoir for *Vibrio cholerae* 01 serotype Ogawa. However, for the case of Beira, the influence of an environmental reservoir on the spatial pattern of cholera incidence, due to *Vibrio cholerae* 01 serotype Inaba, is harder to confirm. Although there is a correlation between cholera incidence and the distribution of certain environmental parameters in space, there is no overall correlation with the temporal pattern of rainfall. In addition, a correlation between the pattern of incidence of cholera and dysentery, and clustering of both diseases in the more urban south of the city, raise the possibility of further influences that affect both diseases. In Gorongosa there is no evidence of suitable conditions for the existence of an environmental reservoir for *Vibrio cholerae* and alternative explanations for an observed difference in the distribution of cholera and bacillary dysentery must be sought, such as the greater communicability of *Shigella dysenteriae* 1. A physical environmental association in Quelimane suggests that cholera is more endemic there than the other two sites where a more epidemic strain, serotype Inaba, has proliferated. Comparison with the distribution of bacillary dysentery supports these findings.

The Spatial Distributions of Cholera and Bacillary Dysentery in the Field Sites

The Spatial Distribution of Cholera and Dysentery in Quelimane

As noted for central Mozambique as a whole in Chapter 4, cholera cases in Quelimane rapidly started reappearing in early January 1992. This followed a period of apparent disappearance since the epidemic that ended in July 1991. This research has used all confirmed cases that were recorded in hospital admissions books until the end of the epidemic in April 1993. This amounted to a total of 2432 cases additional to the 1179 cases recorded for the period July 1990 - July 1991 which were used for earlier work in Quelimane (Collins 1992). Cases of bacillary dysentery started to appear in Quelimane in November 1992, almost simultaneously with reports of some cases in rural areas such as Mopeia and the districts of Tete province bordering Malawi (MSF 1992b). In many areas, including the City of Quelimane, the dysentery epidemic overlapped with the latter stages of the cholera epidemic. Detailed data are missing for the first part of the epidemic due to problems in diagnosis and the status of bacillary dysentery as a WHO non-recorded disease. Policy decisions from the Ministry of Health later in the year meant that the disease was eventually recorded in the same detail as cholera. For this research a continuum of 2022 well-registered cases have been extracted for the period 1st January 1994 - 31st July 1994.

Figure 5.1 shows that the spatial pattern of cholera incidence across the sub-areas of Quelimane is not uniform. The coefficient of variation for incidence rates between sub-areas is 70.1 per cent. A significant difference between the observed and expected rates of incidence based on the rate of incidence for the overall site was confirmed by computation of the chi-square statistic ($p<0.005$). Areas of higher incidence range across the north-western facing flank of the city, and a small area of the inner south-eastern flank, with the highest rate of incidence occurring in communal unit Manhawa which had 327 cases per 10,000 people. Figure 5.2 reveals a different spatial pattern to rates of incidence of bacillary dysentery which recorded a coefficient of variation of 87.5 per cent between sub-areas. In this instance, areas of higher incidence range across most of the south-eastern communal units of the city.

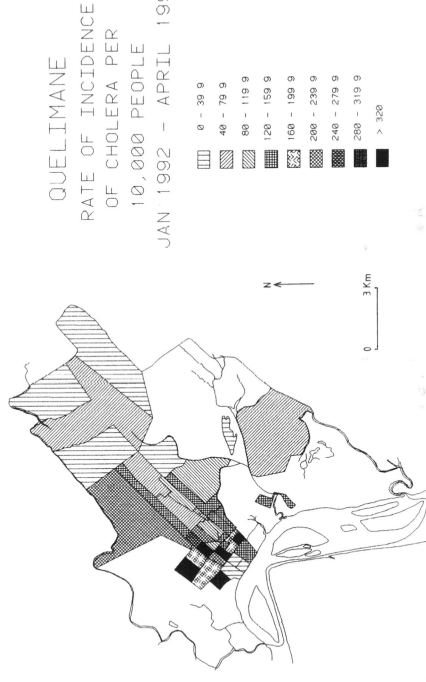

Figure 5.1 Spatial distribution of rates of incidence of cholera per 10,000 people at Quelimane

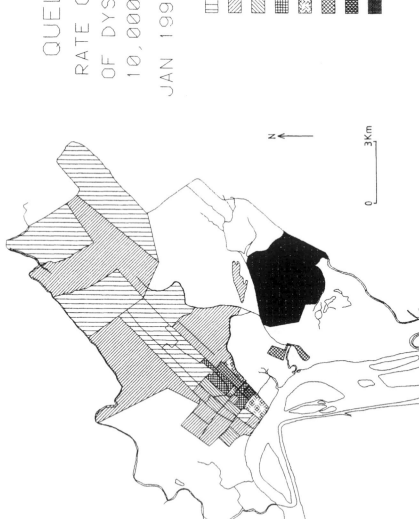

Figure 5.2 Spatial distribution of rates of incidence of bacillary dysentery per 10,000 people at Quelimane

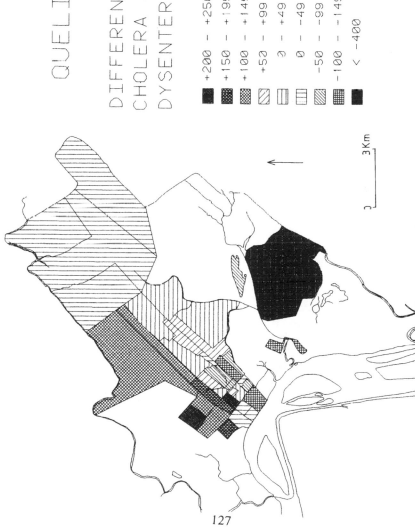

QUELIMANE

DIFFERENCES BETWEEN
CHOLERA RATE AND
DYSENTERY RATE

+200 - +250 Cases of cholera per
+150 - +199 10,000 more than cases
+100 - +149 of dysentery per 10,000
+50 - +99
0 - +49
0 - -49
-50 - -99 Cases of cholera per
-100 - -149 10,000 less than cases
< -400 of dysentery per 10,000

3Km

Figure 5.3 Differences between rates of incidence of cholera and dysentery at Quelimane

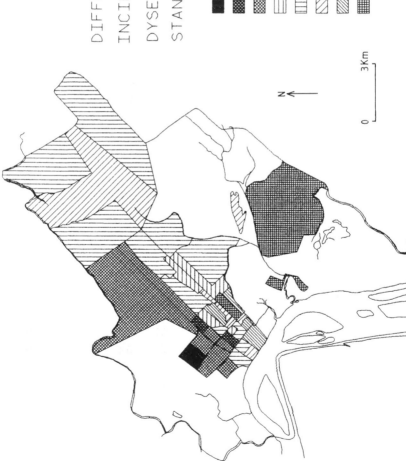

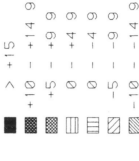

Figure 5.4 Differences between standardised residuals for cholera and dysentery calculated from observed and expected rates of incidence at Quelimane

The magnitude of difference between the spatial distribution of rate of incidence for the two diseases is apparent in Figure 5.3, which represents the product of subtracting the cholera rate from that of dysentery. Further statistical investigation confirms no significant correlation between sub-area incidence of the two diseases (r=0.27), computation of the Lorenz curve producing an index of dissimilarity of 33.8. However, the index of dissimilarity is not exceptionally high, and the distributions require further investigation to assess in what way they vary from one another. A chi-square test of independence on rates of incidence of cholera with those of dysentery suggests some form of non-random association (p<0.005). The following analysis further investigates the relationship between the two patterns of incidence using a technique based on standardised morbidity ratios.[1]

Potential discrepancies that may be caused by using simple correlation statistics are reduced by calculating the observed and expected rates of incidence independently for each disease at each Communal Unit and then contrasting the resultant standardised residuals. Observed rates for each sub-location and each disease are related to rates of incidence for the entire population, which were 169 per 10,000 for cholera and 121 per 10,000 for dysentery.[2] The differences between the cholera and dysentery residuals, represented in Figure 5.4, not only confirm that the two diseases are dissimilarly distributed, but also emphasise that the patterns tend towards reciprocal homogeneity. In summary, the pattern of disease by communal unit in Quelimane was found to be distinctly clustered in favour of higher incidence of cholera in the north-western flanks and higher incidence of dysentery in a large part of the other areas.

The Spatial Distribution of Cholera and Dysentery in Beira

The periodicity of the Beira cholera epidemic was similar to that of Quelimane save for recorded cases starting and ending a few weeks later. However, excluding 40 cases in the last five months, all 1,395 cases extracted from the hospital admissions books were confirmed by the

---

[1] This has been adapted from similar principles used for Standardised Mortality Ratios (SMR's), advocated by Howe (1972) and Jones (1981), and widely applied to census surveys. It has been used here to compensate for the limitation in comparing rates of incidence of different diseases that have been calculated from different epidemic periods.

[2] The standardised residuals for each Communal Units is calculated by $O-E/\sqrt{E}$, where O = observed rate and E = expected rate.

hospital laboratory as being due to *Vibrio cholerae* 01 serotype Inaba rather than the serotype Ogawa identified in Quelimane. The first cases of bacillary dysentery associated with the current epidemic in Sofala province were reported by MSF in the northern districts bordering Tete province for December 1992 (MSF 1993d). Cases of dysentery were reported to be on the increase in Beira by the city health department as early as October 1992 (Noticiário Epidemiologíco 1993), but there is no absolute confirmation available whether these earlier cases of dysentery were due to *Shigella dysenteriae* 1 or some other pathogen causing the symptoms of bloody diarrhoea. The first main surge of cases in Beira confirmed as being associated with *Shigella dysenteriae* 1 are indicated by the hospital as occurring in December 1992. However, crisis conditions in the hospital and diagnostic confusion in the early stages of the epidemic meant that up to 1000 assumed initial cases were not considered accurate enough for the purposes of this research. Only later cases of bacillary dysentery, confirmed by laboratory analysis at the Ministry of Health in Maputo as being due to *Shigella dysenteriae* 1, and accurately recorded in the registration book were used. This amounts to the total of 2,325 cases that were recorded between 10th February 1993 and 8th August 1994.

Figure 5.5 shows the spatial distribution of incidence of cholera at Beira and Figure 5.6 the spatial distribution of bacillary dysentery. In both instances higher rates of incidence occur in and around the more urban southern part of the city. Correlation of the rates of incidence between the two diseases is significant using the product-moment parametric test ($r=0.68$ $p<0.01$). The index of dissimilarity derived from the Lorenz curve is a relatively low value of 23.1. Regression of the total cases of dysentery on the total cases of cholera is significant ($r^2=63.0$ $F=34.0$ $p<0.01$) and reveals sub-locations that fall outside of the 95 per cent confidence intervals generated by this association (Figure 5.7). Regression of the dysentery rate on that of cholera (Figure 5.8) is also significant ($r^2=46.4$ $F=17.3$ $p<0.01$).

The spatial analysis of residuals in both instances display a non-random pattern with contiguous blocks of sub-areas (Figures 5.9 and 5.10). Positive standardised residuals, indicating areas with higher rates of cholera not correlating with the dysentery rate, are indicated on Figures 5.9 and 5.10 and are concentrated in one area. Negative standardised residuals, indicating areas with higher amounts of cases and higher rates of dysentery per 10,000 people, not correlating with that of cholera, occupy the large outer bairros. The exceptions are Bairro 4 (Chaimite) at the core of the city

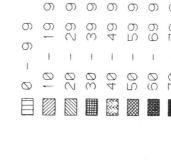

BEIRA

RATE OF INCIDENCE OF
CHOLERA PER 10,000 PEOPLE
FEBRUARY 1992 – MAY 1993

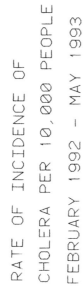

0 – 9 9
10 – 19 9
20 – 29 9
30 – 39 9
40 – 49 9
50 – 59 9
60 – 69 9
70 – 79 9

3 Km

N

0

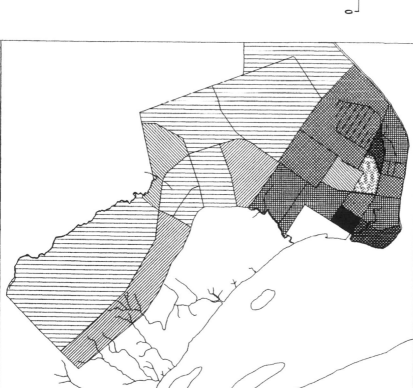

Figure 5.5 Spatial distribution of rates of incidence of cholera per 10,000 people at Beira

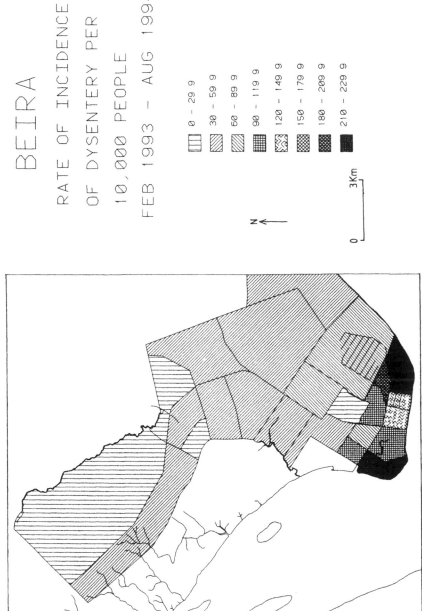

Figure 5.6 Spatial distribution of rates of incidence of bacillary dysentery per 10,000 people at Beira

132

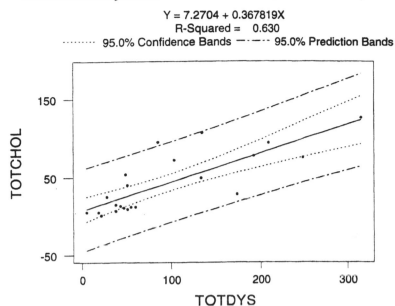

Figure 5.7 **Regression fit of total cases of dysentery per bairro on total cases of cholera per bairro at Beira**

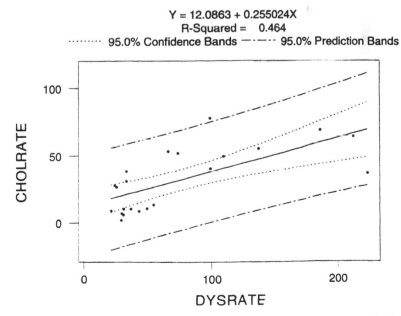

Figure 5.8 **Regression fit of dysentery rate per bairro on cholera rate per bairro at Beira**

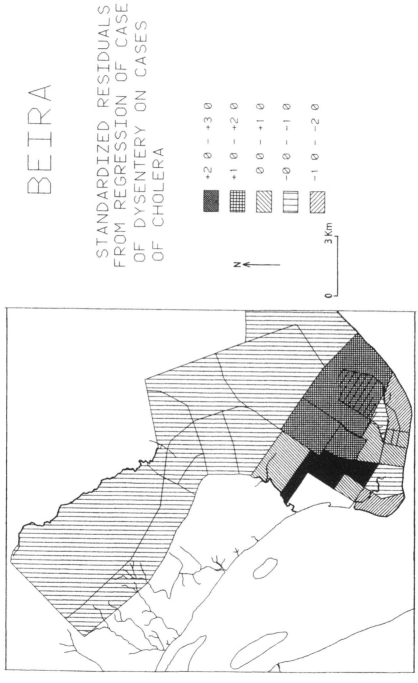

Figure 5.9 Spatial distribution of standardised residuals from regression of total cases of dysentery per bairro on total cases of cholera per bairro at Beira

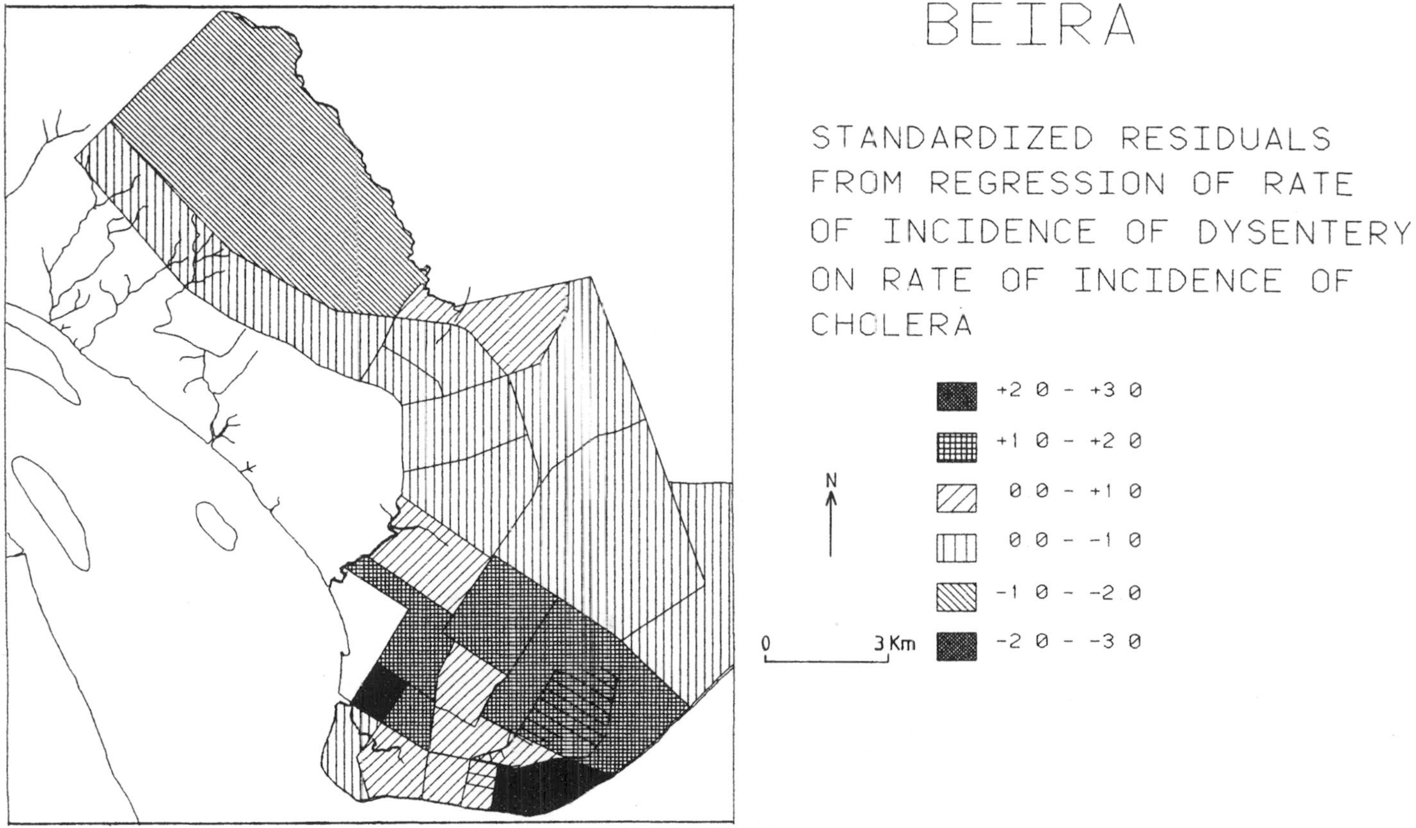

Figure 5.10 Spatial distribution of standardised residuals from regression of dysentery rate per bairro on cholera rate per bairro at Beira

BEIRA

STANDARDIZED RESIDUALS
FROM REGRESSION OF RATE
OF INCIDENCE OF DYSENTERY
ON RATE OF INCIDENCE OF
CHOLERA

+2 0 – +3 0

+1 0 – +2 0

0 0 – +1 0

0 0 – –1 0

–1 0 – –2 0

–2 0 – –3 0

N

0   3 Km

with a small negative residual, and Bairro 1 (Estoril), a planned residential part of the city that has the largest negative residual. The residual maps are a useful background for considering factors that differentially influence incidence of cholera and dysentery for a few sub-locations. However there is no clear indication of the overall variation between the two diseases that was found for the case of Quelimane.

Cholera and Bacillary Dysentery in Gorongosa

Suspicion of the presence of cholera amongst the registered cases of diarrhoea in Gorongosa was reported in October 1992. A major outbreak was confirmed through laboratory analysis in November 1992 (MSF 1992a). MSF and the hospital estimated that during the first weeks and up until 20th November there were 552 cases with over 150 deaths. For this research, however only 211 well registered cases that followed this period have been extracted from hospital records. This represents all the cases in the relatively short period between 20th November 1992 and 22nd December 1992, after which the cholera epidemic ended.

Staff at the hospital said that the first symptoms of dysentery appeared as the cholera waned with 35 cases in December 1992 and 28 in January 1993. As described in Chapter 3, there appears to have been conflicting accounts of how many cases there were from in and around the town. Consequently, for this part of the analysis in Gorongosa it has only been possible to use 43 confirmed cases of dysentery from the hospital admissions book for the period 14th January 1994 until 25th March 1994. This low number of confirmed and recorded cases of dysentery was inadequate for comparison with the spatial distribution of cholera as was done for Quelimane and Beira. However, by grouping sub-areas it has been possible to gain an impression of a difference in distribution. Also of interest here is the further information generated from a comparison between cholera and dysentery using the 68 Gorongosa questionnaires which indicate that 47 per cent of those interviewed had cholera and 54 per cent dysentery during the previous three years. 34 per cent said they had suffered from both diseases in the last three years.

Figure 5.11 represents the spatial distribution of incidence of cholera in and around Vila de Gorongosa calculated from the 211 hospital recorded cases and government supplied population figures. Higher rates of incidence are found in the centre of the town. By grouping *bairros* into the broader categories of centre, inner and outer zones, the total percentage of

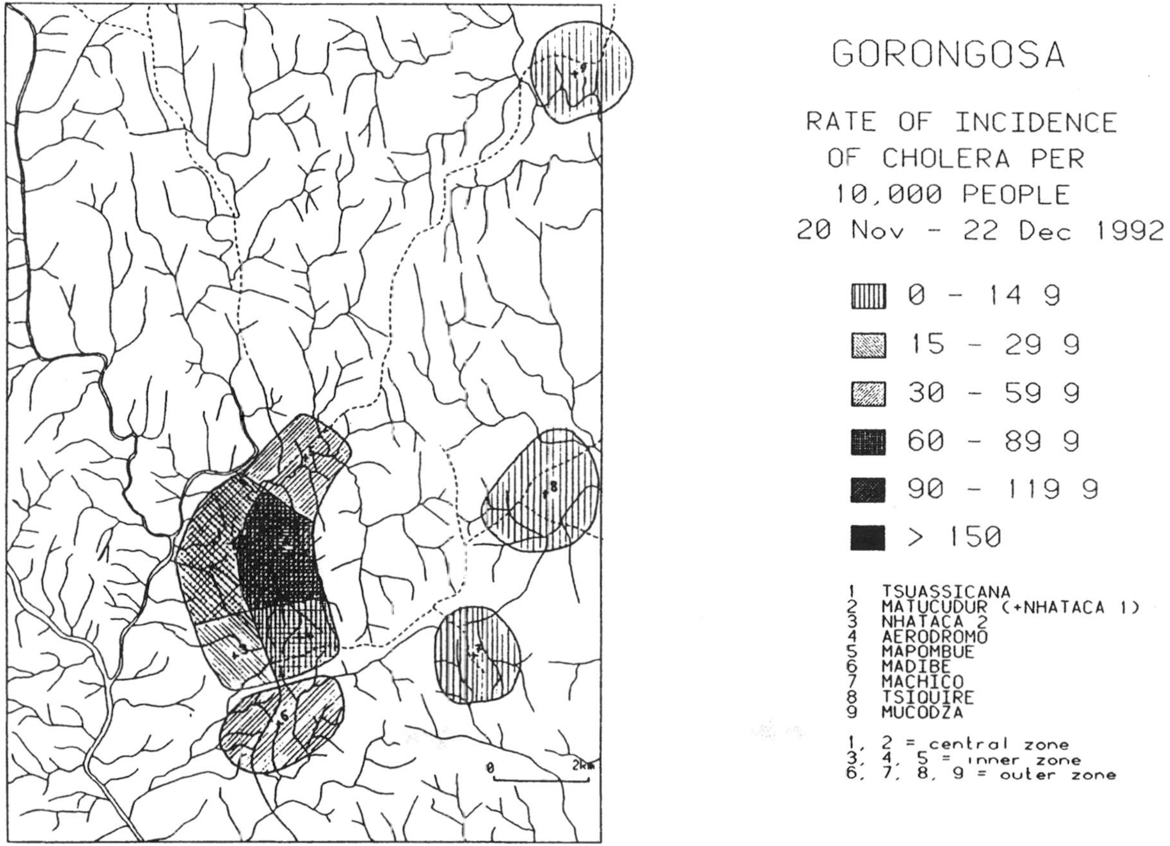

GORONGOSA

RATE OF INCIDENCE
OF CHOLERA PER
10,000 PEOPLE
20 Nov - 22 Dec 1992

0 - 14 9
15 - 29 9
30 - 59 9
60 - 89 9
90 - 119 9
> 150

1 TSUASSICANA
2 MATUCUDUR (+NHATACA 1)
3 NHATACA 2
4 AERODROMO
5 MAPOMBUE
6 MADIBE
7 MACHICO
8 TSIQUIRE
9 MUCODZA

1, 2 = central zone
3, 4, 5 = inner zone
6, 7, 8, 9 = outer zone

Figure 5.11 Spatial distribution of rate of incidence of cholera in and around Vila de Gorongosa

137

Table 5.1   Distribution of cases of cholera and small sample of dysentery by zone at Gorongosa using hospital data

	CHOLERA		DYSENTERY	
	Cases	% of total	Cases	% of total
Central Zone	106	(51.0)	15	(34.9)
Inner Zone	87	(41.8)	19	(44.2)
Outer Zone	15	(7.2)	9	(20.9)
Total	208	(100)	43	(100)

Table 5.2   Distribution of cases of cholera and dysentery on the basis of questionnaire responses at Gorongosa

	CHOLERA			DYSENTERY		
	Cases	Sample	% of sample	Cases	Sample	% of sample
Central Zone	17	36	47.2	19	36	52.8
Inner Zone	5	15	33.3	9	15	60.0
Outer Zone	10	17	58.8	9	17	52.9
Total	32	68	-	37	68	-

cases for each zone can be compared with those derived from the small sample of dysentery cases described above. The data presented in Table 5.1 shows a greater contrast between outer and central zones of Vila de Gorongosa for cholera than for the case of dysentery.

The results in Table 5.2 from questionnaire responses on prevalence of cholera and dysentery in the area have also been used to investigate possible differences in the pattern of incidence. However, the results do not reflect the pattern revealed by the hospital records with the outer zone registering a higher percentage of people with cholera than the inner zone.

The percentage who had dysentery was almost the same for inner and outer zones. In the case of Gorongosa the data therefore suggests that distance to the hospital, or some other factor, accounts for an artificially low amount of hospital registered cases from the outer fringes of the study area. It is also possible that some of the outer zone cases first had cholera whilst still taking refuge in the central zone during the later part of 1992.

In the light of existing information on differences in the pathogenesis of cholera and dysentery, one further explanation for these results is the greater communicability of *Shigella dysenteriae* 1 causing it to be more homogeneously distributed in Gorongosa. However, the data available are insufficient to confirm or contradict suggestions of an association between higher incidence of cholera and specific areas. In any case the transient situation that most people experienced in and around the town, such as being displaced towards the central area for safety, but having to make frequent return visits to the outer areas for supplies, means there may be reduced grounds for associating patterns of incidence with the nature of individual *bairros*. This is considered in greater detail in Chapter 6.

Cross-sectional Association of Incidence of Cholera and Dysentery with the Physical Environment

Association of Incidence of Cholera with Favourable Environmental Reservoirs for Vibrio Cholerae 01

The results from research in Quelimane in 1991 found that from a matrix of 13 measured variables, sampled at 81 water sources, higher conductivity was the environmental feature displaying the closest association with the spatial distribution of rates of incidence of cholera. Soil pH was also indicated as being a probable associating phenomenon (Collins 1993). The strongest confirmation of physical environmental influences on the distribution of incidence of cholera in the current study of three field sites was again presented by the case of Quelimane. A total of 82 samples were analysed for the survey of the city in January 1994 and a further 73 analysed for the survey of the city in June 1994. Samples taken from the city's sporadic tapped water supply which comes from the common source of the Licuar 50 km away were excluded from the physical environmental analysis since they produced little variation, were often not in use, and were not representative of local environmental conditions.

Figure 5.12 reveals a spatial pattern to the average conductivity values for communal units calculated by the survey of well water samples carried out in January 1994. Figure 5.13 reveals the spatial pattern of pH values for the same period calculated by averaging the well water and soil samples within each communal unit. For this purpose the 82 well water samples and 44 soil samples, located next to the well sites, have been used. In both instances, areas of higher conductivity and pH are again consistent with areas of higher incidence of cholera. The association is not perfect. For example pH values above 7.0 are also found on the inner south-eastern flank of the city where some relatively lower cholera rates were recorded. Also, the correlation coefficient for incidence of cholera and average pH shows a lower level of significance for the second period of 1994 ($r=0.40$ $p<0.05$). However the correlation coefficients between rate of incidence of cholera and average conductivity derived from the first ($r=0.51$ $p<0.01$) and second ($r=0.55$ $p<0.01$) sampling period in 1994, and average pH ($r=0.57$ $p<0.01$) gained from the first sampling period in 1994 are all significant at the 99 per cent confidence level.

Of note moreover is that none of the other environmental parameters measured in the current study, such as turbidity, faecal coliforms, soil density and water level, showed any significant relationship. In the earlier work the parameters of turbidity, water pH on its own, ammonia, nitrate, faecal coliforms, water level, soil type and water temperature also did not correlate significantly with rate of incidence of cholera. The work in 1991 had also found a strong correlation between rate of incidence of cholera and population density ($r=0.71$ $p<0.01$) but that the regression equation remained significant with the inclusion of conductivity ($r^2=62.0$ $F=21.2$ $p<0.01$). No other variable could be successfully included. The spatial distribution of residuals from the regression of population density on rate of incidence (Figure 5.14) revealed a positive secondary factor in the north-western flank of the city that was suggested as higher salinity. The current research clearly confirms the spatial association between areas of higher incidence of cholera and areas with higher conductivity, though the positive correlation with population density, shown in Figure 5.15, is now reduced ($r=0.51$ $p<0.01$). Clustering of well water sites recording a conductivity of more than 2,500 μs during the 1994 survey, in comparison to the distribution of those of less than 550 μs, is apparent in Figure 5.16. This pattern is again consistent with the hypothesis that there is an association between higher incidence of cholera and a brackish environment in that part of the city.

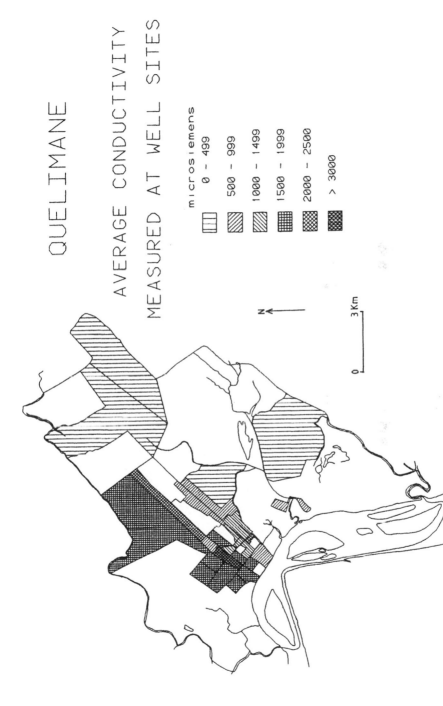

Figure 5.12 Spatial distribution of average conductivity per Communal Unit at Quelimane

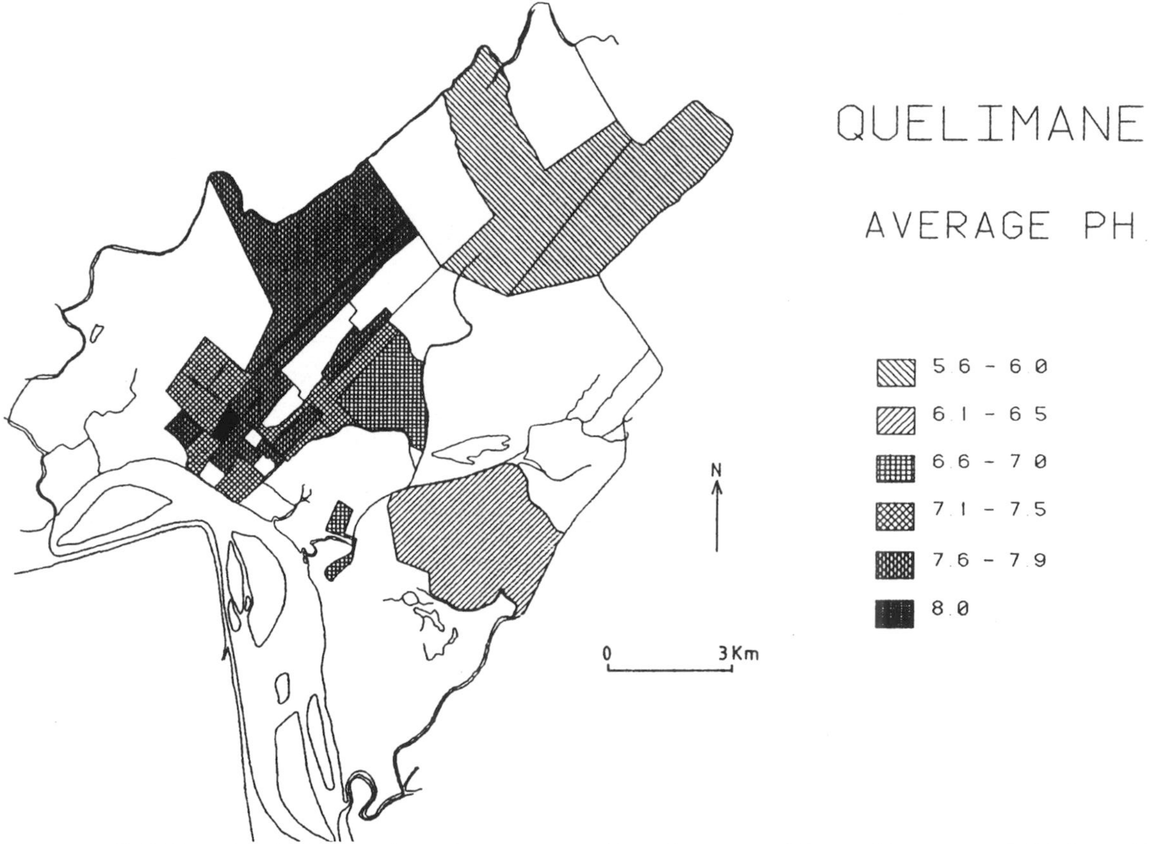

QUELIMANE

AVERAGE PH

56 - 60
61 - 65
66 - 70
71 - 75
76 - 79
80

N

0   3Km

Figure 5.13 Spatial distribution of average soil and water pH per Communal Unit at Quelimane

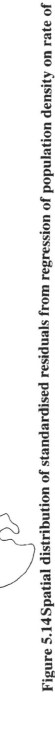

QUELIMANE

STANDARDIZED RESIDUALS FROM
REGRESSION OF POPULATION
DENSITY ON RATE OF INCIDENCE
AND LOCATIONS OF WELLS WITH
SIGNIFICANTLY HIGH AND LOW
CONDUCTIVITY READINGS

STANDARDIZED RESIDUAL

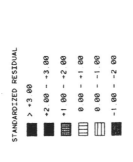

■ > +3.00
■ +2.00 - +3.00
▦ +1.00 - +2.00
▥ 0.00 - +1.00
▥ 0.00 - -1.00
▦ -1.00 - -2.00

* WELLS WITH SIGNIFICANTLY HIGH (99%level) CONDUCTIVITY READINGS

+ WELLS WITH SIGNIFICANTLY LOWER (99%Level) CONDUCTIVITY READINGS

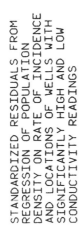

N←

0 ————— 3Km

143

Figure 5.14 Spatial distribution of standardised residuals from regression of population density on rate of incidence of cholera at Quelimane, 1990 - 1991

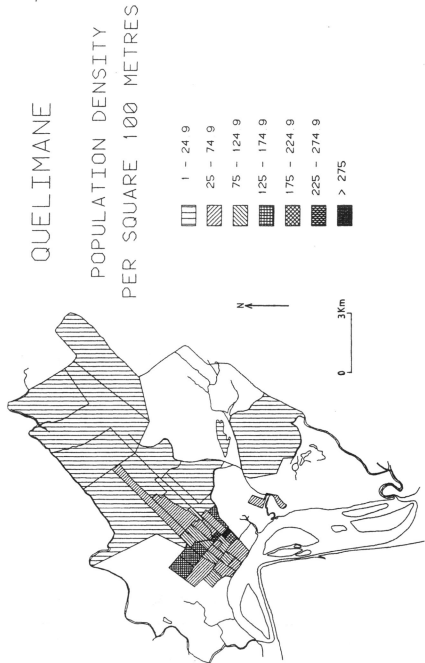

Figure 5.15 Population density at Quelimane

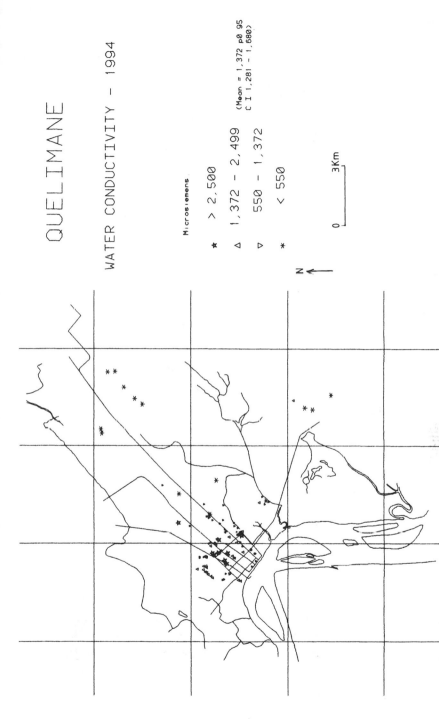

Figure 5.16 Clustering of high and low conductivity readings at Quelimane in 1994

145

In the case of Beira, the overall physical environmental conditions were found to differ from those of Quelimane. The average conductivity and pH, using the 134 well water samples and 64 soil samples, is lower (Table 5.3) and therefore in a general sense less favourable to the preferences of endemic *Vibrio cholerae 01*. Despite the overall conditions appearing less supportive of a physical environmental niche for cholera than for the case of Quelimane, the distribution of environmental conditions at the level of sub-areas is again revealing. Figures 5.17 and 5.18 show that areas of higher conductivity and higher pH occur around the core region in the south of the city of Beira with the more rural and

Table 5.3   Average pH and conductivity readings (microsiemens) at Quelimane, Beira and Gorongosa

	Quelimane	Beira	Gorongosa
Average pH	7.5	6.4	6.4
Average Conductivity µS	1358	863	280

peripheral areas representing zones with lower values of both. As with Quelimane, the strongest statistical correlations between rate of incidence of cholera and the physical environmental parameters by sub-areas was average conductivity ($r=0.65$ $p<0.01$) and average pH ($r=0.83$ $p<0.01$). The correlation with population density (Figure 5.19) was only just significant at the 95 per cent confidence limit ($r=0.44$ $p<0.05$). The other environmental variables do not correlate.

A comparison of the distribution of more saline environments (Figure 5.17) with the distribution of positive and negative residuals from the regression of incidence of dysentery on incidence of cholera (Figure 5.10) shows that the areas where cholera is higher than expected correspond with those recording high conductivity. The exceptional Bairro No 1, Estoril in the south-east of Beira, which has a lower than expected rate of incidence of cholera, but much higher than expected rate of incidence of dysentery, has the lowest average conductivity readings in the southern part of the city. The pattern is to some extent repeated for the case of averaged pH

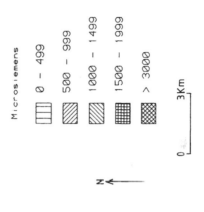

BEIRA

AVERAGE CONDUCTIVITY
MEASURED AT WELL SITES

Microsiemens

▥	0 – 499
▨	500 – 999
▨	1000 – 1499
▦	1500 – 1999
▩	> 3000

N

0   3Km

Figure 5.17 Spatial distribution of average conductivity per bairro at Beira

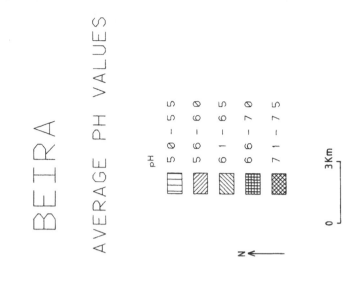

BEIRA

AVERAGE PH VALUES

pH

	50 - 55
	56 - 60
	61 - 65
	66 - 70
	71 - 75

N

0 _____ 3Km

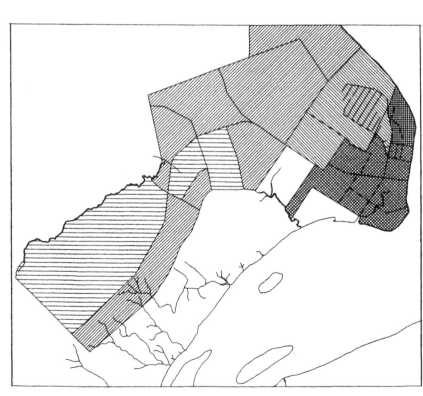

Figure 5.18 Spatial distribution of average pH per bairro at Beira

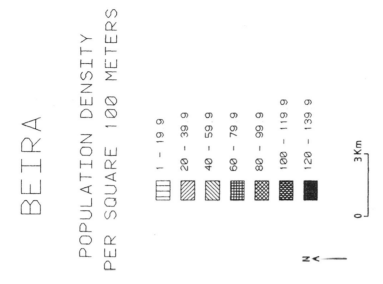

BEIRA

POPULATION DENSITY
PER SQUARE 100 METERS

	1 – 19 9
	20 – 39 9
	40 – 59 9
	60 – 79 9
	80 – 99 9
	100 – 119 9
	120 – 139 9

0   3Km

N

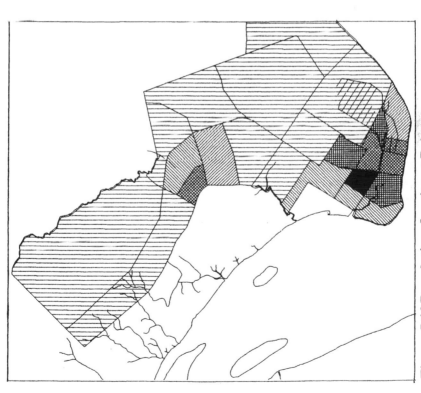

Figure 5.19 Population density at Beira

values. This combination of results suggests it is likely that there is a similar environmental factor at work as has been proposed for the case of Quelimane. However, the main confounding result in this assertion, for the case of Beira, is that incidence of cholera and dysentery tend to converge at the primary level of analysis, both being broadly concentrated in the southern more urbanised part of the city. Whilst absence of higher than expected incidence of cholera in the northern half of the city is explainable by the acidic fresh-water environment in those areas, absence of dysentery in the same areas suggests either, spatially coincidental factors that affect dysentery, or more influential factors applicable to both diseases.

In Gorongosa, values derived from a sample of 28 locations indicate that there is no saline environment and that the average pH is relatively acidic throughout that area. The role of an environmental reservoir, with favourable conditions of salinity and pH, in shaping the pattern of incidence of cholera is therefore not applicable in that location. Detectable differences in the distribution of the two diseases must therefore consider other factors in this instance, such as the greater communicability of dysentery indicated as a possible explanation in the previous sub-section.

The Distribution of Dysentery and Absence of a Physical Environmental Association with Shigella Dysenteriae 1

Observation of the distribution of dysentery has provided a further key to interpreting the association of physical environmental parameters and incidence of diarrhoeal disease. In the case of Quelimane, the distribution of higher and lower incidence of dysentery has been shown to be almost the opposite to that of cholera. No significant correlations exist between the rate of incidence of dysentery and population density, conductivity or pH, nor any of the other physical environmental variables. This supports the hypothesis that favourable environmental reservoirs are important in the case of *Vibrio cholerae* 01 but not in the case of *Shigella dysenteriae* 1. The lack of a clear association with population density in this instance could be a further reflection of the greater communicability of dysentery. It may also be that having arrived after cholera, the people on the side of the city that had been more affected by cholera were more immune to further diarrhoeal disease epidemics. However, this is regarded as unlikely since there is no clear pathogenic evidence that one bacterial disease can provide immunity against another.[3]

In Beira, there is no significant correlation of dysentery with average pH, average conductivity or population density at the 99 per cent level. Average pH alone becomes significant if using the 95 per cent confidence level ($r=0.53$ $p<0.05$). The contrast between the spatial association of cholera with environmental factors and the lack of association of dysentery and environmental factors is visible through observation of the residuals from the regression of rate of incidence of dysentery on rate of incidence of cholera (Figure 5.10). The area occupied by the positive residuals from the regression equation, indicating zones with unexplained higher cholera rates, are closely coincident with the areas of higher conductivity, and to a large extent, higher average pH. The areas with negative residuals, indicating zones where there is unexplained higher dysentery rates, are away from the zones with higher pH and conductivity. An exception is the case of Bairro 1 (Estoril) which has the highest rate of dysentery and is also the exceptional part of the southern part of the city in terms of its very low conductivity and pH.

In conclusion, the hypothesis of a spatial physical environmental influence on incidence of cholera is consistent with these results. Should the physical environmental reservoir not be influential on the distribution of incidence of cholera, there would be more reason to expect a closer resemblance to the distribution of dysentery. This is because both are faecal-oral bacterial diseases that cause diarrhoea, have been similarly associated with 'underdevelopment' and poverty, and have affected many of the same sub-regions of continents. In the context of these similarities, many approaches to diarrhoeal disease have not differentiated between individual pathogenic causes. However, the results of this first part of the analysis already reveal some distinct variations that support assertions of

---

[3] Despite earlier indication of 90 per cent protection against rechallenge with El-Tor of either Ogawa or Inaba serotypes presented by Levine *et al.* (1981), Clemens and Sack *et al.* (1990) have more recently found that immunity is not necessarily provided by one serotype of El Tor cholera over another. One of the notable features of the recent emergence of *Vibrio cholerae* 0139 is also that previous infection with the El Tor serotypes does not provide immunity (Swerdlow and Reis 1993). At least one study in more general terms proposes that recent diarrhoea morbidity actually predisposes to persistent diarrhoea amongst the same people (Sazawal and Bhan *et al.* 1991). Further to this it can be argued that the numbers of infected people in all sub-areas represent fractions of overall populations such that many more would not, in any case, have gained immunity.

the relevance of local environmental factors in the distribution of incidence of cholera, but not of dysentery.

The variation in patterns of association for the three urban zones shows that physical environmental influences on cholera are likely to depend on the ecological context of the location and specific pathogenesis. Cholera attributable to serotype Ogawa is associated with environmental factors in Quelimane, but no explanation for the dysentery distribution is apparent. In Beira, the association with the same environmental factors and cholera incidence due to serotype Inaba remains consistent, but lacks the additional confirmation applicable to Quelimane since the distribution of dysentery is not fundamentally different. The closer association of the two in this instance may therefore indicate a more general factor that is affecting both diseases, such as the intensity of urbanisation in the southern part of the city. In Gorongosa, where there is no evidence of physical features that disproportionately influence cholera, there exists the possibility that the differences in distribution between the two diseases relate to greater communicability of dysentery. Further evidence for the above assertions is provided through analysis of the spatio-temporal dimensions of disease distributions.

Spatio-temporal Association of Incidence of Cholera and Dysentery with the Physical Environment

Appearance, Disappearance and Reappearance: Observations on Epidemicity and Endemicity of Cholera and Bacillary Dysentery

Precise definitions of endemic as opposed to epidemic cholera are difficult to formulate. However, as a guideline, Miller *et al.* (1985, p261) have stated that cholera can be said to be endemic in an area where cases occur 'not necessarily continuously, but regularly and without evidence of reimportation on each occasion, and a seasonal pattern is usually observed'. As described in Chapter 4, cholera arrived in Africa in the 1970s as an epidemic disease. In the years that followed some countries became endemic for cholera with outbreaks each year while others remained cholera-free or only experienced a few imported cases. Glass and Claeson *et al.* (1991) define the most endemic countries as those with more than 8 years of cholera and indicate Mozambique, Zaire, Nigeria, Liberia and Cameroon as falling into this category for the period up till 1990.

The appearance and disappearance of endemic El Tor cholera is dependent on the *Vibrio* being able to find a means of survival for longer periods. Two recently authenticated explanations exist. Firstly, cholera presents a large amount of symptom-free cases (Sepulveda and Gomez-Dantes 1992) and therefore may be incorrectly presumed absent from the community for short periods. Secondly, some areas may have environmental reservoirs within which the *Vibrio* is able to survive in a dormant non toxigenic form for prolonged periods should there be suitable physiological conditions (Drasar 1992, 1996; Colwell and Huq 1994). Each of these may involve an ability for the pathogen to adapt, favouring serotypes that have been present for longer.

Resurgence of major disease outbreaks occurs when suitable conditions are created for the reactivation of the pathogen, such as those caused by local environmental changes and/or a deterioration in the overall resistance of people occupying an area. On the other hand, importation of a new serotype may also cause severe epidemic conditions since it is confronted with little immune resistance in the community. In such circumstances it is less likely to show such a strong correlation with the distribution of geophysical conditions (such as pH and salinity), but this may emerge as it becomes endemic in the environment with more time.

The unravelling of the epidemicity and endemicity of cholera and dysentery in the field can provide some useful indications of probable influences on patterns of incidence. On the basis of background information on specific pathogens (Chapter 1), the field sites (Chapter 4), and the results presented so far in this chapter, incidence of cholera in Quelimane appears to be associated with endemic disease maintained by local environmental conditions. The pathogenic particularities of Beira's 1992 cholera epidemic suggests it was part of a more recent epidemic wave of the disease and therefore environmental reservoirs can be expected to be less of a factor in that instance. This would help to explain why the distribution of the Beira cholera epidemic had a greater similarity with that of the *Shigella dysenteriae* 1 epidemic.

Seasonality of the Epidemic Curve and Rainfall

Figure 5.20 reveals a significant correlation between the pattern of incidence of cholera and rainfall at Quelimane ($r=0.59$ $p<0.01$) for the epidemic period between June 1990 and May 1993. The first surge in cholera incidence in 1990 occurred as the driest part of the year was approaching and peaked during the driest month. High incidence was maintained during the rainy months but dropped off as the rains declined. The subsequent epidemic peaks occurred in January 1992 and December 1992 corresponding with the start of the rains for the next two years. The correlation between rainfall and incidence of cholera becomes much stronger during this period ($r=0.80$ $p<0.01$).

The relationship between recorded incidence of cholera and rainfall at Beira for the period January 1992 - May 1993 is shown in Figure 5.21. The first peak in incidence followed the arrival of rains in 1992. The second major epidemic peak occurred at the same time as the following year's rains. Other parts of the epidemic curve do not associate at all resulting in no overall correlation ($r=-0.10$), save for during the dry months between June and September. Also included in Figure 5.21 is the recorded monthly incidence of dysentery from January 1993 until July 1994. This displays no correlation with rainfall at all ($r=-0.03$), initially peaking during the rainy season during the decline of cholera and then consistently cutting across the pattern of rainfall. The results of the rainfall analysis are important in that it reveals a further physical environmental parameter that is more associated with incidence of cholera in Quelimane than in Beira, and that lacks an association with dysentery. The following discussion assesses specific reasons for these patterns of association.

The epidemic peaks of diarrhoeal disease incidence have been largely associated with the wet season. An explanation for a surge in diarrhoeal disease with the onset of rains is that faecal contamination is washed into drinking water supplies, such as rivers and open wells. A local saying is 'a chuva vai acordar a cólera' (the rain will awaken cholera). Old and leaky piped water supplies also become more susceptible to contamination at this time as pathogens become more readily diffused in the wet earth around underground pipes. Of interest here is the deterioration of water quality in terms of total coliforms, faecal coliforms and faecal streptococci in wells, rivers and springs during the wet season that was quantified by Lindskog and Lindskog (1988) in rural Malawi. A similar pattern was recorded by Moore *et al.* (1965) in Costa Rica, Feachem *et al.* (1978) in Lesotho and Barrell and Rowland (1979) in Gambia. The impact of the wet season may be genuinely suspected as also being a factor in Beira where flooding by rainwater is particularly bad in some of the most densely populated Bairros, such as Chipangara and Munhava (Figure 4.9). This is also the case in Quelimane where flooding is worst in the Communal Units of

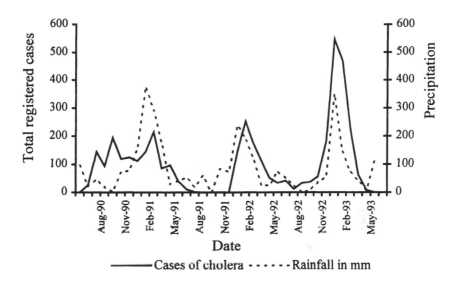

Figure 5.20 The relationship between incidence of cholera and rainfall at Quelimane

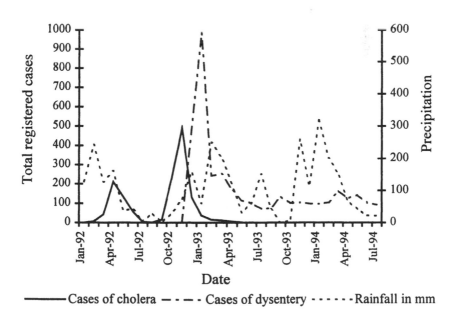

Figure 5.21 The relationship between incidence of cholera, dysentery and rainfall at Beira

Manhawa and Aeroporto (Figure 4.8) which had swelled to capacity during the period of peak population displacement in the 1980s.

However, the stimulus for early phases of epidemics has been less clear since sometimes incidence of cholera has started to appear during a dry period. In Mozambique, the 1992 drought interfered with the drinking water supply of both cities. In the case of Beira, the piped Pungwe water source was turned off on the grounds of becoming too saline to drink, and in the case of Quelimane the piped Licuar water supply dried up altogether. Concerning this it can be pointed out that the worst year for cholera in Mozambican history, 1992, was also the year of its worst drought. During a drought more people end up using fewer wells, which have reduced volumes of water. Under these circumstances, contamination might be suspected to increase. However, continuous replenishment of the well water through its bottom could also be considered beneficial since filtration of bacteria is enhanced. Of interest here is that Wright (1986) in Sierra Leone recorded a gradual increase in pollution during the dry season, which was interpreted as an increasing concentration of bacteria as water volumes decreased. Meanwhile, Sandiford *et al.* (1989) found a combination of both phenomena. Whilst there was an overall correlation between higher rainfall and faecal contamination in rural Nicaragua, during the dry period they found that protected wells had higher average levels of contamination than others. This was presumably due to intense usage of a diminished quantity of water.

Levels of faecal coliform contamination measured in this research during two periods of the year indicated that contamination in wells generally decreased as water levels lower during the drier period except for the case of Gorongosa where the results for the two periods were more similar (Table 5.4). On the basis of these results, the start of a cholera epidemic in a dry period looks less likely to be related directly to an increase in well contamination. However, a further explanation for seasonal patterns that requires attention is that, rather than increases in contamination, physiological conditions of an environmental reservoir become more favourable to the disease pathogen during times of reduced water levels. Should this be the case, it would explain why resurgence of endemic cholera takes place in the dry period prior to its subsequent proliferation during the rainy period.

This explanation applies to the case of Quelimane where it is suggested that during drought the groundwater supply became more brackish due to a saline intrusion, thus creating more areas with favourable

Table 5.4   Average quantities of faecal coliforms cultured from water samples taken at two times of year

	QUELIMANE		BEIRA		GORONGOSA	
	n	FC	n	FC	n	FC
PHASE 1 Wetter	92	574	110	788	28	215
PHASE 2 Dryer	84	401	113	337	20	285

Notes:

FC = Average number of faecal coliforms per 100ml water.

n = Number of water samples successfully cultured. (Samples from sporadic supply from taps and standpipes connected to pumping stations have been ignored)

conditions for *Vibrios* adapted to those conditions. This would explain why the first epidemic of 1990 started during an exceptionally dry period. As suggested above, subsequent heavy rainfall caused contaminated water to be spread to more sites and secondary transmission was enhanced by faecal material being spread around areas of habitation. Since the local physiological conditions of certain areas are already suitable for survival and increased toxigeneity of *Vibrio cholerae*, contamination was spread around in a medium ideal for its success. This contributes to explaining why the subsequent epidemic peaks occurred during times of maximum rainfall. Whereas flooding is also likely to be influential in the case of Beira, the presence of a more epidemic serotype and a different complex of local factors has meant that the rainfall effect has not become apparent to the same extent that it has in Quelimane. In Beira, the evidence of a predisposing environmental terrain as the principal determining factor on the distribution of the disease was less pronounced and therefore the rainfall effect on local physiological conditions became less evident.

The indication that dysentery is not so affected by rainfall serves as further confirmation of the associations described above. Dysentery is much less likely to be a disease that becomes endemic in the physical environment and it is therefore to be expected that it will have more in common with the less endemic cholera events. This is confirmed by its lack of association with seasonal rainfall in either town.

Environmental Influences on Spatial Diffusion and Persistence of Cholera and Bacillary Dysentery

A further aspect of the analysis of physical environmental association has been to observe the spatial distribution of the diseases by sub-area for each month of the epidemics using time sequence mapping. During the early analysis of cholera in Quelimane in 1991 this showed that in its initial stages the main focus of incidence of cholera moved from one side of the main urban area to the other. This change was towards areas identified as environmentally preferable to the longevity of *Vibrio cholerae*. The disease spread from the location of the initial reported incidents in Chirangano, with the densest population, to the opposite side of the main urban area of Quelimane (Figure 4.4). It was this north-west facing flank of the city, Manhawa, that had the higher rate of incidence throughout the rest of the epidemic. This area also had the highest rates of incidence throughout the latter epidemic analysed by this research, indicating that the pattern established during the advanced stages of the earlier epidemic was maintained. Hence the area in and around Manhawa, namely Communal Units 1, 2, 3, 4, 10 and 12, accounted for 81 per cent of cases in the first month of the new epidemic (Figure 5.22). This reduced to just 27 per cent by the last month of the epidemic as the disease became more dispersed through secondary transmission.

Without clear referencing of the early stages of the dysentery epidemic in Quelimane it is not possible to execute a complete analysis of diffusion and persistence as has been achieved for the cholera epidemic. However, using the well registered batch of cases between January 1994 and August 1994, it has been calculated that, at the peak of the epidemic in January 1994, 45 per cent of all cases occurred in the seven Communal Units (5,7,13,20,27,29,36) around the south-eastern flanks of Quelimane, a focus distinctly different from that of cholera. This percentage remained at between 39 per cent and 47 per cent for the entire January to August period.

Figure 5.23 displays the monthly percentages of total cases of cholera per sub-area for the five *bairros* of Beira with highest overall incidence of cholera for the period February 1992 - May 1993. These are the contiguous areas of Bairros 2, 3, 6, 7, and 9. Figure 5.24 shows the five *bairros* that had the highest overall incidence of dysentery for the period February 1993- July 1994. Three of these were the same as the areas with the highest incidence of cholera. In both cases (most clearly in the case of dysentery) the monthly percentages of cases indicate that the diseases persisted at a relatively even rate in the high incidence *bairros* of Beira. This indicates that once disease selected these zones its distribution did not shift around in response to more favourable environmental niches, as was suggested for the initial cholera outbreak in Quelimane. It also indicates that, unlike cholera in Quelimane, secondary transmission has not altered the weighting of cases occurring in these areas as the disease persisted.

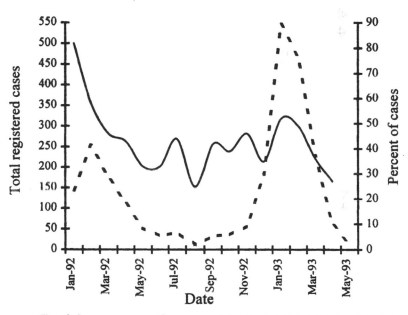

- - - Total Cases ————Communal Units 1,2,3,4,10,12 as % of total

Figure 5.22 The temporal relationship between recorded cases of cholera and percent of cases occurring within Communal units 1,2,3,4,10,12 on north-western flank of main urban zone of Quelimane between January 1992 and May 1993

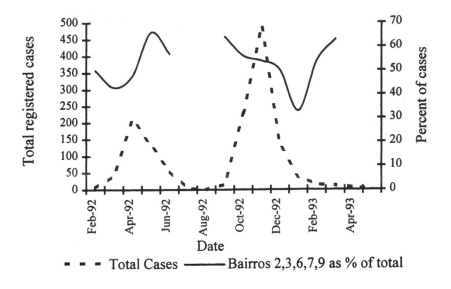

Figure 5.23 **The temporal relationship between total recorded cases of cholera and percent of cases occurring within Bairros 2,3,6,7 and 9, the 5 locations with the highest amount of cholera cases for the period February 1992 - May 1993**

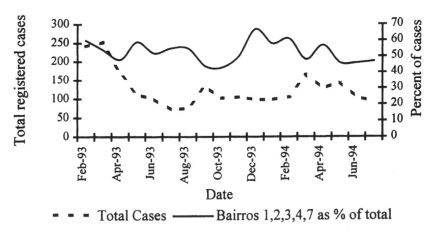

Figure 5.24 **The temporal relationship between total recorded cases of dysentery and percent of cases occurring within Bairros 1,2,3,4, and 7, the 5 locations with the highest amount of dysentery cases for the period February 1993 - July 1994**

The Spatio-temporal Differences of Environmental Variables Measured at the Field Sites

Coefficients derived from correlating the results of two periods of environmental data collection in Quelimane and Beira in 1994 are presented in Table 5.5. Even though the second period of the research has not always used exactly the same sites as the first, the results show a general continuity in the association between variables for the two periods. This suggests a high degree of reliability in the survey methods and techniques, including selection of representative sample sites, and provides more confidence to some of the associations that have been presented in this research. It is also of key interest in that it reveals that there was relatively little environmental change between the two periods that affected the correlation of the variables. This may to some extent be explained by a lack of extreme seasonal differentiation between the two periods that were used but also provides evidence that the spatial distribution of distinct environmental characteristics is not ephemeral. The associations between distinct sub-areas with favourable conditions for *Vibrio cholerae* and higher incidence of cholera are supported by this result since the disease has been shown to persistently proliferate in the same areas.

A closer examination of changes in the status of individual environmental parameters between different periods has been possible by considering those water sample sites that were re-identified during different visits (Table 5.6). In the case of Quelimane, it was also possible to extend the comparison to data for sites that were used during the 1991 survey, although this was limited to only 17 locations since many of the wells used for the smaller 1991 sample had been filled in or become dilapidated.

The results show that water pH and conductivity readings were similar between the two sampling periods in 1994 at Quelimane, Beira and Gorongosa. However, changes had occurred to the water of the Quelimane sites sampled in 1991 with the result that readings did not correlate well. This is an indication that over this longer time period the local physical environment at individual sites in Quelimane changed, though not linearly. For example, there was a decrease in conductivity (all but three samples), but an increase in pH (all but three samples) between the earlier and later tests. It could be argued that this is accounted for by a diminution in the saline intrusion with better rainfall (causing lower conductivity readings)

Table 5.5 Correlation coefficients from environmental data sampled at two times of year in Quelimane and Beira

	Depth to water		Faecal coliforms		Conductivity		Water pH		Turbidity		Population density		Dysentery rate	
	Q	B	Q	B	Q	B	Q	B	Q	B	Q	B	Q	B
Cholera rate	-.22	.35	.11	.32	.51	.65	.57	.83	-.30	-.03	.51	.44	.27	.68
	-.25	*.39*	*-.24*	*.49*	*.55*	*.62*	*.40*	*.82*	*-.34*	*-.19*	*-*	*-*	*-*	*-*
Dysentery rate	.37	.26	-.08	.00	-.25	.20	-.15	.53	-.22	.14	.31	.21		
	.26	*.59*	*-.06*	*.44*	*-.17*	*.26*	*-.28*	*.53*	*-.05*	*-.20*	*-*	*-*		
Population density	.01	.21	-.18	.16	.48	.74	.40	.61	-.17	-.24				
	-.08	*.11*	*-.34*	*-.12*	*.49*	*.66*	*.29*	*.55*	*-.25*	*-.26*				
Turbidity	.11	-.14	-.10	.19	-.17	.04	-.40	.03						
	.29	*-.04*	*.03*	*.19*	*-.18*	*-.09*	*-.36*	*-.02*						
Water pH	-.03	.04	.17	.24	.54	.49								
	-.18	*.04*	*-.08*	*.16*	*.49*	*.62*								
Conductivity	-.27	.05	.09	.30										
	.37	*.03*	*-.08*	*.16*										
Faecal coliforms	.04	-.12												
	.36	*.26*												

City	Depth to water		Faecal Coliforms		Conduct-ivity		Water pH		Turbidity		Pop Density		Dysentery Rate		Cholera Rate		Soil Density	
	Q	B	Q	B	Q	B	Q	B	Q	B	Q	B	Q	B	Q	B	Q	B
Soil pH*	-.19	.13	.30	.35	.58	.37	.70	.70	-.23	.04	.48	-.08	-.20	.08	.62	.23	.15	-.27
Soil den*	.11	.05	-.04	-.09	.02	-.38	.17	-.27	-.23	-.03	.02	.60	.06	.17	.17	.41		

Notes:

Q = Quelimane B = Beira

Upper figures are for the first phase of data collection completed in early 1994. The lower figures (in *italics*) are the result of the second phase of data collection carried out in the same locations towards mid-1994.

*Soil pH and soil density were sampled only once.

Shaded figures are significant in excess of the 99% confidence level using Pearson's product-moment two tailed values and allowing for changes to sample size. A total of 73 samples were used for Quelimane and 134 for Beira, these figures being subject to small variations for individual variables and the availability of sample sites for reanalyses during the second period of data collection. In the case of correlating two variables measured through water analysis, the results of the 73-134 water samples have been used. For correlation with population density, cholera rate and dysentery rate, averaged water analysis values per sub-area of each city has been used. This meant that for these variables between 22 and 39 sub-areas have been used.

163

Table 5.6 **Analysis of change in environmental variables using repeat sites sampled on different occasions**

	Turbidity	Water pH	Conductivity	Faecal coliform	Depth to water
Quelimane	0.17	0.68	0.96	0.50	0.90
Mar 94 + Jul 94	n=75	n=76	n=76	n=74	n=59
Quelimane	0.03	0.36	0.47	0.45	0.71
Jul 94 + Aug 91	n=17	n=17	n=17	n=17	n=13
Beira	0.12	0.82	0.64	0.15	0.82
Jan 94 + Jun 94	n=65	n=66	n=66	n=60	n=64
Gorongosa	0.99	0.70	0.96	0.19	-
Feb 94 + Jun 94	n=18	n=18	n=18	n=18	-

Note:
Shaded figures are significant in excess of the 99% confidence level using two tailed values.

and increase in loss of organic content through leaching (causing more alkali ground conditions).

A further result of interest is that quantities of faecal coliforms between different sampling periods do not correlate at Beira and Gorongosa, and at Quelimane do not correlate so well as pH and conductivity. This reflects the earlier results displayed in Table 5.4. However, whilst levels of faecal coliform contamination varies for different times of year, it has already been shown to not correlate spatially with incidence of cholera or dysentery for either (Table 5.5). Ironically, it is this variable that is most frequently used in health and water contamination studies. The results support the contention that faecal coliforms are not an accurate indicator of the spatial distribution of diarrhoeal disease hazards, despite their usefulness in indicating a general context of poor standards of hygiene.

Turbidity is a further measure that is widely used in water analysis studies, displays variation between different periods, and which consistently does not correlate with incidence of cholera or dysentery in this study. Further to this, the results indicating that coliform counts do not correspond to the spatial distribution of incidence in these faecally contaminated areas is consistent with there being further factors that shape the distribution of cholera and dysentery. In the case of Quelimane these have been indicated as physiological factors, such as higher pH and salinity, that assist the improved survivability and toxigeneity of endemic *Vibrio cholerae*. In Beira these are also likely to be important but, as indicated by clustering of cholera and dysentery in the urban south of the city, pathogenesis, and lack of rainfall association, are less likely to be the principal explanation for the distribution of incidence of the disease. In Gorongosa, there is no evidence of endemicity of cholera and concordantly no evidence of associating physiological factors.

6 Pattern and Process in Diarrhoeal Disease Incidence: The Role of Resettlement, Forced Displacement and Environmental Change

This chapter presents the results from demographic and sociogeographic research carried out in the three field sites at the same time as the environmental associative analysis described in the previous chapter. The first section assesses the age and sex distribution of cases of cholera and dysentery, and concludes that differences in age and sex distributions of both diseases are consistent with the interpretation of results presented in Chapter 5. The second and main part of the chapter then turns to influences on the spatio-temporal relationship between population displacement and incidence of cholera and dysentery. These include the role of environmental changes induced by displacement that favour disease pathogens, as well as differences in susceptibility and socio-economic status amongst displaced people (c.f. Collins 1993a, p337). The influence of local environmental circumstances and role of the key factors of water supply, sanitation, fuel and cultivation in environmental health issues are considered for different locales.

Age and Sex Distributions as an Indication of Differences in Influence on Incidence of Cholera and Dysentery at the Field Sites

The age profile of incidence of diarrhoeal disease can provide an indication of the endemicity or epidemicity of the pathogen responsible. If a disease has become endemic in a community, then some immunity to the pathogen can be acquired (Vogel 1992). Since infants have not had time to develop biological resistance they are more likely to experience higher incidence.

167

However, with a new epidemic disease where all the community experiences the pathogen for the first time, the expected age distribution is a closer reflection of the age structure of the population. This was noted by Mulholland (1985) in deciding that cholera in a Sudanese refugee camp was more epidemic than endemic. A further factor that can affect this trend for the very young is the protection available through breast feeding (Clemens *et al.* 1990; AHRTAG 1993), which can delay infection until weaning (Ahmed *et al.* 1993).

There are two reasons why this research has chosen to include an analysis of the age distribution of cases. Firstly, it is important to establish whether there are age differences between the diseases and sites that need to be taken into account in assessing the role of environmental and demographic factors. For example, large differences in age profile between cholera and dysentery at the different sites would suggest a need to control

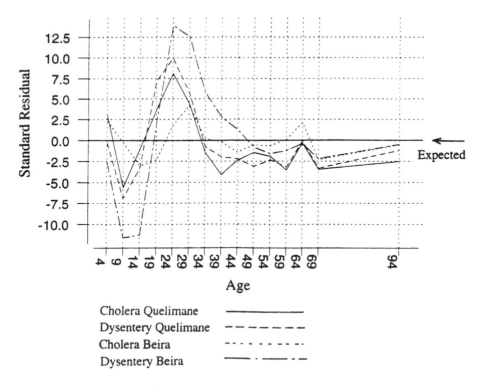

Figure 6.1   Standardised residuals of age of cases of cholera and dysentery against the age distribution of Sofala Province

for age in assessing the spatial distribution of the diseases. Secondly, analysis of differences in age profiles of the diseases provides an opportunity to further verify conclusions drawn in Chapter 5, namely that cholera at Quelimane was more endemic than cholera at Beira, and cholera at Beira more so than dysentery at both sites.

Strong correlations were found between the age distributions of incidence of cholera and dysentery at Quelimane and Beira using the data derived from hospital admission books (r=0.76-0.96 p<0.001). The age data for Gorongosa were not considered adequate for the same analysis since figures for infants with dysentery did not include many who were thought to have been redirected to an emergency paediatric feeding centre alongside the hospital. Though the results indicate that age does not significantly interfere with the comparison of environmental, demographic, and structural factors presented in this thesis, smaller variations between the diseases and sites deserve some attention. Analysis of residuals from regression indicated ages when one disease had unusually higher or lower numbers of cases compared to that of the other. Residual differences could also be derived by comparing each distribution independently against an expected age distribution based on groups of five years. This was eventually preferred since it provided similar comparative information with the added relevance of comparing disease by age group against the population pyramid for Sofala Province (Figure 4.11).[1] Figure 6.1 shows that in each case the age distribution of disease cases deviates significantly from this representative age distribution. This was confirmed using chi-square analysis (p<0.001).

The age distributions of both diseases are characterised by lower than expected numbers of cases between ages 5-15. This reflects greater resistance to communicable disease during the period of life called the 'golden age of resistance'. A comparative decline in resistance and accompanying opportunism of disease pathogens following 'the golden age of resistance' is therefore a possible explanation for the higher than expected number of cases that occur during the 20's age group. Higher

---

[1] The expected number of cases for each age group was computed from the division of the number of people in each age group by the total population multiplied by the total number of cases of a disease in that age group. The standardised residuals were calculated by O-E/$\sqrt{E}$, where O = observed and E = expected number of cases for each age group. The generalisation was made that the population pyramid for Sofala approximates to that for other areas. No population data for age groups of less than five years were available at the time of carrying out this research.

than expected cases of cholera in Quelimane in the 0-4 age group confirm suggestions of the endemicity of serotype *Ogawa* in that location, since it can be argued that subsequent age groups have established some resistance against the pathogen. In Beira, higher than expected amounts of cholera cases also occurred in the 0-4 age group but the distribution subsequently reflects the age structure of the population more closely. This in turn suggests less resistance to serotype Inaba, and its association with a more recent epidemic. The overall epidemic nature of dysentery is confirmed by the fact that there were not higher than expected numbers of cases in the youngest age group. The greater magnitude of variation that is displayed by dysentery (in particular at Beira) may relate to the fact that it is more sensitive to variations in immunity and resistance between different age groups.

The sex distributions of the diseases are also considered of interest, since similar rates of incidence between the sexes might be expected where disease is endemic. The rationale here is that the influence of an environmental reservoir is less likely to be gender specific than the human reservoir, which can be subject to both biological and socio-economic differences in susceptibility. However, the complexity of gender differentials in incidence of diarrhoeal disease is also recognised. For example, Sørensen and Dissler (1986) reported a significantly higher number of females in the age group 15-44 who developed cholera in Sudanese camps, unexplained by age structure of the camp. This differs from what is found in most epidemics where incidence is higher amongst males (Feachem 1981; Lasch *et al.* 1984). Sørensen and Dissler (1986, p280) mention that higher incidence among males in the 19th century was explained by their greater mobility.

The sex distribution of the two diseases is shown in Figure 6.2 and Table 6.1. Chi-square tests using 2×2 contingency tables showed that there were significantly more males than females for both cholera in Beira and dysentery in Beira and Quelimane (p<0.001). The greatest difference was for dysentery at Beira, followed by dysentery at Quelimane. By way of contrast, for cholera at Quelimane there is no significant difference between the number of males and females (p>0.05). These results are consistent with the hypothesis that immunity and resistance on account of sex plays less of a role amongst cases of the endemic disease at Quelimane.

In Gorongosa there are also approximately equal numbers of male and female cases of both cholera and dysentery, but it must be noted that

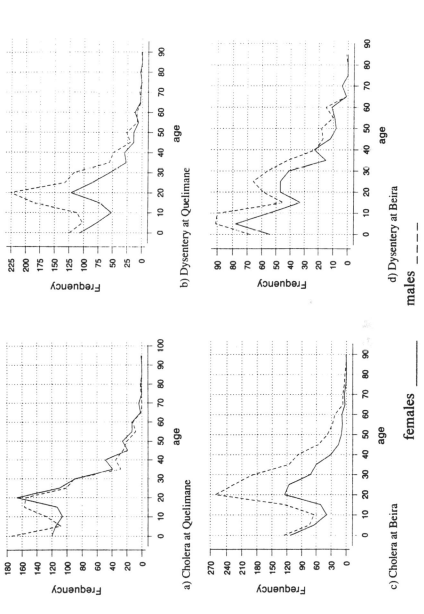

Figure 6.2 (a,b,c,d) Age by sex distributions of incidence of cholera and dysentery at Quelimane and Beira

a) Cholera at Quelimane

b) Dysentery at Quelimane

c) Cholera at Beira

d) Dysentery at Beira

females _____   males _ _ _ _

171

Table 6.1   **Incidence of cholera and dysentery by sex in Quelimane, Beira and Gorongosa**

	QUELIMANE		BEIRA		GORONGOSA	
	Male %	Female %	Male %	Female %	Male %	Female %
CHOLERA	51.4	48.6	57.3	42.7	48.8	51.2
	(n = 2122)		(n = 1392)		(n = 211)	
DYSENTERY	62.7	37.3	65.7	34.3	48.8	51.2
	(n = 1923)		(n = 2320)		(n = 43)	

Note:
Shaded percentages indicate those where differences between numbers of males and females are significant in excess of the 95% confidence level using chi-square analysis on pairs of proportions.

Gorongosa has significantly more women than men in total, such that proportionately there is again a higher level of male incidence as at Beira. Local government figures show that there were approximately 1.72 females for each male in Gorongosa during six months sampled during 1993 and 1994 (Administração do Distrito de Gorongosa 1994), compared to a near equal ratio of 1.07 females per male in Beira in 1991 (Comissão Provincial do Plano de Sofala 1992) and estimated ratio of 0.96 females per male in 1994 (Comissão do Plano de CECB 1994). There were 0.96 females per male in Quelimane in 1991 (Comissão Provincial do Plano de Zambézia 1991). In the case of Quelimane, it was also possible to calculate that there was no more than 0.16 per cent variation in proportions of males to females between sub-areas.

Comparison of the proportions of male to female cases for sub-administrative areas with the proportion of male to female cases for an overall site found no significant differences for cholera in Quelimane, Beira or Gorongosa. However, there were significantly more male cases than expected for dysentery in communal units 10 (Aeroporto) and 29 (Liberdade) at Quelimane (Figure 4.8) and for Bairros 4 (Chaimite) and 6 (Esturro) at Beira (Figure 4.9). There are no clear explanations for these exceptions, the main importance of the results remaining that across 64 out of 68 (94.1 per cent) sub-areas gender differentials do not influence the spatial-temporal distribution of these diseases. Though age and sex are recognised here as important aspects of studies on infectious diseases the above results suggest it unlikely that they significantly interfere with the overall analysis of environment, health and displacement described in this chapter.

The Distribution of More Recent Settlement in Quelimane, Beira and Gorongosa

A key hypothesis outlined in Chapters 1-3 was that disproportionately higher incidence of cholera and dysentery can occur amongst displaced people due to increased biological and socio-economic vulnerability to infection. Additionally, it has been suggested that displaced people can experience greater exposure to disease environments after emergency resettlement (Mulholland 1985; Shears and Lusty 1987) and that environmental changes caused by displacement and resettlement may exacerbate levels of cholera incidence (Collins 1993, p336). Comparison of incidence of the diseases between more recently settled and more established residents of the field sites enables assessment of the association between population displacement, local environments and incidence of cholera and dysentery. Representation of the spatial distribution of the more recently settled population using the sub-areas of the cities has enabled comparison with the spatial distribution of the diseases and environmental characteristics determined in Chapter 5.

Questionnaire interviews recorded the number of years that households had lived at their current location to determine the approximate distribution of more recently settled residents (Table 6.2). The use of a 10 year upper limit for classifying residents as more recently settled was used since beyond this period it would not be likely that questions of immunity, susceptibility, adaptation and integration would be relevant. The ten year cut off point was also considered suitable as this divided the population into those who were present before 1984, about which time some of the most intensive disruption causing population displacement in rural Mozambique was under way, and those who had moved to their current residence during or after this disruption. However, requesting the specific number of years at current location meant that it has also been possible to make comparisons using shorter time periods. Table 6.2 shows that about half of the sample at all sites have been resident for less than ten years,

Table 6.2   Number of years that respondents were resident at their current location

Years	QUELIMANE			BEIRA			GORONGOSA			ALL		
	No.	%	Cum%	No.	%	Cum%	No.	%	Cum%	No.	%	Cum%
0-5	128	44.6	44.6	139	37.1	37.1	19	27.9	27.9	286	39.2	39.2
5-10	41	14.3	58.9	45	12.0	49.1	15	22.1	50.0	101	13.8	53.0
10-15	28	9.8	68.6	67	17.9	66.9	13	19.1	69.1	108	14.8	67.8
15-20	27	9.4	78.1	53	14.1	81.1	6	8.8	77.9	86	11.8	79.6
20-25	25	8.7	86.8	48	12.8	93.9	5	7.4	85.3	78	10.7	90.3
25-30	11	3.8	90.6	9	2.4	96.3	4	5.9	91.2	24	3.3	93.6
30-35	14	4.9	95.5	9	2.4	98.7	3	4.4	95.6	26	3.6	97.2
35-45	9	3.1	98.6	3	0.8	99.5	2	2.9	98.5	14	1.9	99.1
45+	4	1.4	100	2	0.5	100	1	1.5	100	7	0.9	100
ALL	287	100		375	100		68	100		730	100	

174

thus providing an added incentive for using this length of time as an upper limit, since it provided larger comparative samples of two groups of people. In the case of Quelimane 59 per cent of the 287 people interviewed lived in their current location for less than 10 years. In Beira this decreases to 49 per cent of 375 interviews and in Gorongosa 50 per cent of 68 interviews.

Distinctive irregularities in the distance-decay curve of annual numbers of resettling people can be identified for each site (Figure 6.3). These correspond to key historical moments. For example, the tail of the curve is broken by a peak at about 20 years back representing the re-organisational movement occurring around the independence period of 1975. The peak at around 12 years back corresponds to activity in the war of destabilisation, which increasingly targeted the rural and peri-urban populations. In the case of Gorongosa, a focal point of the war on several occasions, this caused additional peaks at about 16 and 9 years back. The particularly low level of resettlement in Beira at about 10 years back

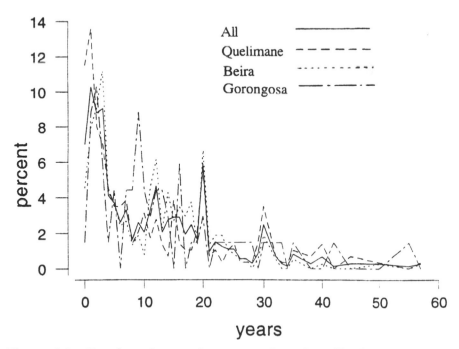

**Figure 6.3   Number of years that respondents have lived at their
current locations in Quelimane, Beira and Gorongosa**

corresponds with the famine years of 1983-1987 when the city was more cut off and forced to survive on its own subsistence activities. The re-emergence of the city as a commercial centre in the 1990s restored the general propensity of the population to relocate. For all areas, the very steep initial decline is exaggerated due to extra movements associated with the post 1992 Peace Agreement era.

In Quelimane 46 of the 287 people interviewed said that they had suffered from cholera and 80 from dysentery within the last three years; in Beira 110 of 375 from cholera and 166 from dysentery, and in Gorongosa 32 of 68 from cholera and 37 from dysentery. These figures reflect much higher incidence rates than those indicated by the data compiled from the hospital registration books. There are several reasons for this. Firstly, except for cholera in Quelimane, only part of the three year period referred to on the questionnaire has been used for the hospital registered cases. Secondly, though respondents were requested to report only confirmed incidence, these were not necessarily registered as such in the hospital records if considered by the staff to be only a mild case of the disease. Mild cases would also have evaded registration through not being referred on to the main Hospital from the local health posts. Thirdly, there are problems of accuracy of response. For example, it is well known that in disaster relief situations people will report ill-health in response to questions on nutrition or disease to not miss out on potential aid distributions or new infrastructural facilities.

Despite limitations in obtaining absolute figures from the sample of questionnaires, the data are adequate for the principal purpose of making a comparison between different groups. The results in Table 6.3 show incidence of cholera and dysentery to be about the same between the people who had been resident for more than and less than 10 years in Quelimane and Beira. Interestingly, in Gorongosa incidence is higher amongst the group that had been resident for more than ten years and particularly in the case of dysentery. Reasons for this difference are sought in the following subsection of this chapter through analysis of possible variations in susceptibility between the longer term residents (established residents) and the voluntary and forced migrants who arrived more recently.

Comparison between shorter periods of residency was also carried out (Table 6.4). This revealed some variation in the number of cases of cholera and dysentery with different periods of residency, but only dysentery at Beira amongst the 3-5 year residents produced a significantly different

Table 6.3 Comparison of incidence of cholera and dysentery between people resident for more than and less than 10 years

| | QUELIMANE | | | | BEIRA | | | | GORONGOSA | | | |
| | CHOLERA | | DYSENTERY | | CHOLERA | | DYSENTERY | | CHOLERA | | DYSENTERY | |
	Prop	%	Prop	%	Prop	%	Prop	%	Prop	%	Prop	%
Less than 10 years resident	27/169	16	46/169	27	51/184	28	82/184	45	16/34	47	16/34	47
More than 10 years resident	19/118	16	34/118	29	59/191	31	84/191	44	16/34	47	21/34	62
All	46/287	16	80/287	28	110/375	29	166/375	44	32/68	47	37/68	54

Table 6.4 Comparison of incidence of cholera and dysentery between subsets of residency period

	QUELIMANE CHOLERA		QUELIMANE DYSENTERY		BEIRA CHOLERA		BEIRA DYSENTERY		GORONGOSA CHOLERA		GORONGOSA DYSENTERY	
	Prop	%	Prop	%	Prop	%	Prop	%	Prop	%	Prop	%*
Less than 1 year resident	4/33	12	6/33	18	3/17	18	5/17	29	0/1	0	0/1	0
1-2 years resident	6/39	15	10/39	26	7/30	23	10/30	33	1/6	17	3/6	50
2-3 years resident	3/23	13	8/23	35	6/34	18	12/34	35	4/7	57	3/7	43
3-5 years resident	5/33	15	8/33	24	20/58	35	35/58	60	3/5	60	3/5	60
5-10 years resident	9/41	22	14/41	34	15/45	33	20/45	44	8/15	53	7/15	47
More than 10 years resident	19/118	16	34/118	29	59/191	31	84/191	44	16/34	47	21/34	62

Notes:

Prop.   Denotes proportion of each residency group reporting having had the disease.

Shaded value is significantly higher than other age groups in the column in excess of the 95% confidence level using chi-square analysis on pairs of proportions.

* Combining of less than 3 years groups at Gorongosa for dysentery produces a significantly lower percentage than the more than 10 years resident group.

result from the other periods of residency (p<0.05). The least variation between the different periods of residency is apparent in the data for cholera at Quelimane. This may be an indication that period of residency is least relevant in the case of the more endemic disease. However, the prime importance of the results at this stage in the analysis is in showing that, except for one period of dysentery at Beira, there has been generally no significant difference in incidence of cholera or dysentery for different periods of residency.

The distribution of the population by period of residence was mapped by sub-areas for Quelimane and Beira. Figures 6.4 and 6.5 shows that there is a distinct spatial pattern to the settlement of people in the last 10 years.[2] Figure 6.4 shows that in Quelimane there are three communal units where over 90 per cent of interviewees arrived within the last 10 years. These areas correspond to those with the highest incidence of cholera. Areas with fewer than 20 per cent correspond with the zones further away from the zones of high cholera incidence including the area of Communal Unit 39 (Madal) where the highest rate of incidence of dysentery occurred.

Analysis using correlation coefficients for all the sub-areas measured (Table 6.5) confirms that the distribution of more recent resettlement across sub-areas of Quelimane correlates significantly with the distribution of cholera incidence but not with that of dysentery. There is a weaker correlation with population density and a series of significant inter-correlations with the key environmental variables of conductivity and pH. By way of clarification of the inter-correlations, Principal Components Analysis (Table 6.6) serves to indicate that more recent resettlement, incidence of cholera, dysentery, population density or the physical environmental parameters.

A synopsis of this initial analysis is that, areas in Quelimane where high percentages of more recently settled people reside are much more affected by cholera, despite the fact that there was no significant difference in rates of self-reported incidence of the disease between more recently settled and established residents in the town as a whole. By way of contrast there is no apparent overall association or spatial correlation between settlement period and incidence of either disease in the case of Beira. In Quelimane, the results suggest that increased susceptibility to infection

---

[2] Sub-areas with only 7 or less respondents have been omitted to avoid possible misrepresentation associated with smaller samples. They are areas with near median values and as such do not alter the main pattern that has been displayed.

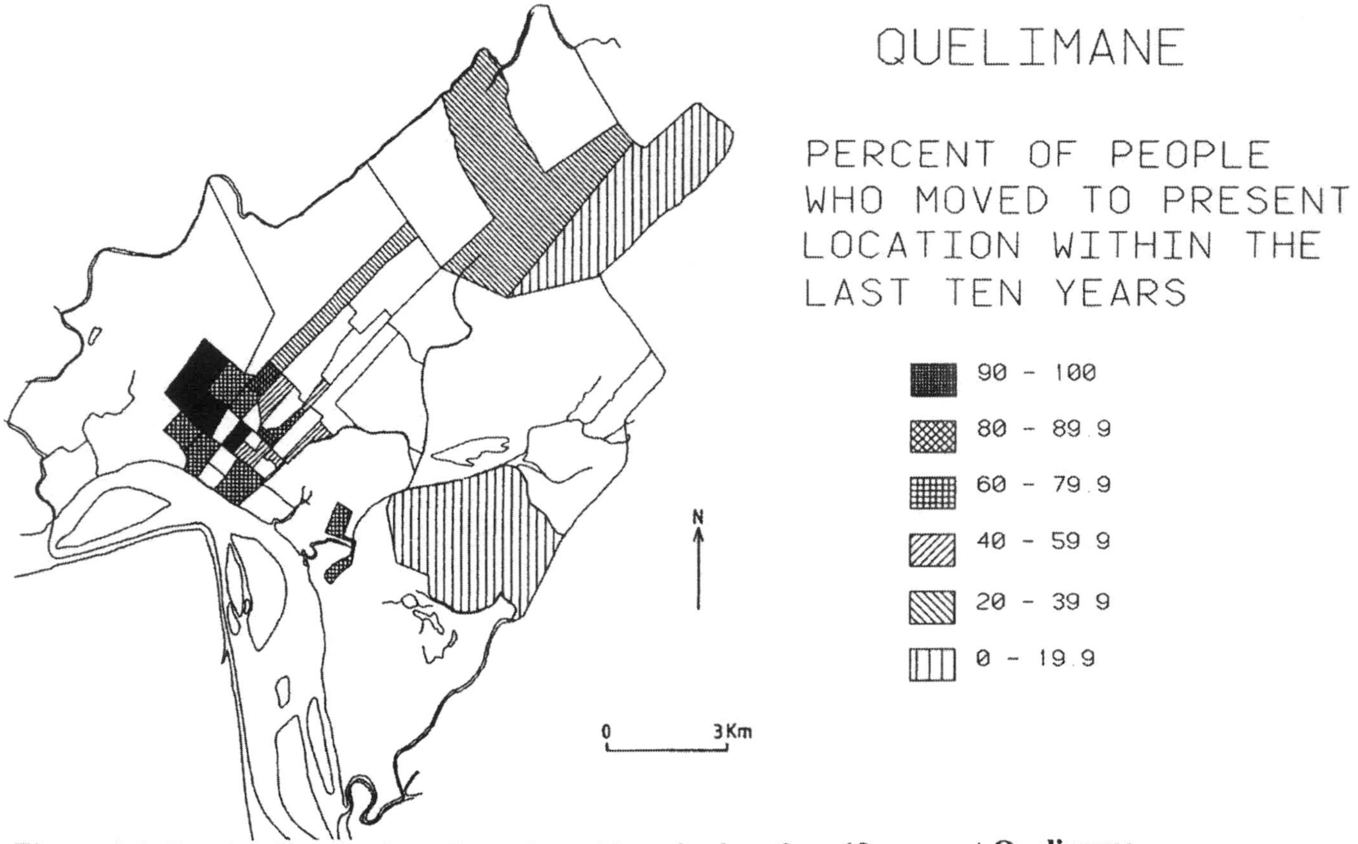

QUELIMANE

PERCENT OF PEOPLE
WHO MOVED TO PRESENT
LOCATION WITHIN THE
LAST TEN YEARS

90 - 100

80 - 89.9

60 - 79.9

40 - 59.9

20 - 39.9

0 - 19.9

N

0   3Km

Figure 6.4 Spatial distribution of people resident for less than 10 years at Quelimane

180

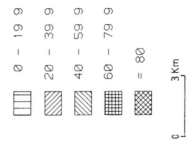

BEIRA

PERCENT OF PEOPLE
WHO MOVED TO PRESENT
LOCATION WITHIN THE
LAST TEN YEARS

0 – 19 9

20 – 39 9

40 – 59 9

60 – 79 9

= 80

0   3 Km

N

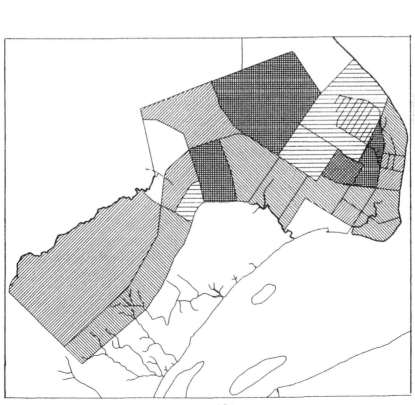

Figure 6.5 Spatial distribution of people resident for less than 10 years at Beira

Table 6.5 Correlation of more recently settled people, rates of incidence of cholera and dysentery, population density, and selected environmental parameters by sub-area at Quelimane and Beira

	Average pH		Average Conduct.		Population density		Dysentery rate		Cholera rate	
	Q	B	Q	B	Q	B	Q	B	Q	B
%of recently settled	**0.65** n=21	**0.15** n=20	**0.51** n=21	**0.20** n=20	**0.34** n=21	**0.05** n=20	**-0.22** n=21	**0.05** n=20	**0.65** n=21	**0.15** n=20
Cholera rate	0.57 n=28	0.83 n=20	0.51 n=28	0.65 n=20	0.51 n=39	0.44 n=22	0.27 n=39	0.68 n=22		
Dysentery rate	-0.15 n=28	0.53 n=20	-0.25 n=28	0.20 n=20	0.31 n=39	0.21 n=22				
Population Density	0.40 n=28	0.61 n=20	0.48 n=28	0.74 n=20						
Average Conductivity	0.72 n=28	0.77 n=21								

Notes:

Q = Quelimane B = Beira

Shaded figures are significant at the 99 per cent level of confidence using two tailed values.

n = Number of sub-areas used.

Table 6.6   **Principal Component Analysis of inter-correlations with more recent settlement at Quelimane**

Eigenvalue	3.277	1.044
Proportion	0.546	0.174
Cumulative	0.546	0.720

Variable	PC1	PC2
% of recently settled	-0.440	0.043
Cholera rate	-0.448	-0.090
Dysentery rate	0.167	-0.886
Population density	-0.335	-0.427
Conductivity	-0.472	0.122
pH	-0.492	-0.084

through recent mobility is not a factor, but that nonetheless, those people who have moved recently have concentrated in areas of high cholera incidence. In this context, the question arises whether displaced people have had to settle in the areas that are already more prone to cholera, or whether their presence has increased the likelihood of cholera occurring in those areas through environmental changes. The history of the area, as described in Chapter 4 suggests that both hypotheses could be supported. Though there is no official documentary record, use of the low lying north-eastern margin of the city by people displaced by the war was tolerated by the local authorities. Other parts of the city were already over-populated, or part of the semi-state owned coconut plantations. Having settled in large numbers in a marginal zone, prone to flooding, further impoverishment of the surface environment occurred, such as a loss of vegetation cover, exposure, alkalinization, and poor sanitation.

The opinion of an older assistant, several long term residents interviewed during the questionnaire survey, and personnel at the local planning office was that devegetation occurred due to a combination of increases in population brought about by incoming displaced people in the 1980s and by the inability of the population to obtain fuel and building material from traditional sources of natural resources in the rural areas. The fact that the area was previously part of the plantation zone suggests that the surface environment was previously similar to that of the plantation areas still in existence at the time of carrying out the survey. These were typically more acidic and less saline.

An increase in salinity in the area was the most likely explanation for several dead mango trees and explains the lack of less halophytic vegetation in this area. Trees are used to build houses (the felling of a remaining palm tree being witnessed while carrying out the survey). In other parts of Quelimane palms form an upper canopy of vegetation under which shrubs and low level ground vegetation abounds. However, though there is evidence for an environmental change having taken place, the causes have been much more contentious. In particular it should be pointed out here that it was unclear to what extent vegetation had been removed by displaced people living in that area or a more general mix of Quelimane occupants. Although the results of the questionnaire survey confirm a very high percentage of displaced people in this area, suggesting their presence was likely to have been a contributing factor, the area is low lying and prone to flood, thus representing an environmentally vulnerable area prior to their arrival.

In Beira, absence of overall higher incidence of cholera or dysentery amongst recently settled people (except for dysentery amongst those resident 3-5 years at Beira), or significant association with areas where there are high percentages of recently settled people, is also consistent with the earlier results. Since the serotype of *Vibrio cholerae* in Beira was less established in environmental reservoirs there were fewer opportunities for primary transmission associated with specific areas of ecological change. Sensitivity of individual diseases to the geochemical environment and increased susceptibility through relocation may become less apparent where there are strong influences from wider reaching structural circumstances affecting the built environment and community. This would help to explain why incidence of cholera and dysentery display a more congruent pattern in Beira than in Quelimane.

Displacement, Resettlement and Susceptibility

The above results, indicating that more recent resettlement is generally not prone to higher incidence of cholera and dysentery, are inconsistent with the existing accounts of disease amongst displaced people in Africa cited in this thesis (Dick 1984,1985; Shears and Lusty 1987; Toole and

Waldman 1993; Toole 1995; Prothero 1994). One possible explanation for this may be the greater diversity of resettlement and displacement associated with the urban areas studied, in comparison to the more specific cases of refugees referred to in the literature on disease and displacement. Despite the overall demographic impact of the war, affecting the majority of Mozambicans (Green 1992), there remain a range of different circumstances under which people have relocated in Mozambique in recent years. To investigate this matter further, the following analysis considers why and from where the more recently settled people moved. This has enabled a comparison of disease incidence and differences in susceptibility experienced by varied categories of migrants.

A Profile of Recent Resettlement in Quelimane, Beira and Gorongosa

Interviewees who were resident for less than 10 years in the same location were asked to indicate from where they had last moved and their main reason for relocating. Table 6.7 reveals that movement was from a wide range of different places both inside and outside of the urban areas. Though the figures cannot be used for a strict comparison, since the areas vary in size, the overall diversity of origins is evident in that there have been moves from most urban sub-areas and many districts. It can be noted here that districts of origin extended beyond the 12 that constitute Sofala Province and 16 that constitute Zambézia Province. The numerous origins suggested at the outset that the recently settled people were likely to have been associated with varied previous circumstances and should not be considered a homogeneous group. Further variations in origin are demonstrated in Table 6.8. These figures show that a significantly greater proportion of recently settled people came from outside the urban area in the case of Quelimane and Gorongosa, but more from inside in the case of Beira.

Classification of different groups of recently settled people was simplified to a cross-tabulation of movements from inside and outside the urban boundary against principal reasons for relocating (Table 6.9). Reasons for leaving a previous location were found to be very varied but could be broadly classified into the categories of voluntary migrations and forced migrations. Voluntary migrations included factors such as marriage, choosing to change job, educational reasons, wanting to be nearer to family or work place, or wanting to improve accommodation. The categorisation required some subjective analysis in assessing the extent to which critically

Table 6.7   Number of areas from which recently settled residents have relocated

| | PREVIOUS SUB-AREAS IDENTIFIED INSIDE URBAN AREA | | PREVIOUS DISTRICTS IDENTIFIED OUTSIDE URBAN AREA |
	Prop.	(%)	No.
QUELIMANE	26/39	(66.7)	26
BEIRA	21/22	(95.5)	21
GORONGOSA	4/7	(57.1)	12

Table 6.8   Number of respondents whose previous residence was inside and outside of the urban area within the last ten years

| | INSIDE URBAN AREA | | OUTSIDE URBAN AREA | |
	Prop.	%	No.	%
QUELIMANE	75/169	44.4	94/169	55.6
BEIRA	113/184	61.4	71/184	38.6
GORONGOSA	5/34	14.7	29/34	85.5
TOTAL	193/387	49.9	194/387	50.1

poor conditions in the previous accommodation may have forced the person to move. Involuntary migrations were sub-divided into those directly uprooted by the war and those resulting from other factors such as extreme overcrowding, a dispute or divorce, rising cost of living, economic destitution and being forced to look for work. In most instances there was little doubt if a person had moved directly due to the war although clearly, various factors were often inter-related.

The results outlined in Table 6.9 show that in all three sites a larger percentage of recent movements are accounted for by the two forcibly displaced categories. A smaller proportion of the forced migrants were directly due to uprooting by war except in the case of Gorongosa where this group constituted the majority. Uprooting by war in the context of this research are cases where people have escaped injury and death, had their home burnt, or where risk of being targeted by armed groups or caught in

Table 6.9 Simplified profile of people resident for less than 10 years, classified in broad terms of origin and cause of displacement

| | QUELIMANE | | BEIRA | | GORONGOSA | |
	From inside city	From outside city	From inside city	From outside city	From inside city	From outside city
	No (%)	No (%)	No (%)	No (%)	No (%)	No (%)
Directly displaced by war	2 (2.7)	17 (18.1)	4 (3.5)	24 (33.8)	2 (33.3)	21 (61.9)
Forced migrants	34 (45.3)	36 (38.3)	68 (60.2)	14 (19.7)	0 (0.0)	0 (0.0)
Voluntary migrants	38 (50.7)	38 (40.4)	33 (29.2)	27 (38.0)	3 (66.7)	8 (38.1)
Unable to determine cause	1 (1.3)	3 (3.2)	8 (7.1)	6 (8.5)	0 (0.0)	0 (0.0)

the crossfire became too great. Most of these have therefore been displaced from rural areas where this was predominant. Though the larger group of other forced migrants is represented by movements from both inside and outside the urban areas there were significantly more of these from within the urban area of Beira. This is partly due to the continued high growth rate and congestion in the urban core of the city, the immediate localised expansion of which is constrained by areas of low lying ground in flood for much of the year.

A further factor behind the necessity to relocate in the case of Beira has been the rapid economic changes that put pressure on people to move out of areas that became too expensive, and a tightening up on housing policy in the former colonial part of the city. Rents have been increasing more rapidly since the State Housing Administration changed its policy in 1991 (Mozambique Information Office 1991). Many of the occupants who moved into or around this accommodation with the departure of the Portuguese are also being encouraged to accept a lump sum to buy housing materials and move out, making way for the *nouveau riche* and rekindled foreign interests. Consequently, approximately 71 per cent of the internal resettlement in Beira has been from the urban core. In Quelimane this type of movement was still barely evident. Instead a large amount of internal relocation (53 per cent) was from environmentally poor areas on the north-western facing flank that has been identified as having significantly higher than average incidence of cholera. In Quelimane forced movements, not directly caused by the conflict, were also reported as being due to congestion (20 per cent of all movement) but additionally by people looking for work or wanting to improve their work conditions (32 per cent). This is not surprising as in the past the City of Quelimane was a centre for finding employment with the large companies that run the coconut and tea plantations. Although earlier on the agricultural sector in Zambézia was based on slavery associated with the *prazo*[3] system, which was a means of establishing Portuguese rule (Vail and White 1980, p8), the later period of colonialism implanted a more structured agricultural sector. The perception of opportunity through formal employment has to some extent survived. In Sofala province much less of a commercial agricultural base was achieved.

---

[3] *Prazo* means 'a period of time' and was used as a system of legitimising ownership of land by settlers and their mixed race descendants, a government priority throughout three hundred years.

Displacement directly related to the conflict represented a significant percentage of people in both Quelimane and Beira. Unsurprisingly they are not the largest group. The cities in Mozambique were never designated resettlement areas for war refugees despite the high number of displaced people that ended up there during the conflict. In Gorongosa, where the overall context has been one of war and population displacement throughout much of the conflict, the survey recorded 37 per cent of the total sample of residents in the town as being forcibly displaced by conflict in the last 10 years. Ninety-one per cent of the displaced arrived from outside of the municipal boundary. However, according to government officials the approximate population of the town at the time of this survey was 59,000, whilst in 1980 the population was calculated by local officials to be only 14,000. Assuming a natural growth rate of 2.6 per cent the population would be only 19,550 by 1993. A large percentage of the extra 39,000 may therefore be considered as being accounted for by displaced people. This is possibly as much as 65 per cent of the population. The low figure of 37 per cent found in this survey is partly because only those moving in the last ten years were included. Though no early official figures exist, and allowing for exaggerations in the present population total provided by a conservative estimation of the natural growth rate, it can be calculated that tens of thousands of people were also displaced to Gorongosa town during the first half of the 1980s.

Incidence of Cholera and Dysentery by Category of Displacement

Data presented in Table 6.10 indicate that the dysentery rate is significantly higher amongst those displaced by war than the other groups at Beira ($p<0.05$-$p<0.005$). There is also a significantly higher cholera rate amongst forced migrants than voluntary migrants at Beira if a lower level of significance is used ($p<0.10$). However, in general, across the three sites, there is no evidence that those forcibly displaced by war have been more affected by cholera or dysentery, although it does appear that those who have moved voluntarily in the last 10 years are generally less affected. This perhaps reflects their higher socio-economic status, which has allowed them to choose residence. The lack of a clear association between displacement and disease at this level also reinforces the suggestion that any spatial correlation between displaced groups and higher disease incidence reflects more pre-existing environmental conditions, or

Table 6.10 Incidence of cholera and dysentery for different types of recently settled people

	QUELIMANE				BEIRA				GORONGOSA			
	CHOLERA		DYSENTERY		CHOLERA		DYSENTERY		CHOLERA		DYSENTERY	
	Prop	%	Prop	%	Prop	%	Prop	%	Prop	%	Prop	%
Directly displaced by war	2/19	(11)	7/19	(37)	10/28	(36)	19/28	(68)	12/23	(52)	12/23	(52)
Forced migrants	10/70	(14)	19/70	(27)	26/82	(32)	38/82	(46)	0/0	(0)	0/0	(0)
Voluntary migrants	15/76	(20)	18/76	(24)	12/60	(20)	20/60	(33)	4/11	(36)	4/11	(36)
More than 10 years resident	19/118	(16)	34/118	(29)	59/191	(31)	84/191	(44)	16/34	(47)	21/34	(62)

Notes:

Prop.   Denotes proportion of each residency group reporting having had the disease.

Shaded value is significantly higher than more than 10 years resident group in excess of the 95% confidence level, and significantly higher than voluntary migrants in excess of the 99% confidence level, using chi-square analysis on pairs of proportions.

environmental change after relocation, than any innate susceptibility of migrant or forcibly displaced groups.

Primary Subsistence of Long-term Residents and Different Categories of Migrant Before and After Resettlement

If migration or displacement on their own do not appear to affect susceptibility to disease, there nonetheless remain other socio-economic factors that do have an effect, and amongst factors, level of primary subsistence are perhaps the more obvious. For example, people who can not afford to re-heat stored cooked food are at risk of infection through its contamination, whilst they are also more susceptible to infection through reduced physical well-being associated with their poverty. Some aspects of primary subsistence that are important in influencing exposure to pathogens and/or reflect levels of socio-economic well-being are the type of water supply used, latrine ownership, type and source of fuel, and cultivation. In addition, people's main activity or form of employment can contribute as a further measure of socio-economic status.

Analysis of large quantities of data collected through the questionnaire survey and collated in summary tables isolated elements of the above variables that were significantly different between the categories of migrant and those resident for more than 10 years. The differences referred to below are those which are significant using chi-square analysis on pairs of proportions and a level of confidence of at least 95 per cent in each instance. This was the first stage in isolating and contrasting potential changes in susceptibility to the diseases experienced by different migrant groups. In addition, an analysis was conducted to see whether current levels of primary subsistence were better or worse than before moving using the same measures of water, sanitation, fuel, and land plot ownership.

Water supply Differences in water supply are important since they can indicate variations in exposure to faecal contamination, which facilitates transmission of disease pathogens (Bartram 1990).[4] Access to certain

---

[4] Although as pointed out in Chapter 2, faecal coliforms do not necessarily serve as an indication of variation in contamination by diarrhoeal disease pathogens, the measure serves as a good indication of general levels of hygiene and socio-economic well-being associated with a water source.

water sources, such as via a private tapped supply is also a reflection of the better socio-economic well-being of its users. Results from the water analysis carried out during this research indicated variation in quality between different supplies (Table 6.11). Definitive guides about what should be the maximum acceptable level of contamination is open to debate. However, in general the high standards of hygiene control of some northern countries are unrealistic targets for Third World countries for the foreseeable future. For example, if using World Health Organization guidelines of 0 faecal coliforms and 0 tubidity in 100 ml of water (WHO 1985, p2) all but 5 out of 111 (4.5%) samples at Quelimane, 24 out of 181 (13.3%) samples at Beira and 7 out of 28 (25%) samples at Gorongosa would be deemed unfit for consumption. The slightly higher percentage at Beira is accounted for by water taken from taps connected to the 'treated' supply, which when functioning occasionally produced uncontaminated samples. The highest percentage of good quality water samples taken at Gorongosa is attributable to successfully installed bore holes and well-preserved springs. Though table 6.11 indicates that there was a widespread problem of poor water quality, it might be argued from the above account that people with greater access to supplies such as bore holes or the 'treated tap water' have a reduced likelihood of contracting a diarrhoeal disease.

Tables 6.12-6.14 shows the usage of each water supply for different categories of resident. Significantly higher percentages of the forced migrants were found to be using the concrete wells and significantly less forced and voluntary migrants the traditional wells at Quelimane (Table 6.12). In addition significantly more voluntary migrants were using the 'treated' tap water. However, the water analysis results (Table 6.11) indicates that the different level of usage of the concrete and traditional wells by different groups at Quelimane is unlikely to have made much difference in terms of levels of exposure to faecally contaminated water, since both well types were of equally poor quality. Though voluntary migrants may have been better off because of greater use of the treated tap supply, there is no evidence that the forced migrants or directly displaced by war group were worse off than the established residents as a result of water supply. No significant differences in use of water supply between categories of residents at Beira (Table 6.13) or Gorongosa (Table 6.14) could be established.

Table 6.15 suggests that households who have relocated at Quelimane have not undergone significant changes in water supply. This is because

Table 6.11 Water quality indicators for different water supplies

	QUELIMANE			BEIRA			GORONGOSA		
	FC	Cond	pH	FC	Cond	pH	FC	Cond	pH
'Treated' tap supply	140	288	7.5	5	154	6.9	-	-	-
Open concrete wells	851	1671	7.4	658	1097	6.4	1277	234	6.4
Closed concrete wells	374	1339	7.3	-	-	-	-	-	-
Oil drum and tyre wells	245	1342	7.2	973	1280	6.0	-	-	-
Boreholes	7	1116	7.0	-	-	-	23	274	6.1
Traditional earth wells	500	1170	6.5	360	255	5.5	-	-	-
Cisterns	624	199	7.7	478	203	7.3	-	-	-
Natural springs	-	-	-	-	-	-	158	293	6.4
Rivers	-	-	-	-	-	-	347	183	7.4

Notes:

FC = Average number of faecal coliforms per100ml water.

Cond = Average conductivity in micro-seimens.

pH = Average pH.

Figures are based on the first survey of 111 water samples at Quelimane, 181 water samples at Beira, and 28 water samples at Gorongosa.

193

Table 6.12 Use of water supply by category of resident at Quelimane

	More than 10 years resident		Voluntary migrants		All forced migrants*		Directly displaced by war		All	
	n	%	n	%	n	%	n	%	n	%
'Treated' tap water	9	16.7	19	40.4	7	15.6	2	20.0	35	24.0
Bore hole	1	1.9	0	0.0	2	4.4	0	0.0	3	2.1
Concrete wells	25	46.3	23	48.9	30	66.7	8	80.0	78	53.4
Traditional wells	18	33.3	4	8.5	3	6.7	0	0.0	25	17.1
Cisterns	1	1.9	1	2.1	3	6.7	0	0.0	5	3.4
Total	54	100	47	100	45	100	10	100	146	100

Notes:

n = number of responses from first phase of questionnaire survey.

* Includes directly displaced by war category.

Shaded values are significantly different from the more than 10 years residents in excess of the 95% confidence level using chi-square analysis on pairs of proportions.

Shaded and underlined values are significantly different in excess of the 99% confidence level.

Table 6.13 Use of water supply by category of resident at Beira

	More than 10 years resident		Voluntary migrants		All forced migrants*		Directly displaced by war		All	
	n	%	n	%	n	%	n	%	n	%
'Treated' tap water	24	21.8	6	17.1	15	21.1	1	5.9	45	20.8
Concrete and tin wells	63	57.3	23	65.7	49	69.0	13	76.5	135	62.5
Traditional wells	18	16.4	6	17.1	5	7.0	3	17.7	29	13.4
Cisterns	5	4.6	0	-	2	2.8	0	-	7	3.3
Total	110	100	35	100	71	100	17	100	216	100

Notes:

n = number of responses from first phase of questionnaire survey.

* Includes directly displaced by war category.

195

Table 6.14   Use of water supply by category of resident at Gorongosa

	More than 10 years resident		Voluntary migrants		Directly displaced by war		All	
	n	%	n	%	n	%	n	%
Bore hole	12	38.7	4	33.3	10	40.0	26	38.3
Concrete wells	1	3.2	0	-	2	8.0	3	4.4
Natural springs	15	48.4	6	50.0	9	36.0	30	44.1
Rivers	3	9.7	2	16.7	4	16.0	9	13.2
Total	31	100	12	100	25	100	68	100

Notes:
n = number of responses from first phase of questionnaire survey.

the transition has been predominantly from traditional wells to concrete wells between which there was little difference in levels of contamination (a few people also previously used rivers and natural springs). However, it is recognised that this result is not definitive since it is based on the contamination levels of different types of water supply sampled at the urban areas rather than supplies that were used before relocating from rural areas. It was beyond the remit of this research to test the water quality of numerous origins of displaced people outside the urban areas.

In contrast to the results at Quelimane, those forcibly displaced in Beira (Table 6.16) experienced a 43 per cent decrease in the use of tapped water, shown in Table 6.11 to be of much better quality than the other supplies at that site. The large shift from using tap water amongst the forced migrants group in Beira reflects the movement of people away from the colonial residential areas due to rising rents associated with structural adjustment. The transition of the forced migrants at Beira was to a greater use of the city's tin and concrete wells, a notoriously bad source of water, recording an average of 973 faecal coliforms per 100 ml during the first phase of the fieldwork with individual cases of up to 2,000 faecal coliforms per 100 ml of water. These wells also recorded higher levels of conductivity than the other sources. Though the results show that all groups of residents are exposed to inappropriate water supply, the forced migrants at Beira have arguably experienced worse conditions than they did prior to relocating.

Table 6.15 Type of water supply used by Quelimane households before and after relocation

WATER SUPPLY	Voluntary migrants		All forced migrants*		Directly displaced by war		Total less than 10 years resident	
	BEFORE n (%)	AFTER n (%)	BEFORE n (%)	AFTER n (%)	BEFORE n (%)	AFTER n (%)	BEFORE n (%)	AFTER n (%)
'Treated' tap water	19 (40.4)	19 (40.4)	10 (22.2)	7 (15.6)	3 (30.0)	2 (20.0)	29 (31.5)	26 (28.3)
Bore hole	1 (25.0)	0 (-)	0 (-)	2 (4.4)	0 (-)	0 (-)	1 (1.1)	2 (2.2)
Concrete wells	7 (14.9)	23 (48.9)	11 (24.4)	30 (66.7)	1 (10.0)	8 (80.0)	18 (19.6)	53 (57.6)
Traditional wells	20 (42.6)	4 (8.5)	20 (44.4)	3 (6.7)	5 (50.0)	0 (-)	40 (43.5)	7 (7.5)
Cisterns	0 (-)	1 (2.1)	0 (-)	3 (6.7)	0 (-)	0 (-)	0 (-)	4 (4.4)
Rivers	0 (-)	0 (-)	3 (6.7)	0 (-)	1 (10.0)	0 (-)	3 (3.2)	0 (-)
Natural springs	0 (-)	0 (-)	1 (2.2)	0 (-)	0 (-)	0 (-)	1 (1.1)	0 (-)
Total %	47 (100)	47 (100)	45 (100)	45 (100)	10 (100)	10 (100)	92 (100)	92 (100)
Average minutes to water supply	13	9	12	12	6	7	12	10
Average number of times collected	2.2	2.0	2.3	1.8	2.6	1.7	2.2	1.9

Notes:

n = number of responses from first phase of questionnaire survey

* Includes directly displaced by war category.

Shaded values are significantly different after relocation in excess of the 95% confidence level using chi-square analysis on pairs of proportions.

Shaded and underlined values are significantly different in excess of the 99% confidence level.

Table 6.16 Type of water supply used by Beira households before and after relocation

WATER SOURCE	Voluntary migrants BEFORE n (%)	Voluntary migrants AFTER n (%)	All forced migrants* BEFORE n (%)	All forced migrants* AFTER n (%)	Directly displaced by war BEFORE n (%)	Directly displaced by war AFTER n (%)	Total less than 10 years resident BEFORE n (%)	Total less than 10 years resident AFTER n (%)
'Treated' tap water	14 (40.0)	6 (17.1)	45 (64.3)	15 (21.1)	2 (12.5)	1 (5.9)	59 (56.2)	21 (19.8)
Concrete/tin wells	17 (48.6)	23 (65.7)	15 (21.4)	49 (69.0)	7 (43.8)	13 (76.5)	32 (30.5)	72 (67.9)
Traditional wells	4 (11.4)	6 (17.1)	8 (11.4)	5 (7.0)	5 (31.3)	3 (17.7)	12 (11.4)	11 (10.4)
Cisterns	0 (-)	0 (-)	0 (-)	2 (2.8)	0 (-)	0 (-)	0 (-)	2 (1.9)
Rivers	0 (-)	0 (-)	2 (2.9)	0 (-)	2 (12.5)	0 (-)	2 (1.9)	0 (-)
Total %	35 (100)	35 (100)	70 (100)	71 (100)	16 (100)	17 (100)	105 (100)	106 (100)
Average minutes to water Supply	2.4	2.5	1.2	2.0	2.6	4.4	1.5	2.1
Average number of times Collected	3.1	3.1	3.5	3.6	3.2	3.6	3.4	3.4

Notes:

n = number of responses from first phase of questionnaire survey

* Includes directly displaced by war category.

Shaded values are significantly different after relocation in excess of the 95% confidence level using chi-square analysis on pairs of proportions.

Shaded and underlined values are significantly different in excess of the 99% confidence level.

Table 6.17 Type of water supply used by Gorongosa households before and after relocation

WATER SOURCE	Voluntary migrants		Directly displaced by war		Total less than 10 years resident	
	BEFORE n (%)	AFTER n (%)	BEFORE n (%)	AFTER n (%)	BEFORE n (%)	AFTER n (%)
'Treated' tap water	2 (16.7)	0 (-)	0 (-)	0 (-)	2 (5.4)	0 (-)
Bore hole	1 (8.3)	4 (33.3)	2 (8.0)	10 (40.0)	3 (8.1)	14 (37.8)
Concrete wells	1 (8.3)	0 (-)	0 (-)	2 (8.0)	1 (2.7)	2 (5.4)
Traditional wells	5 (41.7)	0 (-)	9 (36.0)	0 (-)	14 (37.8)	0 (-)
Natural springs	1 (8.3)	6 (50.0)	0 (-)	9 (36.0)	1 (2.7)	15 (40.5)
Rivers	2 (16.7)	2 (16.7)	14 (56.0)	4 (16.0)	16 (43.2)	6 (16.2)
Total %	12 (100)	12 (100)	25 (100)	25 (100)	37 (100)	37 (100)
Average minutes to water supply	8.4	7.7	4.3	4.9	5.7	5.8
Average number of times collected	2.9	2.2	3.0	2.4	3.0	2.3

Notes:

n = number of responses from first phase of questionnaire survey

Shaded values are significantly different after relocation in excess of the 95% confidence level using chi-square analysis on pairs of proportions.

Shaded and underlined values are significantly different in excess of the 99% confidence level.

By further way of contrast the displaced at Gorongosa experienced an improvement in water supply after resettlement since they made a transition from using rivers and traditional wells to using spring water and bore holes (Table 6.17). Their use of these sources was almost equal to that of the long term residents indicating there was no discrimination as a result of being a forced migrant. Whilst rivers in the Gorongosa area were found to harbour up to 958 faecal coliforms per 100 ml, contamination of bore holes was often as low as 0 faecal coliforms per 100 ml. This also applied to some of the better protected spring water supplies. Although there have been shortages of water during the drought of 1992, there was no evidence that any one group suffered disproportionately poor access to water supply during that time. The average distance travelled to collect water was similar between different groups before and after relocation at each site with the maximum average travelling time for any one group not exceeding 12 minutes.

Latrine ownership Ownership of a latrine is important since those without a latrine are more likely to be exposed to health hazards associated with open air defecation (Feachem and Bradley *et al.* 1980, Pacey 1980). The overall level of faecal contamination of the environment in urban areas caused by open air defecation impacts on incidence of diarrhoeal disease because secondary transmission of pathogens is increased (Cairncross and Feachem 1983). This is also affected by socio-economic status since most of the poorer households cannot afford the necessary materials to build a latrine.[5] It is estimated that the number of people in urban areas of developing countries without access to adequate sanitation increased during the 1980s (World Bank 1992). Use of latrines in urban areas is deemed one of the most effective ways of reducing incidence of diarrhoea (Daniels and Cousens *et al.* 1990). For example, with reference to five rigorous studies on improved sanitation, Esrey and Feachem *et al.* (1985) calculate that a median 36 per cent reduction in incidence of diarrhoeal disease morbidity can be achieved. They estimate this to be more than can be expected from improvements in either water quantity or quality although it should be mentioned that there still remains some debate about

---

[5] Construction of a latrine in most urban areas of coastal Mozambique requires purchase of building blocks and a moulded concrete slab. Simpler designs in Quelimane and Beira are not possible because of the low lying and water-logged terrain.

the validity of generalising these guidelines.[6]

Analysis of the results in Table 6.18 indicates that at Quelimane, voluntary migrants and those directly displaced by war more frequently owned a latrine than established residents and forced migrants. In contrast, at Beira all categories of migrants were significantly less likely to own a latrine than established residents. At Gorongosa forced migrants were significantly less likely to own a latrine. In other words, there is an increased likelihood of poor sanitation amongst migrants at Beira, and amongst forced migrants in particular at both Gorongosa and Beira. However, there is no evidence of there being any greater sanitation hazard amongst forced migrants at Quelimane where overall latrine ownership is higher.

Table 6.19 shows that in Quelimane there was no significant difference in latrine ownership before and after relocation. Meanwhile in Beira there was a significant 21.1 per cent decrease in latrine ownership after relocation for the forced migrants. These results indicate that in Beira the displaced groups suffered the loss of an asset and failed to gain circumstances similar to the long term residents. Further to this, where forced migrants from sparsely populated rural areas previously did not use a latrine, the disease hazards are likely to have been far less than those resulting from open air defecation in congested and flood prone areas of Beira. The contrast in the level of ownership of latrines amongst forced migrants and established residents in Beira, a feature that does not occur in Quelimane, suggests greater exposure to disease hazards and marginalization of this group at Beira. For example, building latrines in confined areas with limited resources requires co-operation of the other people who live nearby. Although in Gorongosa a significantly lower percentage (12 per cent) of those directly displaced by war own a latrine compared to established residents (58 per cent), this did not represent a significant deterioration in latrine ownership for displaced people since ownership of a latrine was low among that group before relocation. Also, the area is much more desiccated than the other sites so that exposed

---

[6] The main shortcomings appears to have been in over applying the findings of individual studies to the varied contexts of disease situations in the Third World. For example, Ahmed *et al.* (1994) in a study on family latrines and paediatric shigellosis in Bangladesh, concluded differently that greater progress could be made by intervention through eliminating unsanitary latrines. Also the improvements that can be made through changes in hygiene behaviour are well established (Khan 1982, Kunstadter 1991, Baltazar *et al.* 1993, Traoré *et al.* 1994).

Table 6.18   Latrine ownership by category of resident at Quelimane, Beira and Gorongosa

	More than 10 years resident		Voluntary migrants		All forced migrants*		Directly displaced by war		All	
	Prop	%	Prop	%	Prop	%	Prop	%	Prop	%
QUELIMANE	36/54	66.7	40/47	85.1	31/45	68.9	9/10	90.0	107/146	73.3
BEIRA	76/110	69.1	15/35	42.9	35/71	49.3	3/17	17.7	126/216	58.3
GORONGOSA	18/31	58.1	9/12	75.0	3/25	12.0	3/25	12.0	30/68	44.0
All	130/195	66.7	64/94	68.1	69/141	48.9	15/52	28.9	263/430	61.2

Notes:

Prop = proportion of responses indicating ownership and use of a latrine using first questionnaire survey.

* Includes directly displaced by war category.

Shaded percentages are significantly different from the more than 10 years residents in excess of the 95% confidence level using chi-square analysis on pairs of proportions. Shaded and underlined percentages are significantly different from the more than 10 years residents in excess of the 99% confidence level.

Table 6.19 Latrine ownership before and after relocation

		More than 10 years resident		Voluntary migrants		All forced migrants*		Directly displaced by war		Total less than 10 years resident	
		Prop	%	Prop	%	Prop	%	Prop	%	Prop	%
QUELIMANE	Before	36/54	66.7	39/47	83.0	31/45	68.9	8/10	80.0	70/92	76.1
	After			40/47	85.1	31/45	68.9	9/10	90.0	71/92	77.2
BEIRA	Before	76/110	69.1	19/35	54.3	50/71	70.4	4/16	25.0	69/106	65.1
	After			15/35	42.9	35/71	49.3	3/17	17.7	50/106	47.2
GORONGOSA	Before	18/31	58.1	8/12	66.7	7/25	28.0	7/25	28.0	15/37	40.5
	After			9/12	75.0	3/25	12.0	3/25	12.0	12/37	32.4

Notes:

Prop = proportion of responses indicating ownership and use of a latrine using first questionnaire survey.

* Includes directly displaced by war category.

Shaded and underlined before and after relocation percentages are significantly different from each other in excess of the 95% confidence level using chi-square analysis on pairs of proportions.

faeces become less harmful. By way of contrast, in Quelimane it did prove possible for the forced migrants to build latrines to the same extent as the established residents. A likely explanation for this lies in a greater degree of overall inter-communal co-operation at that city, a theme that is explored further in Chapter 7.

Fuel Adequacy of fuel supply is important in the context of disease prevention in that it influences ability to boil contaminated water and to cook food adequately. Surprisingly little research has focused on the association between specific disease infection and adequacy of fuel for cooking during epidemics, despite awareness of a crisis in availability (Leach and Mearns 1988; Munslow 1988) and recent recommendations that its provision be part of emergency aid packages (LaMont-Gregory 1995). Again, availability of fuel reflects socio-economic status in urban areas, since there is currently a heavy dependency on individual purchasing power to obtain it. The alternative is a lengthy trek to a rural area to harvest fuel independently, which uses up valuable time and energy needed for other survival activities.

Tables 6.20 and 6.21 show that between different groups of residents in both Quelimane and Beira there is no significant difference in the type of fuel used, whether it is obtained from the local market or personally harvested. However, relocation has been associated with a significant increase in the use of wood and charcoal by the forced migrants at Beira (Table 6.22). There has also been an increase in the use of the local markets (signifying a decrease in personally harvesting fuel) amongst forced migrants at both sites (Table 6.23). The increase in use of wood and charcoal by the forced migrants at Beira has been partly a result of a significant decrease in use of electricity, gas, diesel and paraffin ($p < 0.05$). As with the change from tapped water to well water, this result applies mainly to those who relocated from the city core due to structural adjustments.

The most significant aspects of these results are that they are a further example of how relocation has altered the circumstances of the displaced groups, making them more like those experienced by the other residents at the place of resettlement. However, whilst not worse off than the longer term residents at the same location, it could be argued that the displaced are worse off in comparison to their previous circumstances because fewer previously had the financial burden of purchasing fuel. A contrary argument is that less time spent collecting fuelwood allows more time to

Table 6.20 Dependency on wood and charcoal as principle fuel supply for different categories of resident at Quelimane, Beira and Gorongosa

	More than 10 years resident		Voluntary migrants		All forced migrants*		Directly displaced by war		All	
	Prop	%	Prop	%	Prop	%	Prop	%	Prop	%
QUELIMANE	33/54	61.1	29/47	61.7	23/45	51.1	7/10	70.0	85/146	58.2
BEIRA	92/108	85.2	31/35	88.6	66/71	93.0	17/17	100	189/214	88.3
GORONGOSA	31/31	100	12/12	100	25/25	100	25/25	100	68/68	100
All	156/193	80.8	72/94	76.6	114/141	80.9	49/52	94.2	342/428	79.9

Notes:

Prop = proportion of households indicating wood and/or charcoal as principle fuel supply using first questionnaire survey.

* Includes directly displaced by war category.

Table 6.21 Use of local market to obtain fuel for different categories of resident at Quelimane, Beira and Gorongosa

	More than 10 years resident		Voluntary migrants		All forced migrants*		Directly displaced by war		All	
	Prop	%	Prop	%	Prop	%	Prop	%	Prop	%
QUELIMANE	41/53	77.4	38/47	80.9	38/45	84.4	6/10	60.0	117/145	80.7
BEIRA	93/108	86.1	28/34	82.4	66/71	93.0	16/17	94.1	187/213	87.8
GORONGOSA	8/31	25.8	4/12	33.3	1/25	4.0	1/25	4.0	13/68	19.1
All	142/192	74.0	70/93	75.3	105/141	74.5	23/52	44.2	317/426	74.4

Notes:

Prop = proportion of households indicating use of a local market as principle means to obtaining fuel supply using first questionnaire survey.

* Includes directly displaced by war category.

Shaded percentages are significantly different from more than 10 years residents in excess of the 95% confidence level using chi-square analysis on pairs of proportions.

Table 6.22 Dependency on wood and charcoal for fuel before and after relocation

		More than 10 years resident		Voluntary migrants		All forced migrants*		Directly displaced by war		Total less than 10 years resident	
		Prop	%	Prop	%	Prop	%	Prop	%	Prop	%
QUELIMANE	Before	33/54	61.1	31/47	67.4	23/45	51.1	7/10	70.0	54/92	58.7
	After			29/47	61.7	23/45	51.1	7/10	70.0	52/92	56.5
BEIRA	Before	92/108	85.2	30/35	85.7	53/70	75.7	15/16	93.8	83/105	79.1
	After			31/35	88.6	66/71	93.0	17/17	100	97/106	91.5
GORONGOSA	Before	31/31	100	12/12	100	25/25	100	25/25	100	37/37	100
	After			12/12	100	25/25	100	25/25	100	37/37	100

Notes:

Prop = proportion of households indicating wood and/or charcoal as principle fuel supply using first questionnaire survey.

* Includes directly displaced by war category.

Shaded before and after relocation percentages are significantly different from each other in excess of the 95% confidence level using chi-square analysis on pairs of proportions. Shaded and underlined percentages are significantly different in excess of the 99% level of confidence.

Table 6.23 Use of local market to obtain fuel before and after relocation

		More than 10 years resident		Voluntary migrants		All forced migrants*		Directly displaced by war		Total less than 10 years resident	
		Prop	%	Prop	%	Prop	%	Prop	%	Prop	%
QUELIMANE	Before	41/53	77.4	31/46	67.4	25/44	56.8	2/10	20.0	56/90	62.2
	After			38/47	80.9	38/45	84.4	6/10	60.0	76/92	82.6
BEIRA	Before	93/108	86.1	27/35	77.2	55/70	78.6	3/16	18.8	82/105	78.1
	After			28/34	82.4	66/71	93.0	16/17	94.1	94/105	89.5
GORONGOSA	Before	8/31	25.8	5/12	41.7	2/25	8.0	2/25	8.0	7/37	18.9
	After			4/12	33.3	1/25	4.0	1/25	4.0	5/37	13.5

Notes:

Prop = proportion of responses indicating a local market as principle source of fuel before and after relocation using first questionnaire survey.

* Includes directly displaced by war category.

Shaded before and after relocation percentages are significantly different from each other in excess of the 95% confidence level using chi-square analysis on pairs of proportions. Shaded and underlined percentages are significantly different in excess of the 99% level of confidence.

be spent profitably on other activities. However, given the level of impoverishment of many of the respondents, it is more likely that greater dependence on purchasing fuel from a local market equates with more regular periods of being unable to afford to cook, representing an increase in the risk of contamination and infection through consumption of food and water. In Gorongosa everybody uses wood for fuel but a significantly higher amount of war displaced harvest their fuel than the other groups who make some use of the local market. The average distance people have to travel to get their fuel in Gorongosa is about the same for all groups (3.5-4.4 km). However this again represents a worsening of conditions for the war displaced since it was also found that they were travelling an average 3 km further than before relocation.

Cultivation and Main Economic Activity

Maintenance of a cultivation plot is a key survival activity in Mozambique. There has often not been the option of purchasing food in a market, either because it did not exist (as during the mid-late 1980s), or because it is too expensive for most people (as during the early 1990s). Informal trading of foodstuffs has occurred throughout, but this also depends on having one's own supply to trade. Hence, in the urban areas as in the rural areas, the *machamba* (cultivation plot) has been integral to sustaining most households' nutritional status, which is a prime defence against diarrhoeal disease (Heikens and Schofield *et al.* 1993). The importance of a land plot also applies to those in formal employment, since all but the highest wages are inadequate for feeding a household.[7] It can be argued therefore that where employment is achieved along with owning a land plot, it indicates a better level of socio-economic well-being. Also, despite Mozambique's commendable attempts to provide education for all, households with members in education are likely to have greater relative socio-economic well-being since this demonstrates that the household is not dependent on participation of these individuals in full time survival strategies.

Data presented in Table 6.24 show that a higher percentage of established residents cultivate land plots at Quelimane and Beira, whilst data in Table 6.25 show that migrants are cultivating less after relocation.

---

[7] At the time of carrying out fieldwork for this research a monthly salary for a state employee of 75,000Mt (£10.00) would supply adequate food for a household of 6 for only half a month.

Table 6.24 Ownership of a cultivation plot for different categories of resident at Quelimane, Beira and Gorongosa

	More than 10 years resident		Voluntary migrants		All forced migrants*		Directly displaced by war		All	
	Prop	%	Prop	%	Prop	%	Prop	%	Prop	%
QUELIMANE	90/109	82.6	36/76	47.4	45/89	50.6	14/19	73.7	171/274	62.4
BEIRA	140/187	74.9	32/60	53.3	50/113	44.3	15/28	53.6	222/360	61.7
GORONGOSA	31/31	100	12/12	100	24/25	96.0	24/25	96.0	67/68	98.5
All	261/327	79.8	80/148	54.1	119/227	52.4	53/72	73.6	460/702	65.5

Notes:

Prop = proportion of households indicating ownership of a cultivation plot using both questionnaire surveys.

* Includes directly displaced by war category.

Shaded percentages are significantly different from more than 10 years residents in excess of the 95% confidence level using chi-square analysis on pairs of proportions. Shaded and underlined percentages are significantly different from more than 10 years residents in excess of the 99% level of confidence.

Table 6.25 Ownership of a cultivation plot before and after relocation

		More than 10 years resident		Voluntary migrants		All forced migrants*		Directly displaced by war		Total less than 10 years resident	
		Prop	%	Prop	%	Prop	%	Prop	%	Prop	%
QUELIMANE	Before	90/109	82.6	50/76	65.8	68/87	78.2	16/18	88.9	118/163	72.4
	After			36/76	47.4	45/89	50.6	14/19	73.7	81/165	49.1
BEIRA	Before	140/187	74.9	42/60	70.0	55/111	49.6	25/27	92.6	97/171	56.7
	After			32/60	53.3	50/113	44.3	15/28	53.6	82/173	47.4
GORONGOSA	Before	31/31	100	9/12	75.0	22/25	88.0	22/25	88.0	31/37	83.8
	After			12/12	100	24/25	96.0	24/25	96.0	36/37	97.3

Notes:

Prop = proportion of households indicating ownership of a cultivation plot before and after relocation using both questionnaire surveys.

* Includes directly displaced by war category.

Shaded before and after relocation percentages are significantly different from each other in excess of the 95% confidence level using chi-square analysis on pairs of proportions. Shaded and underlined percentages are significantly different in excess of the 99% confidence level.

211

In the case of Quelimane this is the only example that suggested a worsening of primary subsistence conditions for recent migrants, although this was not found to be significant for those directly displaced by war. The greatest decrease in plot ownership was for those directly displaced by war at Beira. Overall, it can be concluded that at both Quelimane and Beira resettlement has caused the loss of a nutritional asset. Also, at both sites resettlement caused a corresponding reduction in the already small amount of people who sell their produce (Table 6.26). For those households there has therefore been an additional worsening of subsistence in terms of loss of income.

The argument that differences in ownership of a cultivation plot has increased susceptibility to disease also needs to take into account the possibility of individuals having additional means of support, such as income from formal or informal employment. Results displayed in Table 6.27 show that fewer respondents of voluntary and forced migrant households with a *machamba* were engaged in additional employment than the established residents, thus providing further support for the argument that the groups of more recent migrants are worse off in terms of economic subsistence. The results in Table 6.27 distinguish between males and females and compare the proportions of each separately to control for the fact that supplementary income generating activities are much lower for women.

Further definitive contrasts in main activity that could be identified between the forced migrants and established residents were that;

- More established residents had formal and informal sector employment (27.1%) than those directly displaced by war (7.1%) at Beira ($p<0.05$).
- More established residents were in education (17%) than those directly displaced by war (3.6%) at Beira ($p<0.05$).
- More of the forced migrants were in the military or unemployed (15.6%) than established residents (0.9%) at Quelimane ($p<0.05$).

The results that significantly fewer of the war displaced were engaged in formal or informal employment and education compared to the other groups at Beira, a distinction, which does not occur at Quelimane, reinforces the earlier results suggesting that the war displaced at Beira rank relatively worse off.

In Gorongosa 100% of established residents and 97% of migrants said they owned a land plot, and if anything the level of cultivation appears to have slightly increased after relocation. Few people claimed to produce

Table 6.26 Proportions of households owning a cultivation plot and selling some of its produce before and after relocation

		More than 10 years resident		Voluntary migrants		All forced migrants*		Directly displaced by war		Total less than 10 years resident	
		Prop	%	Prop	%	Prop	%	Prop	%	Prop	%
QUELIMANE	Before	4/42	9.5	8/30	26.7	10/34	29.4	2/8	25.0	18/64	28.1
	After			5/23	21.7	4/21	19.1	1/6	16.7	9/44	20.5
BEIRA	Before	6/84	7.1	3/25	12.0	1/31	3.2	1/14	7.1	4/56	7.1
	After			0/21	0.0	1/33	3.0	0/10	0.0	1/54	1.9
GORONGOSA	Before	0/31	0.0	0/9	0.0	1/22	4.6	1/22	4.6	1/31	3.2
	After			0/12	0.0	0/24	0.0	0/24	0.0	0/36	0.0

Notes:

Prop = proportion of households who own a cultivation plot and sell its produce using first questionnaire survey.

* Includes directly displaced by war category.

Table 6.27 Ownership of cultivation plot and supplementary income generating activity

		More than 10 years resident		Voluntary migrants		All forced migrants*		Directly displaced by war		All	
		Prop	%	Prop	%	Prop	%	Prop	%	Prop	%
QUELIMANE	Men	19/38	50.0	8/35	22.9	4/39	10.3	2/4	50.0	31/112	27.7
	Women	2/71	2.8	3/41	7.3	2/50	4.0	2/15	13.3	7/162	4.3
BEIRA	Men	35/97	36.1	3/16	18.8	11/53	20.8	1/11	9.1	49/166	29.5
	Women	2/91	2.2	0/44	0.0	3/60	5.0	1/17	5.9	5/195	2.6
GORONGOSA	Men	2/9	22.2	0/2	0.0	1/8	12.5	1/8	12.5	3/19	15.8
	Women	0/22	0.0	0/10	0.0	0/17	0.0	0/17	0.0	0/49	0.0

Notes:

Prop = proportion of responses indicating a main income generating activity in addition to household ownership of a cultivation plot using both questionnaire surveys.

* Includes directly displaced by war category.

Shaded percentages are significantly different from more than 10 years residents in excess of the 95% confidence level using chi-square analysis on pairs of proportions. Shaded and underlined percentages are significantly different from more than 10 years residents in excess of the 99% confidence level.

214

enough to be able to sell any of their produce during this period. Those that did sell some produce before being displaced ceased to do so after resettling. In addition to cultivation the only other responses recorded for main activity at Gorongosa were 6.5% of established residents and 12% of people directly displaced by the war who considered themselves unemployed and 3.2% of established residents and 12% of people directly displaced by the war who indicated they were in education. On this account there is no grounds to suggest the circumstances of those directly displaced by war were different to the circumstances of long term residents.

Susceptibility through Settlement

It has been indicated above that although forcibly displaced groups may have become more susceptible to disease, in most instances this has not led to disproportionately higher incidence of cholera and dysentery at the field sites. Instead exposure of all residents to local environments appears to be the predominant influence in determining the distribution of disease incidence. In the case of dysentery in Beira, being directly displaced by war exaggerated susceptibility primarily because of resettling into worse circumstances than those experienced before displacement. Some accounts, such as that by Moore *et al.* (1993) on the health of displaced and resident populations of central Somalia during the 1992 famine, put the emphasis more on the process of displacement. However, increased exposure to disease risk following displacement is also already recognised as a further important factor in explaining refugee ill-health (Dick 1984; Mullholland 1985; Shears and Lusty 1987; Moren *et al.* 1991). Typically this includes overcrowding in camps and resettlement centres, being in locations that are unable to provide adequate subsistence (food aid may not provide adequate variety in diet), and being in a local environment which is not conducive to good hygiene, sanitation, and water supply (flooding, salinity and alkalinity can be included in this). In this way the natural and modified environments where displaced people relocate can increase their exposure to disease pathogens and present conditions conducive to reducing resistance to infection.

Data presented in this chapter suggest that in Beira, being forcibly displaced made a significant difference to susceptibility to dysentery (and to a lesser extent cholera), in that defences provided through basic subsistence were disproportionately reduced. This creates a window of opportunity for communicable diseases to gain an advantage. However in this instance such an analysis only serves to reinforce the view that the conditions at the place of resettlement were the paramount cause. Whilst clear indications of the role of the local physical environment in influencing the distribution of incidence of endemic cholera at Quelimane have been presented in Chapter 5, data presented in this chapter has not shown any difference in incidence caused by the process of displacement. These results support the argument that pathogenicity and location were stronger influences on diarrhoeal disease epidemics at the field sites than susceptibility brought about by population movement.

7 Socio-economic and Political Change and Incidence of Cholera and Bacillary Dysentery

The results of the environmental and demographic research presented in the last two chapters have suggested that the distribution of cholera in Quelimane can be explained a function of specific localised environmental conditions that favour the persistence and virulence of the disease pathogen. However, in Beira this was less apparent, suggesting a greater role for contextual factors. This chapter explores a range of underlying socio-economic, administrative and behavioural factors that influence incidence of cholera and dysentery in the different areas. Firstly, the relationship between health and urban infrastructure is addressed, secondly the health implications of structural adjustment are considered, and thirdly the role of changing behaviour within the affected communities is discussed.

Examination of the role of these factors contributes further to understanding the relative importance of the micro-environmental and demographic influences identified earlier. It also provides a response to the demand that disease ecology integrate an understanding of the underlying as well as immediate causes of ill-health through analysis of disease and 'development' (Hughes and Hunter 1970), the underdevelopment of health (Stock 1986), and the political ecology of disease (Mayer 1993). Understanding of the underlying influences on ill-health in different locales contributes to a more *realistic* identification of sustainable policies for reducing the risk of high incidence of cholera and dysentery.

Infrastructural Changes and Environmental Health in Urban Mozambique

There is a growing awareness that rapid urbanisation, increases in the number of urban poor, and many of the changes in urban environments of developing countries have a negative effect on health and will continue to do so in the foreseeable future (Hardoy and Cairncross *et al.* 1990; WHO 1991a; Harpham and Tanner 1995). However, despite much speculation, little detailed work has been carried out to determine the role of infrastructural changes and policy shifts on incidence of specific diseases.

A general overview of the health effects of urbanisation in the Third World is provided by Hardoy and Satterthwaite (1991) who review the massive scale and range of environmental problems and the role and limitations of interventionist policies. Bergstrøm and Ramalingaswani (1991) refer to the importance of the extensive breakdown of infrastructure and services in slum areas that create conditions conducive to the resurgence of diseases previously believed to be under control. Harpham and Lusty *et al.* (1988), Harpham (1994) and Tanner and Harpham (1995, p35) stress the role of urbanisation and an increasing poverty in urban areas as precursors to poor health status, but accept there remain many gaps in our knowledge in the field of urban health research.

The issues surrounding structural adjustment programmes and their affect on health in some developing countries have also been introduced, both in general terms of health and well-being (Anyinam 1989; Cooper-Weil *et al.* 1990; O'Connor 1991; Tumwine 1992; Loewenson 1993), and in brief accounts of broad association with cholera (Donovan 1991; Labonte 1992). However, it has been suggested that, apart from the likely decrease in health status caused by an increase in poverty amongst low-income urban populations, there is currently little specific evidence of the impact of structural adjustment on health (Cooper-Weil *et al.* 1990, p8; Harpham 1994, p120). Further to this, research that assesses the specific disease consequences of behavioural changes resulting from development policies has been limited.

Housing and the Emergence of a Habitational Crisis

The spatial distribution of housing conditions is an important feature of the built environment that warrants attention in the analysis of incidence of cholera and dysentery. This is because the conditions of people's housing and basic services are both physical determinants of health and generally reflect the social-economic vulnerability of the resident. Differences in habitation in the main cities of Mozambique are typical of many colonial cities in that there is a dense urbanised core of colonial houses and blocks of flats and congested surrounding suburbs of more makeshift housing. In Beira the makeshift housing consists of reed, wattle and tin shacks in low lying rice producing zones and in Quelimane more typically of wattle and coconut palm leave huts in and around low lying rice producing zones, salt flats and coconut plantations. In Gorongosa a handful of old concrete buildings from the colonial era are surrounded by baked mud and grass huts. However, the distribution of housing conditions and occupants in Mozambique's urban areas is complex and requires further historical analysis.

During the latter part of the colonial period in Beira there was a rapid increase in building in and around the urban core along the coast and port area. Many modern blocks of flats were erected in the down-town area and large mansions continued to be erected along the coastal strip, named Estoril after its equally salubrious counterpart in Portugal. The suburbs of wattle housing and shacks located on low lying ground near to the core of the city remained clearly defined zones throughout that period. Despite evidence of attempts to improve services to those areas in the dying days of colonialism, mainly through a limited amount of strategically placed standpipes, they remained desperately impoverished areas. The main thrust of the last colonial Master Plan in 1965 was primarily concerned with linking the coastal areas with the new highway and ways of developing them for tourism (Tegelman and Kalsi *et al.* 1987). In Quelimane, there is a much smaller area of old colonial housing that is concentrated around the central business district. The smaller size of the city and primary function as a service centre for the province of Zambézia, contrasts with Beira's earlier function as an international port and tourist centre. Other than in the concrete part of the city, the rest of Quelimane's housing is similar to that found in the rural areas. Unlike at Beira there are few large apartment blocks or hotels. The function of Gorongosa town was primarily as a small district administrative centre and transit point for agricultural produce. Its classification as an urban area occurred only recently due to the swelling of its population during the war.

At independence the majority of the quarter million Portuguese settlers in Mozambique, most of whom were concentrated in the residential quarters of the cities, left the country. Fear of nationalisation and loss of property and personal wealth, of encountering bloodshed in revenge attacks similar to what had occurred in the Belgium Congo, and inability to accept the legitimacy of a truly Mozambican President were some of the reasons for the mass exit (Munslow 1983; Azeveo 1992). The exodus of most of the professional workforce created a large gap in the management of the country's infrastructure and left many European style buildings unoccupied.

Though FRELIMO were not slow to define their policy, there were few trained people who were able to implement it. Up to 85 per cent of doctors, engineers, surveyors and planners had left.[1] Nationalisation of rented housing occurred in 1976. The evacuated European style housing often became occupied by people from rural and semi-rural areas unfamiliar with how to maintain modern European buildings. In some instances the services to houses and tower blocks had been sabotaged by the exiting Portuguese. Further deterioration of the 'concrete' environment arrived with near siege conditions caused by the war of destabilisation that arrived just a few years later. In Beira during this period electricity would be cut off for up to eight months at a time and the piped water supply halted because it depended on electric pumps. Similar siege conditions occurred at Quelimane, though arguably the infrastructural impact was less since overall the city was not so dependent on these services. For example, apartment blocks, the water distribution network and the sewage system, all of which were dependent on maintenance and electricity were more extensive at Beira.

At Quelimane, save for the central core of the city, a more rural lifestyle had prevailed and hence there was less dependence on the services that were sabotaged. Hazards to health increased as drains in and around the concrete cities became blocked due to insufficient water being used to flush toilets. When the electricity supply did return, much of the pumped water to these areas was lost through leaks which could not be repaired due to a lack of parts. Another feature of the urban environment was the increase in numbers of people inhabiting one building. For example, an upstairs maisonette which formerly housed one family typically became home to up to four or more families. The net effect of this deterioration in

---

[1] This figure is based on unpublished estimates made by Skillshare Africa (formerly I.V.S), who have been working alongside the Mozambican Government since shortly after Independence to 'gap fill' missing skilled and professional personnel with 'Cooperantes' who train local staff.

habitation in the old colonial parts of the cities was that by the mid 1980s it was not necessarily correct to define the wattle suburbs as the poorer zones of the city as a more homogenous state of poverty ensued.

The events of recent years have seen the emergence of a third stage in the distribution and relative quality of housing conditions in the main cities of Mozambique. This has been disproportionately more prominent in Beira than in Quelimane. The first signs of this change arrived with the introduction of the Programma de Reforma Economica (PRE) in 1987, which marked the beginning of the International Monetary Fund's intervention in Mozambique. At a local level this meant that the food rationing system was phased out and that prices for basic supplies rose. The local unit of currency, the metical, which for some years had no purchasing power at all, achieved some value as official exchange rates were brought more into line with the black market one.

There was also an increase in foreign interests in the country. This was particularly pronounced in the case of Beira because of the refurbishment of the port and the Beira Corridor, a vital outlet to the sea for Zimbabwe and Zambia, and a necessary feature of the wider ideological conflict in Southern Africa supported by SADCC (Southern Africa Development and Co-ordinating Committee)(Gibb 1987; Amin *et al.* 1987; Smith 1988). This managed to attract EEC funding and direct involvement of national development agencies such as SIDA (Swedish International Development Agency) and FINIDA (Finnish International Development Agency). It marked the start of the period in which highly paid 'experts', mainly European, used large amounts of money to not only refurbish the port and elements of the Beira Corridor, but also to erect compounds of luxury housing for themselves in some of the city's best remaining open sites. Other foreign interests opted for the total refurbishment of old housing.

A further surge of activity in urban Mozambique arrived with UNOMOZ (United Nations Operation in Mozambique) who came to oversee the Peace process and the lead up to elections. More existing buildings were renovated and rented out at high rates. Some of the wealth from this succession of activities made its way into the hands of local entrepreneurs who have not only gained an advantage in remaining settled in the concrete city, but have also acquired the wealth to be able to purchase land plots and build houses away from the centre. However, these processes have been very selective of individual buildings and land plots, and consequently many slums in the centre of town that still reflect conditions of absolute poverty and a serious health hazard are close to the fully serviced houses and apartments. As a result of this third change in housing status in the city there are therefore noticeably greater contrasts in human well-being over small areas than ever before.

The close spatial proximity of environmentally poor and relatively good quality housing is of further relevance to understanding the disease distributions used in this research. Since bacillary dysentery caused by the pathogen *Shigella dysenteriae* 1 is much more communicable than cholera caused by *Vibrio cholerae* it has had more impact in the dense urbanised concrete parts of the city of Beira. People from both poorer and better off households have been affected by this disease. In terms of disease ecology, it is reasonable to suggest that disease attracted by the conditions of the poor households reaches a level at which the entire vicinity is at risk. An apparent overall increase in wealth in the concrete city is therefore not matched by a decrease in dysentery. With cholera, however, targeted exposure of a household to a contaminated source and exposure to greater quantities of bacteria is the more likely mode of contracting the disease, and therefore the close contact of the immediate neighbourhood can be less of a hazard. This is particularly evident should the cholera pathogen be more endemic in the physical environment as suggested for Quelimane, since there is a greater likelihood of primary transmission from an environmental origin than through predominantly secondary transmission associated with new and virulent strains. Indeed in Quelimane little association between higher incidence of cholera and its smaller down town concrete area was established.

Water Supply in the Context of Urban Development

The ongoing inadequacy of water supply services in the cities of Third World countries is being addressed by international policy making aimed at the reform of urban water utilities. The dominant trend at present has been to expand the private sector's role (World Bank 1992; Briscoe 1993). However, the gradual establishment of market-oriented economic policies since 1987 (which accelerated in the 1990s), has had a mixed effect on water supply for the inhabitants of Beira and Quelimane. Overall, at the time of carrying out this research, new approaches were failing both to overcome the shortcomings of the colonial period, or to enhance aspects of relative progress achieved during the post independence period. One map of estimated needs for new water sources, produced using data supplied by Agua Rural (Rural Water), classifies the entire country as falling into the three categories of acute need, great need or considerable need (MSF 1994, p77). This research corroborated this rather drastic assessment for the cases of Quelimane, Beira and Gorongosa through water quality analysis (Table 6.11). Changes in development perspectives are particularly well reflected by the distribution and management of a water supply.

In colonial times the piped water supply that was pumped around the more European parts of the Mozambican cities, sufficient for bathrooms containing showers, flush toilets and bidets, was billed to individuals or workplaces according to readings taken from external meters outside houses. In some parts of the concrete areas this procedure continues. In the suburbs where most of the population lives there were limited amounts of communal standpipes for which no bill was made. Many of the residents of these zones interpret this as having therefore been a period of free water supply. However, it could be argued that this was paid for by the taxes of those in formal employment.

After independence FRELIMO confirmed that water to the suburbs was free of charge and maintained only a nominal fee for water supplied to households in the concrete areas. As many of the meters fell into disrepair (and there were now no replacements) many of these households also ended up with no water bill. The recent policy shift towards marketing the water supply is therefore a new concept for most Mozambicans and has met with considerable practical and administrative difficulties. For example, despite the improved output of tapped water in Beira since the end of prolonged power cuts, some of the high density inner suburban bairros of wattle, reed and tin shacks had no supply at all during the entire period of the research described in this book. Key informants, identifiable as those living next to the standpipes and therefore generally up to date with the comings and goings of the water supply, provided explanations.

In two incidents the *responsável* (literally translates to responsible person), who became the private renter of the tap under the new system, had disappeared with the money that the local population pay him to cover the bill required by the water company, who responded by cutting off the water supply. In a high population density zone of Quelimane the water was turned off when the meter for a key standpipe fell into disrepair. Each stand pipe must have a functioning meter and taps if it is to be allowed to operate. Under the new system it was unclear whether the renter of the tap or the company were responsible for making the repairs and there was added confusion with the percentage of payments that were set aside for maintenance purposes. In another instance the company arrived with the new parts to renovate a standpipe but proclaimed that under the present system these must be paid for on the spot. Nobody paid and the water supply remained disconnected. A return visit just prior to publishing this book revealed that this situation has persisted until the present. There are now almost no functioning public standpipes in Beira.

In many other instances informants said that, with the rising cost of living, they could not afford to pay for water at all, and therefore settled for using only well-water. However, inspired by the new emphasis on purchasing power the owners of some of the better wells in Beira were also making independent charges. Since the groundwater quality in these coastal zones varies over very short distances some households benefit from digging their own well and striking fresh water whilst others encounter water too saline to drink. They are therefore forced to make use of whatever other sources they can find nearby and often end up using more contaminated ones. At some of these the owner stopped using it himself if he has managed to arrange access to an alternative cleaner supply elsewhere. Under these circumstances, contrasts in access to better quality water within small areas is a function of its environmental distribution, the level of co-operation between households, and often on one's ability to pay.

The salt water from some of the poorer wells can be used for washing in extreme circumstances but uses up excess amounts of soap, an extremely expensive commodity for many. In these circumstances people prefer to use small amounts of fresh water which may have further adverse health implications. This is because deficiencies in water quantity for washing is associated with decreased levels of hygiene and higher incidence of secondary transmission of diarrhoeal disease (Feachem 1977; Cairncross and Feachem 1983). Most typically, the emphasis on water quantity is made with respect to water-washed diseases with which shigellosis is generally included (as discussed in Chapter 2) the categories of water-washed and water-borne have been meant in a broad sense and are disputable depending on specific situations). Cholera, considered more of a water-borne-disease, has been traditionally associated with water quality and quantity. Using this criteria it would follow that the higher ratio of dysentery in some of the more built up areas of Beira was also aggravated by gross shortage of water since there was no tapped water supply for long periods and only a scattered distribution of accessible wells.

A successful strategy used by the unserved people for obtaining tap water during the post-Independence years was to simply request it from houses and flats in the old colonial part of the city. This option has however become problematical in the last few years as many of those houses have become privately owned once more. The functioning taps, where entire neighbourhoods of unserved people collected drinking water free of charge, have often disappeared behind high walls and access is denied. The households at which the people are still able to collect water, and where the owner does not charge, have diminished in number with the consequence that there are long queues starting before dawn each day at those remaining. People who used this system previously are also forced to opt for the contaminated open wells. This situation has developed much more in Beira than it has in Quelimane since privatisation of property and commodification has been much greater in the larger and more urban of the two cities. The added irony in Beira is that there has been considerable input to improve the output of the water supply in recent years and for the first time in more than a decade the principal buildings and housing on the distribution network have a twice daily supply that lasts several hours. Thus in Beira, for some, improvements in the infrastructure and a new style of water management have created an improved quality of life and defence against ill-health, but for the majority of others things at the best remain the same, and in some instances have deteriorated.

Almost no sealed tube-wells exist in Beira since it has always been considered a major city within which a piped water supply is more appropriate. Agua Rural, the company responsible for implementing sealed tube-wells concentrated its efforts in the rural districts of Sofala. The analysis of water quality and use in Gorongosa carried out during the fieldwork for this research suggests that a good number of these have been successful in the semi-rural context and could be used more in and around larger urban environments as a back up strategy for periods when there is no tapped water. A further reason for not using tube-wells in Beira has been the underlying geology. Sands, silts and clays in a littoral zone are not ideal for sinking the wells. However, the main reasons must be attributed to non-environmentally based policy decisions since in Quelimane, where the sands and silts are much finer and therefore even less appropriate, tube-wells have been established that manage to bring up good water.

At the time of carrying out the research described in this book, over half of the tube-wells in Quelimane were not functioning due to problems with maintenance. Seven of those used during the 1991 survey were found to be inoperable by 1994. Explanations given by the locals living next to these were similar to the reasons for the breakdown of the standpipes. The parts for tube-wells are expensive, do not get paid for and responsibility is no longer assumed by the state. A further comment here is that NGO projects often pay more attention to rural areas where it is easier to 'pioneer' a water project and generate quick results to please donors, rather than unravel the complexities of the urban situation. This is despite the fact that urban areas are now estimated to account for at least one quarter of the global disease burden (World Bank 1993; Harpham and Tanner 1995, p7).

Given the rapid increase in population which is occurring in many Third World cities and coincident limitations in urban infrastructural development it is probable that urban health problems will greatly outweigh rural health problems in the future (WHO 1991a, p5). In the case of Mozambique, Ministry of Health figures for cholera (Aragon and Chambule *et al.* 1993, p17) indicated in excess of 74 per cent of cases in Sofala, 50 per cent in Zambézia, and 41 per cent nationally to have occurred in urban areas. Even if taking into account the likelihood that the proportion is artificially skewed towards urban cases due to the greater amount of people which may get registered in an urban context, these figures suggest that there is unlikely to be a case for addressing urban health problems with any less urgency than rural areas. One possible way in which increasing urbanisation might be reversed is if water supply and health become so bad that it causes out migration, as has been occurring in New Delhi, India, during the mid 1990s.

Market led policies did little to aid an even distribution of sealed tube-wells in Quelimane. In the Communal Unit with the highest population there was only one, which turned out to be amongst the oldest in the city, but was kept in use by the careful maintenance of a motivated local resident. One tube-well for that area was inadequate since long pauses in pumping are necessary to allow the water to replenish. Meanwhile some new tube-wells are beginning to appear, but most of the time sit idle in the back yards of houses where the owner has purchased his own. Specific projects financed by international NGO's have established others, but these tend to be sited where a project is focusing its own activities. Hence standpipes are often associated with a school, agricultural scheme, church mission or mosque. Access for the general population is dependent on the good will of individual caretakers. Contributions of general assistance for well construction from NGO's pass through the state company. This was set up in the past to enable co-ordination and co-operation in NGO activities aimed at improving the general availability of a good water supply for everybody. However, the latter shift in policy meant that NGO input in urban areas was translated into a centralised market for clean water supply dependent on ones ability to pay for pump parts.

Sanitation and Urban Infrastructure

This sub-section comments more specifically on the extent to which the combination of poor sanitation and infrastructural circumstances exacerbated high levels of incidence of cholera and dysentery at different locations. Though poor sanitation has undoubtedly been a part of the cycle of secondary transmission of cholera and dysentery, considerable variation exists in the numbers of people not using sanitation facilities between the different urban centres studied. The questionnaire survey reported in Chapter 6 showed that of those interviewed, approximately 26 per cent in Quelimane, 42 per cent in Beira, and 56 per cent in Gorongosa did not have any sanitation facility at all (Table 6.18). A confirmation of the accuracy of these results was provided by a subsequent survey carried out by AFRICARE using clusters of samples and obtaining a figure of 45 per cent without latrines in Beira (AFRICARE 1994). Whilst the higher figure for Gorongosa is to be expected in a more rural setting, the Beira figure is exceptionally high for an urban area and can be considered a major health hazard. One explanation for this situation is that poor sanitation in Beira is compounded by additional problems relating to the city's location and development which have contributed to a particularly serious level of infrastructural collapse. Some similar problems apply to Quelimane, but it could be argued that overall infrastructural collapse has had less affect.

The growth of Beira into one of Mozambique's main urban areas was primarily due to its location as a port at the mouth of the river Pungwe which was an easily accessible outlet for produce from central provinces and the rapidly developing interior of southern Africa (Muchangos 1989). The economic activities associated with the port and railroad were further supplemented by large scale tourism to the European residential areas along the coast. This started to decline in 1965 with UDI (Unilateral Declaration of Independence) in Rhodesia and completely halted in 1975 with the mass departure of the Portuguese at Independence. The previously labelled *Bairros Indígenas* (Indigenous suburbs) that appear in and around the city core on old city plans were originally occupied by a large labour pool that serviced the European city. The beginnings of an outer residential zone had begun in Manga and a large area of small holdings for low intensity agricultural practices at the outer limits of Inhamizúa.

The relative wealth of its earlier years stimulated much economic investment in the infrastructure of the built environment. A large part of the main city area was raised up by sand infills and extensive measures were taken against coastal erosion and to counteract flooding from the sea and rainfall. Drainage was facilitated by a system of large open channels that exited through a sluice system into the sea. The greater part of the city was designed to be dependent on artificial protection requiring extensive maintenance. This meant that the city was particularly susceptible to decline during the post-Independence period when more attention was paid to ruralisation. Economic instability and administrative weaknesses assisted in this demise, and sanitation has been a particularly poignant example. Much of the more modern piped sewage system for the concrete city was never completed. Some parts of a very early outflow system consist of a large open drain that forms the central reservation of a long avenue of three and four storey apartment blocks.

Quelimane has had much less of a concrete infrastructure to depend on. Most residents have always lived in traditional huts save for the central business district and a relatively small zone of Portuguese residential zones that lie immediately adjacent on the north and east sides. There is therefore little evidence that the decline of services to the former core of the city would have radically altered the circumstances of most residents. Sanitation for most of Quelimane's dense population has been predominantly through use of traditional latrines and this has continued up to the present day.

With much of Quelimane and Beira being at about sea level and a water table sometimes only a few inches below ground level, conventional latrine projects, aimed at the majority population with no piped sewage system, have had very limited success. Though there have been developments in latrine designs that address this difficulty (Winblad and Kilama 1986), little progress has been made in these cities. The layout of the urban areas is an added problem since very dense housing, with little room for latrine development, is surrounded by rice paddies and other cultivation, forcing many people to search for places to defecate elsewhere. In some parts of Beira the edge of the main incoming surfaced road (technically the Beira Corridor) was being extensively used as a mass open latrine. There is some justification for this since the road is raised up and the faeces dry out, removing some of the pathogenic content. It was preferable to it festering in the damp undergrowth and being washed around amongst the low lying neighbourhoods to the immediate north-west and south-east of the road.

The main areas for defecation in the former European part of Beira, for the majority without flush toilets, has been in vacant plots awaiting construction and along the coastal margin. These options are being reduced as nearly all the vacant plots become sold off and the beach is increasingly used for recreational purposes. In other *bairros* of wattle, reed and shacks away from the main road people without latrines use the margins of the drainage canals (Figures 7.1a, 7.1b and 7.1c). The sluice mechanism at the main outlet to the sea has not functioned for many years and the high tides regularly flood this area by way of the drainage channels, causing widespread contamination in and around the housing. A further concern highlighted in Chapter 5 is the process of salinisation and alkalinisation caused by flooding of these areas by sea water. This results in a lethal combination of critically poor sanitation and stagnant pools of water with more favourable geo-ecological conditions for enhancing the survival and virulence of *Vibrio cholerae*. Impoverishment of habitat around the artificial drainage canals due to the malfunctioning of the sea outlet, provides a further example of how Beira's built environment can be seen as an underlying health hazard. Overall, the city of Beira suffers from not having the means to cope with an infrastructure it has inherited from an earlier development perspective, instead being forced to pursue strategies more typically associated with rural areas. The grandiose plans for the city's development in colonial times were aimed at serving the needs of a small population of non-indigenous occupants rather than protecting the long term needs of the majority population.

The Grand Hotel, Beira

The story of the Grand Hotel in Beira encapsulates some of the themes described above. The Grand Hotel is a structure of palatial proportions and was known as one of the biggest hotels in Southern Africa during the 1950s (Figure 7.2). It catered for large quantities of tourists from neighbouring countries and from around the world. Its decline started with the demise of tourism in the 1960s. By independence in 1975 it was already closed.

A few years after Independence it was ordered by the then president Samora Machel to be used for the popular task of housing the homeless and destitute. Occupants and local residents recall that large quantities of

(a)

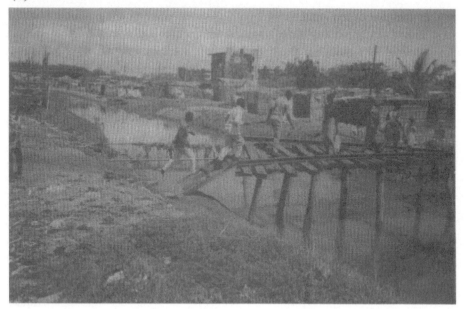

(b)

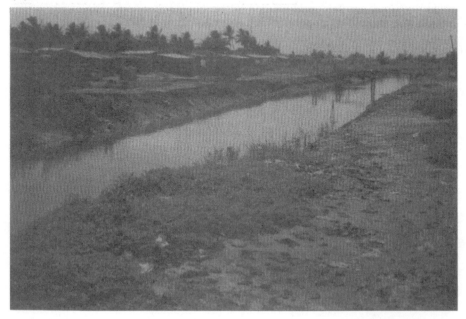

(c)

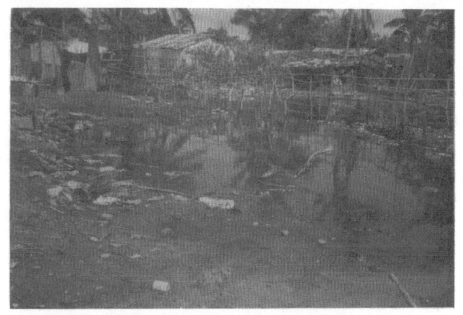

Figure 7.1 (a, b, c) Drainage canals and inhabitation at Beira

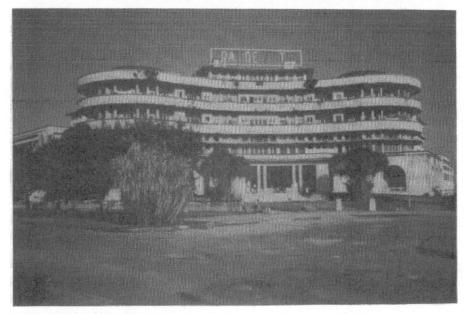

Figure 7.2   The Grand Hotel, Beira

homeless people were confronted by luxurious rooms and chandeliers when they were allocated their places. However, the ensuing problems of the city have produced a situation of absolute poverty in this building as bad as any that can be found in Beira. Though services were originally supplied there has not been water or electricity for years and the occupants are unable to dig a well or grow food. The water situation further worsened when nearby vacant plots containing open wells were privately purchased and fenced off. Several plans to restore the Grand Hotel to something of its former status, whilst resettling the occupants in the process have fallen through. State plans to resettle the current occupants on land plots have not occurred as local government is now forced to concentrate its efforts on selling plots to a long list of applicants with money to construct a house. The housing plots are in short supply and becoming increasingly expensive. In sum, the social agenda that prevailed in the early years after Independence no longer takes precedence and the current market oriented decision making appears to fall short of providing a solution.

The Health Implications of Structural Changes at the Field Sites

There is growing concern about the limited gains and, in certain instances, negative effects of structural adjustment policies on incidence of ill-health in Third World Countries (Tumwine 1992; Loewenson 1993; Wildt *et al* 1993; Grant 1993; Costello and Woodward 1993; Poore 1993; Asthana 1994; Mole 1994). Although policy changes stem from a common ideology upheld by global institutions, their outcomes are likely to vary dependant on the historical context and local conditions within which they are being implemented. Individual analysis of vulnerable locations is required to verify these relationships. This sub-section outlines the context in which structural adjustment has affected health in the areas under study and assesses the implications for incidence of cholera and dysentery.

Health Care in Mozambique

The idea of effective medical care as a form of social control was first introduced in Mozambique with the colonial administration's *Boletim da Assistencia Médica aos Indigenas* in 1928 (Shapiro 1983). This document pointed out that a permanent health service could become an essential factor in the occupation of the colonies. However in the years that followed there is little evidence that the Portuguese managed to gain the hearts and minds of the people through health care. During the subsequent period the main contribution to health and social welfare was in developing large city hospitals. In the case of Beira these were named the 'European Hospital' and the 'Indigenous Hospital', which was built much later. Despite the names it appears there was not a strict form of apartheid, as existed in neighbouring countries, but rather a more complex delineation of privilege based on status through degree of assimilation into the structures of greater Portugal. However, the system was fully discriminatory in the sense that there was virtually no provision for people in rural areas or for the poor who could not afford to pay for medical treatment.

In Quelimane the hospital was divided into 4 classes with the lowest for the 'barefooted' (Webb 1984). It has been asserted that the rudimentary preventive service that existed was to protect settlers from common infectious diseases, ensure only minimum standards of hygiene, and that the overwhelming emphasis was on curative and technological medicine (Walt 1984). More than two-thirds of the country's doctors worked in the capital and nearly all doctors in civilian practice were in the three main cities where not more than 10 per cent of the population lived (Walt 1984, p2). Hanlon (1983) points out that in the late 1960s Portugal began building rural health posts to appease international opinion and counteract some of FRELIMO's support. However this was already too late to have much effect before the final push towards Independence arrived in the early 1970s.

FRELIMO's interests in PHC (Primary Health Care) grew out of the armed struggle, and in particular training nurses to work with its forces. Health workers who have remained in their profession and talk openly about that period say that this assistance was extended to the local population in the liberated zones and was a key area in which the popular campaign for Independence was represented. The theme of health care as a focus for national progress benefited from the personal emphasis put on it by Samora Machel who was formerly a nurse in the colonial health care system, and by FRELIMO recognising the merits of active involvement of people in their own health care as a lesson learned during the liberation war (Walt 1984, p6; Saul 1985).

After Independence, health care was nationalised and proactive policies set in motion a large scale effort to bring health to the people. The achievements of the period until the early 1980s were substantial with more services being made available to more people through a steady output of newly trained health workers. Though only basically qualified, they enabled rudimentary PHC to be implemented. Over ten per cent of national expenditure was on health, much higher than most countries in Africa, and for the first time there were trained medical personnel in every district (Melamed and Walt 1984). Medical personnel in Mozambique claim that a major struggle during that period, which to a lesser extent still remains, was to change awareness of the importance of PHC amidst the legacy of the previous higher status awarded to curative medicine.

The ongoing internal struggle and advances in health care were increasingly disrupted during the 1980s by the war of destabilisation waged by RENAMO and its external supporters. Besides causing Mozambique to spend larger amounts on rebuilding infrastructure and defence instead of further expanding health programmes, the health service itself became a direct target as it was symbolic of FRELIMO ideology. During the period 1982-6 nearly the entire rural health and education services were eliminated through killing and kidnapping of staff and destruction of buildings and equipment (Cliff and Noormahomed 1988). Health personnel were still at risk of being attacked in some parts of the country as late as 1992, prior to the signing of the Peace Agreement in Rome.

The popularity of FRELIMO's health programme before its destruction in the rural areas may be partly testified to in that RENAMO was establishing a similar structure in its areas in western Zambézia during the early 1990s (Wilson 1992). Evidence of some of the effectiveness of the state's PHC programme is clear from the health surveys conducted in this research. For example, in the district of Gorongosa in the interior of central Mozambique, where there has been only limited external input since the end of the conflict, 66 out of 68 (97.1%) people interviewed included ORT (oral rehydration therapy) when asked what they use if they have diarrhoea. This compares with approximately 44% use of ORT for the developing world and nearly 50% for Sub-Saharan Africa (UNICEF 1995, p25). Though many of those interviewed would have gained knowledge of this through recent attendance at the local Hospital which benefits from the assistance of the NGO Medicins Sans Frontières, the high percentage also reflects the input of earlier work carried out by the state.

The legacy of the Primary Health Care movement in Mozambique is that politics and health have not been separate and that health policy was seen as an overall strategy to create a just society (Saul 1985; Munslow 1985). Maintaining motivation amongst low paid health personnel and community mobilisation to pursue this aim were dependent on achieving a momentum of progress. Though brave attempts were continuously made to maintain a presence in district capitals, and city hospitals carried out some of their tasks, even with no electricity supply and limited water, much of the progress that had been made was destroyed. As the war progressed there were additional burdens of mass forced migrations, famines, and droughts. Against this background, and with disease epidemics proliferating out of control external assistance in Mozambique increased towards the end of the 1980s.

Structural Adjustment and Health: Recent Influences

Though Mozambique has been experiencing institutional and infrastructural changes throughout its history, the most recent structural adjustment policies have been a match for any in bringing about significant alterations to services in urban areas. The driving force behind these changes came about as a result of the *Programa de Reforma Económica* (Economic Recovery Program), which was implemented in 1987 following the intervention of the International Monetary Fund. Stock (1995, p349) comments on the nature of structural adjustment programs which 'reflect to some extent the political, economic, and social realities of the individual countries' but points out that 'much more striking is the uniformity of policy direction'. This has been the case in Mozambique, where existing state mechanisms and bureaucracy, such as the National Health Service, survive alongside new initiatives in privatisation. The view from the World Bank is that the policy works as long as the country makes sufficient reforms (World Bank 1993), pointing to a selection of apparently more successful countries. It responds to well-documented failures by pointing out that they represent cases that need more reform, not less (The Economist 1994). However, the signs of failure through worsening conditions at local level are viewed by others as evidence that the policies are inappropriate and have reversed some of the better aspects of the previous systems they tried to reform (Tumwine 1992; de Wildt and Sogge *et al* 1993; Costello and Woodward 1993).

Hanlon (1991) describes how in Mozambique the Economic Recovery Programme came about as a result of FRELIMO's decision in 1983 to improve its relations with western countries and curb further support for the opposition, RENAMO. As the country was pushed further and further into a crisis of war and famine external interventions were accelerated to ensure that aid would be forthcoming. The first stages of intervention by the IMF started during 1987. Hanlon argues strongly that this has been a negative development, representing a threat to the sovereignty of Mozambique. He suggests, for example, that external debt swaps with parastatal companies' assets and privatisation in favour of former owners are the economic hallmarks of the structural adjustment program. This has forced the best technicians to move away from the state apparatus and created a competitive and selfish labour market, whilst the economy was put on the brink of collapse because the companies couldn't sell their products and buyers couldn't buy because they were too expensive. The prices couldn't be lowered because their main costs were imported. Hanlon (1991, p178) also noted that structural adjustment had led to cuts in expenditure on well digging, and to undermining of the National Health Service through cuts in the health budget.

In the urban areas of central Mozambique studied for this research, there have been two noticeable influences on health care emanating from the recent changes. One is related to the administration of the national health service, the other to the co-ordination and participation in health issues amongst the local community. This is explained in more detail below.

Some of the more qualified and experienced health personnel that worked for the national health service transferred to NGO organizations where they could earn larger salaries paid in foreign currency, as hinted at above by Hanlon (1991). They were envied by those who remained in the state service and general morale was reduced amongst the low paid state health workers. The advice to the government has been to improve on its own pay structure. However, in implementing this, complex problems within workplaces arose. In the past employees maintained their positions for varied reasons of which qualifications was only one. For example, those who were *serventes* (servants) for the Portuguese stayed in their positions and became clerks and office staff, attending their basic schooling by night. Others were rewarded with employment for their commitment to the struggle for independence. Their wages remained low whilst increasingly higher wages went to those returning from education in Maputo or overseas who are often younger and need to be prevented from leaving their posts. It was some of these newly formed distinctions and general discontent with wages that lead to strikes amongst lower paid health workers in 1991 (Mozambique Information Office 1991).

Medicines are now purchased, encouraging an emergent economy that is conducive to increases in corruption. Some of the old bureaucratic processes for obtaining treatment emanating from colonial times were never removed by FRELIMO. However the situation is worse now that charges are added for these stages of bureaucracy. Money is handed over simply to receive the results of a medical test for a serious disease such as malaria. When consumables for a test become limited, the remaining few can also be sold unofficially for a higher price. Amongst much of the population it is often unclear which parts of the health procedure are to be paid for and which parts are still free. The implicit message from the top that health is to become a marketable commodity has circulated at all levels within the health service and community and is legitimising actions that were at least officially regarded as taboo in the past. It has frequently been a common sight to see medicines such as injectable penicillin being sold alongside local produce on open air market stalls. The medicines which are sold on market stalls are often out of date and sometimes carry little advice on what they are really for or how they should be administered. Uncontrolled use of antibiotics can have a negative medical effect by contributing to increased drug-resistance in the wider community, and in the case of the antibiotics used for treating dysentery may cause further illness, such as severe hemolytic uremic syndrome (HUS) (Bin Saeed *et al.* 1995; Al-Qarawi *et al.* 1995). There have recently been some additional concerns about drug-resistant tuberculosis and how resistance has contributed to the current pandemic of that disease.

The full extent to which the marketing of health affects cholera and dysentery is unclear since basic treatment in the form of a bed and ORT during an epidemic is generally still available free at specially established wards that have been receiving targeted NGO assistance. However in Quelimane it was not uncommon to be stopped in the street by severely sick people asking for money to buy the antibiotics for advanced dysentery with a prescription for the local chemist in their hand. However, the greatest limitations of a top down health care structure in dealing with incidence of cholera and dysentery are apparent where the former health care strategy was at its strongest. This was in dealing with environmental health problems through representation and participation amongst local communities.

Groupos Dinamizadores (Dynamising Groups) were originally set up in every locality and provided a forum for articulating demands and introducing new policies. Their aim was to increase the participation of the population in the democratic solution of its problems (Lappé and Beccar-Varela, 1980 p40, Walt 1984, p8) in which anything from noisy neighbours to infidelity or local hygiene could be addressed. Though it appears the cadres of FRELIMO later introduced a more politicised rhetoric into these, in a strategy to formulate a front against reactionary groups, and that eventually they became less popular, people interviewed in 1994 still made positive reference to them in terms of community participation. Until the late 1980s, work places had regular meetings during which everyone from the cleaner to the director, and in most instances the foreign *co-operante*, had a voice. The reduction of this type of community participation and organisation has implications for hygiene and preventative health care in and around the *bairros*. A characteristic comment from one resident was 'Before we had more co-operation. Brigades would go around cleaning the place. Now each person does his own thing. He works only for himself'. Others indicated that they felt disenfranchised by the government, since neither national or local government cares any more about what goes on in the *bairros*. Their argument was further supported by the fact that they see less government activity (and more foreign projects) in the area.

Traditional health care practices have remained throughout these transitions in health policy. During FRELIMO's earlier period of Primary Health Care expansion, these practices were to a large extent discouraged. This was more because of concern about the profit making methods of some traditional doctors rather than concern about the medicine that was used. However, restrictions on the use of traditional doctors were ignored and the state largely abandoned its earlier emphasis in later years. A symbolic policy was eventually instigated to investigate the medicines for their scientific value and incorporate the better aspects into the state health system (Barker 1984).

Though traditional medicine has been found to have some useful remedies, practices in some areas have been dangerous for treating cholera and dysentery. For example health workers in Quelimane explained how some traditional doctors in Zambézia were telling mothers to not give their children anything to drink when they had severe diarrhoea. This practice leads to certain death through dehydration. However the local health service got to hear about it and spread the word that children with diarrhoea should drink and that young coconut milk was the best. It has helpful electrolytes that the stomach needs to replenish and is totally free of contamination. This advice was able to become part of the traditional doctor's advice to clients. The contact they maintain with people who do not use the health posts is now recognised as useful for disseminating health information. However, by way of contrast, new problems with the informal sector are being created by the massive increase in the sale of modern medicines on the black market controlled by anonymous individuals with purely financial objectives.

Many of these issues are important in understanding the effects of wider policy changes since they demonstrate how community based Primary Health Care can be undermined by extraneous and institutionalised decision making. Several changes in policy emphasis in recent years have arguably done little to improve community level approaches. Though sometimes well intentioned, a lengthening list of institutional policies and guidelines in Primary Health Care are likely to further limit what can be achieved at community level in extremely poor urban neighbourhoods, such as those described in this book. For example, the increase in selective primary health care (SPHC), popular because interventions can be arranged on a massive, resource-efficient scale does little about conferring health decision making to communities. It also begs the well-established question associated with top down decision making of what problems should be targeted and who is doing the selecting?

Whilst health care in itself is not the central focus of this book, some of the field results that have been obtained can contribute to a debate about which health care approaches might be more appropriate. For example, data from the household survey accompanying this work suggested that for large numbers of people, ability to pay for health care was limited. During the household survey, many residents recounted that they had no income or money at all. The World Health Organization report that recent local studies in Mozambique (location not specified) indicated that approximately one-third of all prescriptions are not filled and that in rural areas only 40 per cent of patients actually pay for their consultation (WHO 1991d, p266).[2] Secondly, there is a limitation in using health care policy which is decided at international level and implemented at national level when health issues vary substantially between urban areas, and even within one city. Thirdly, interventions which fail to maintain the continuity of

---

[2] One way round the problem of inability to pay has been to implement exemption policies (McPake *et al.* 1992, p36). In the case of Mozambique this is called the social fund. In the initial analysis this appears to represent further bureaucratic hurdles in differentiating between individual well-being since overall standards of living are very low. However, further research would be needed to fully investigate the effectiveness of exemption policies in the health care system.

positive aspects of previous policies risk causing a sense of disenfranchisement amongst state employees and local communities. Since Primary Health Care has been so closely associated with Mozambique's former liberation struggle and a national symbol of progress in earlier years, the overwriting of the principles of 'health for free' and 'equity' can be viewed as a challenge to institutional integrity, or in Hanlon's overall more structural assessment, the sovereignty of Mozambique.

Some initiatives have directly confronted the need to redirect resources back into the community. The need to make health care self financing by marketing drugs and health care within the community to compensate for government cuts in expenditure was one of the central tenets of the Bamako Initiative of 1987 (Phillips 1990; McPake *et al.* 1992), principles that were gradually accepted in Mozambique (WHO 1989, 1991). However, whilst such an initiative can be applauded for retaining a focus on seeking solutions more centred on the community, in the context of Mozambique this version of marketing health care still represents a distraction from major issues of importance to poverty and disease ecology. This is because it shifts the emphasis of health care towards curative medicine which is often not the main need and which in some instances may be barely required at all.[3] However, there are some accounts of limited success of this particular initiative in some countries.

McPake *et al.* (1992) present a mixed picture of issues relating to quality, affordability, payment mechanisms, cost recovery, and the role of communities, but conclude that much looks promising about the Bamako Initiative. Perhaps of more importance than their overall assessment of some progress, might be that there was substantial variation between the 5 countries in all aspects investigated and therefore that 'blanket statements...are not warranted' (p56). Comments on health care made in the context of infectious disease epidemics in central Mozambique will also only to some degree apply to other locations. However, one common principle in financing health care anywhere, relates to *prioritisation* in national and international finance. For example, it is now almost public knowledge that much could be achieved in some of the worst affected parts

---

[3]One example is ORS(Oral Rehydration Salts) for treating diarrhoea, provided in sachets and which under the Bamako Initiative are to be sold. Meanwhile, it is well established that a comparative treatment is simply to dissolve a handful of sugar and two pinches of salt in boiled water. A more appropriate approach might therefore be through educating people to make their own, rather than use marketed products.

of the world by simply writing off international debt and reducing expenditure on defence.

Overall this sub-section concludes that initiatives that are not responsive to and structured around the reality of emergent health problems in local communities cannot be a solid base for genuine improvement. However, there is no contradiction in asserting that the state should maintain its responsibility in making adequate health care resources available for all through prioritisation of national expenditure towards improving health.

Other Issues Concerning the Health Impacts of Structural Adjustment

Education The significance of education in influencing ill-health in the Third World is well established (Blacker 1991). The deterioration of education systems due to structural adjustment has therefore been identified as an additional health problem (Tumwine 1992; Asthana 1994). In Mozambique similar principles apply to the education system as have been outlined for health care (Mole 1994). The decline in the overall effort to provide a proactive system that aims to provide education to all rather than just those that can pay for it has implications for health. Firstly, because increases in school fees through adjustment have the effect of consolidating low economic status and low education in the same groups of people, health risks for those groups are intensified. Secondly, because education along with health care has been one of the relative achievements of the past it is important to maintaining a positive outlook in the community, itself a defence against ill-health. Formal education has been particularly relevant where it has been used to disseminate vital information about health and sanitation (Webb 1984; Smith 1984).

In considering the role of education, the education of women is of particular importance. This is because a decreasing level of education for women could become synonymous with an increasing health risk since women are still largely the guardians of water, cooking and the children's level of sanitation. The historical background is that the numbers in schools trebled after independence and despite ongoing customary and social constraints on women there were increases in female attendance (Walt 1984). Rising fees in schools will mean that when poorer families can't meet school expenses fewer children are selected for education. Though no data exists for Mozambique, it is likely that this will provide a selection advantage against women as in circumstances of poverty parents often prefer to pay for a boy to be educated.

Local Economy A further influence of structural adjustment which deserves attention relates to the effects of rapid changes in economic activity on local disease ecologies. The wind down of the war made it possible to transport goods and there has been greater liberalisation on what and where produce can be sold. Whilst overall this has created greater availability of essential items for those with purchasing power there have been some local threats to environment and health. Some indication of the changes that have taken place are reflected at macro-economic scale. In 1992 Mozambique's Gross Domestic Product (GDP) per capita was US$60, by far the lowest in Africa[4] (The Economist 1994). However in June 1994 it was registering a GDP growth rate of 19 per cent, the fastest in all Africa (BBC Focus on Africa News 1994). Though GDP may have limited meaning for some subsistence communities, in Mozambique it meant a major impact on the consolidation of urban areas as market centres, with sprawling zones of open air trading and large concentrations of human activity. However, there has been no compensating provision for quality control of food products and no water and sanitation programme to accompany this surge of human activity in these areas.

The markets also present a health hazard for transmission of diarrhoeal diseases through contaminated food products. A study by Koo *et al.* (1996) has demonstrated the role of street vendor food handling and hygiene in transmission of a newly introduced epidemic strain of *Vibrio cholera* in Guatemala in 1993. In the last four years large areas of Beira, and to some extent Quelimane, have become sprawling market zones attracting large numbers of people despite individual traders often only having a very small amount of produce, such as a couple of kilograms of sweet potatoes or a few cans of Coca-Cola purchased from a larger supplier.

At the broader scale uncontrolled harvesting of natural resources for quick profit is increasing human vulnerability to future health risks. For example large scale deforestation is now occurring in the district of Gorongosa (and many other parts of Mozambique) to supply hardwood timber to international companies. Though this is carried out by private

---

[4] Example GDP figures per capita in Sub-Saharan Africa in 1992 range from US$4,450 in Gabon to $2,790 in Botswana, $1610 in Namibia, $1,030 in Congo, $600 in Angola, $290 in Zambia, and $110 in Tanzania which was the second lowest after Mozambique.

companies the government is party to the process because it is paid a percentage which it vitally needs for, amongst other things, paying off debts. Legislation on flora and fauna that does exist is widely ignored, the situation being compounded further by entrepreneurs who managed to exploit the existence of an unofficial dual administration between the government and RENAMO, which survived well after the end of the war. The situation became so out of control that loggers have even cleared parts of the 'protected' Gorongosa National Park, though recently the zone within which much of the clearing of hard wood occurred has become classified as a 'buffer zone', rather than the National Park *per se* that was delineated on earlier maps.

Some parts of the district's ecology are both unique and if disrupted could provoke particularly severe environmental degradation, such as on and around the steep sided Sierra de Gorongosa mountain range. There are already strong arguments for including that area into the National Park or a wider conservation zone but these are reinforced when the likely health consequences of these changes are considered. Ironically the conflict in Mozambique had protected some areas from being logged since land mines and ambushes made them too dangerous for vehicles to enter. Deforestation finally arrived on the agenda as an issue of wider concern at the recent debates on future land policy, where one agriculture official warned that at the current pace logging would 'destroy the hardwood forests of Sofala province as a meaningful renewable resource within five years' (AIM 1996d, p3). A further factor that requires close investigation in that area is non-traditional and out of season forest burning. This is carried out to extract game meat and is spurred on by the huge profits which can now be made by selling it to the cities.

A direct link between widespread environmental degradation at Gorongosa and ill-health has not yet been accurately established in terms of specific disease incidence.[5] However, existing knowledge of the importance of primary subsistence in protecting against ill-health, described in Chapter 6, would suggest that shortages of fuelwood, erosion of land surfaces, reduced scope for cultivation and siltation of water supply, all process that are provoked by devegetaion, would cause a reduction in quality of life and greater vulnerability to disease infection.

---

[5] A future assessment would require, amongst other investigations, specific research to determine the consequences of increasing denudation of this upland landscape on rainfall and groundwater levels.

Changing Contexts, Changing Behaviour, and Health

This subsection provides some evidence that structural changes in Mozambique have encouraged changes in community behaviour and that these have influenced incidence of diarrhoeal disease in urban areas. Since social cohesion has implications for community involvement in reducing risk of infection from disease, its changing characteristics at different places is likely to be important in assessing varied contextual influences. Some of the data presented in Chapter 6 and further information presented in this sub-section suggest that the level of internal community co-operation of different areas has played a role in defining disease locales. As such, this raises the likelihood of some influence on health as having resulted from structural influences on community behaviour.

Some evidence of differences in community co-operation between the field sites is evident from the response to the survey questions which enquired whether the respondent helped their neighbour when they were ill, and who helped them when they were ill (Table 7.1). The first question was followed by asking how help was administered to confirm the validity of the response. Almost 80 per cent of people in Quelimane indicated that they helped their neighbour as opposed to 52.6 per cent in Beira and 20.6 per cent in Gorongosa. In Quelimane only 0.7 per cent said that nobody helped them when sick whilst in Beira this was 44.9 per cent and in Gorongosa 55.9 per cent. In Quelimane 50 per cent said that help included assistance from their neighbours, whilst in Beira this was 22 per cent and in Gorongosa only 5.9 per cent. The differences indicate a distinct possibility of there being a variation in positive and negative behaviours that may reduce defences of certain communal areas to disease. It supports the earlier indications in Chapter 6 that there is greater inter-personal co-operation in Quelimane than in Beira and Gorongosa.

It can be argued that greater co-operation and co-ordination could be observed in Quelimane than in Beira because there was less commodification of basic survival requirements. Also, the uneven distribution of housing, differential access to water and contrasts in vulnerability through local environmental disasters such as flooding are more pronounced in Beira. The newly emerging market is also much more developed in Beira and, second to Maputo, it is widely recognised as

Table 7.1 Internal community assistance during illness

		QUELIMANE		BEIRA		GORONGOSA	
Question	*Answer*	No.	(%)	No.	(%)	No.	(%)
Do you help your neighbour when they are ill?	Yes	120	(79.5)	119	(52.6)	14	(20.6)
	No	31	(20.5)	107	(47.4)	54	(79.4)
Who helps you when you or your family are ill?	Family only	59	(38.8)	66	(29.1)	24	(35.3)
	Neighbours included[a]	76	(50.0)	50	(22.0)	4	(5.9)
	Neighbours not included[b]	16	(10.5)	9	(4.0)	2	(2.9)
	Nobody	1	(0.7)	102	(44.9)	38	(55.9)

Notes:
[a] Respondents indicating that their neighbours are amongst those who offer help.
[b] Respondents indicating that their neighbours are not amongst those who offer help.

having the highest crime rate in the country.[6] Though a high crime rate can to some extent unite people's resolve to take to action there is an overall negative affect on community continuity since suspicions begin to develop between different neighbourhood groups. Increases in corruption, crime and selfishness in the work place have been mentioned by Hanlon (1991) as part and parcel of Mozambique's restructuring and a change apparent to people who worked in local state structures before structural adjustment. Quelimane managed to maintain much greater continuity with its own development, over and above the fact that it is a smaller city, in that it escaped much of the rapid infusion of 'aid' and commercial activity (much of it foreign) that descended on Beira at the end of the 1980s.

Divisions in wealth exacerbated by new found opportunities for a few people can have a negative influence on behaviour if members of a closely integrated community cease to co-operate with each other on issues of

---

[6] Though no official data for this assertion is available, this statement is based on information offered by residents (and first hand experience) in 5 of Mozambique's cities. This assessment was also frequently made by Beira residents during consultation with local authorities and individuals. Crime in this context primarily refers to theft and violence for financial gain.

prime importance, such as sanitation. Though the official state community organizations which co-ordinated people into work parties for cleaning campaigns, and groups for health education have gone, more of what they represented is still apparent in Quelimane than in Beira. For example, in Quelimane it is still considered taboo to charge people to take water from a well outside your house, since the concept of communal ownership lives on, a situation that has weekend in Beira. Whereas in Beira there was no direct response to the fact that the water supply was cut to a large area of two *bairros*, in Quelimane direct action was taken. For example, two instances were found where local households got together and connected up their own hose pipe to the underground piped water supply without the water company knowing about it. When it was eventually discovered another one was established in someone else's back yard. These served all the people of that part of the *bairro*. Though this is illegal it may further serve to demonstrate how the local community at Quelimane is more prone to banding together to address a problem.

The concentration of wealth into the hands of a few also has infrastructural implications relating to ownership of land and water that are affecting many peoples' access to basic amenities they depend on. Access is lost to wells which disappear behind walls and fences, and unused areas of waste land that were used for defecation, previously available to everybody, are less available as more plots are privately owned and become fenced off. Privatisation of land plots in some instances has also removed the possibility of a cultivation plot. In the past the *Conselho Executivo* (City Council) had a policy of tolerance regarding cultivation of plots that were not occupied by a house.

One further factor that deserves some mention in comparing the sense of community in the two cities is ethnic origin, which is much more diverse in Beira than Quelimane. Data collected in the household survey revealed that in addition to Portuguese there were eight household languages in use in Beira, three in Gorongosa, and only one in Quelimane. This can be extended to two in Quelimane if the closely related Lomwe sub-dialect of Chuabo from Alta Zambézia is included. There is evidence that in colonial times racism and 'tribalism' caused a diminished sense of community in Beira. The best record of this is available as a collection of personalised accounts provided by elderly residents (José 1989). Besides racism by Portuguese, English and Afrikaans residents, there are accounts of community tensions between indigenous tribal groups leading in some instances to large scale street fights and deaths (Mucacho in José 1989, p189).

One of FRELIMO'S biggest campaigns when it came to power in 1975 was to create a sense of national unity. Speeches by the late president Samora Machel referred to the need to stamp out racism, tribalism and sexism (Munslow 1985). Visitors and foreign employees to the country regularly comment on the relative achievements of this in contrast to several of its neighbouring countries. Since Independence, the government has been able to boast that its members represented all the main racial and ethnic groups. In more recent years, the main opposition party RENAMO has also made this claim.

Despite these achievements, there is greater evidence of a reappearance of some 'tribalism' in recent years than at any other post-independence period, and this is more apparent in Beira than other parts of the country.[7] One example of this was a major split within the widely attended catholic church of Beira in 1994, over whether the languages masena or mandau should be used in Mass. Whilst many churches have grown used to using combinations of languages, some church leaders tried to promote mandau as the official language. Political differences have also been strongest in Beira, where significantly higher support for opposition parties has been achieved in comparison to all other parts of the country (AIM 1994). It is the birth place of the opposition leader Alfonso Dlakama, and for many years was home to Jonas Savimbi, leader of Angola's opposition group UNITA. Whereas the centre of the country has always been the opposition's home region, the demise of support for the government in that area has caused the political situation in Mozambique to become more regionally polarised and less of an ideological dispute than ever before.

As Quelimane represents a city that has suffered fewer of the mechanisms whereby community co-operation is reduced, then it might be expected that an extension of the trend of greater co-operation would apply to the smaller district capital of Gorongosa. However, the comparison is not entirely valid since the level of direct war disruption has been so much greater in Gorongosa. The result in Table 7.1 showing that the majority of people said that nobody helped them when ill and that they did not help others may have been affected by the recent tradition of aid delivery to that

---

[7] This point is made purely by way of comparison with previous years and is not intended to imply that tribalism is a prime concern in Mozambique.

area. This is because of the perceived need to advertise a situation of need to survey personnel. However, a local custom of not interfering in your neighbour's misfortunes was presented as a further explanation by a resident from birth who works for the local health service.

Doubts about limitations in community co-operation in Gorongosa did not apply to water supply. Innovation in creating techniques to obtain good water were better than in the cities, although some advantages were provided by the natural environment. The dire circumstances of Gorongosa during the war which restricted the population from getting to the main rivers, and the drought of 1992, meant that necessity became the mother of invention. For example, a common solution for obtaining clean water is submerging half an oil drum in the bed of a small stream with the top above the water level. The water is scooped from the oil drum and clean water filters up through the stream bed to replace it (Figure 7.3a). In another instance an underground source of water was harvested by inserting a banana stem into the side of cut away earth to directly tap it (Figure 7.3b). The water falls from a height into the bucket avoiding intermediary contamination. In other instances creative use of two levels of water collection where being employed by sculpturing the banks of streams and using the upper level solely for drinking water (Figure 7.3c). All of these examples were found to harbour no or comparatively low levels of faecal coliforms, and had good water quality conditions of a slightly acidic pH, and low conductivity.

The importance of culture and behaviour and its significance in health was also demonstrated by care seeking behaviour. The questionnaire surveys found that traditional medicine was still held in high esteem, despite it being discouraged after independence. Whilst 81 per cent of all those interviewed had used modern treatments for diarrhoea, 42 per cent of all those interviewed still made supplementary visits to the traditional healer. This demonstrates the strength of alternative local perspectives despite hundreds of years of external influence. Regardless of differences in opinion over the merits of the remedies that are used, there is arguably an important role for traditional structures in enhancing a community's sense of well-being through emphasising its own solutions to health problems. To date, external interventions have largely dictated the changes in approach for local areas and have had the capacity to cause a negative affect on behaviour with consequent implications for health issues. This theme was reflected at the wider scale in President Chissano's call to officials in Beira to seek internal solutions to problems rather than wait for

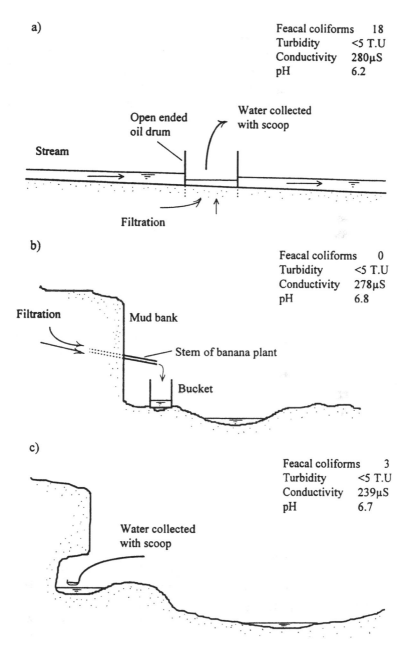

a)

Feacal coliforms   18
Turbidity   <5 T.U
Conductivity   280μS
pH   6.2

Open ended oil drum

Water collected with scoop

Stream

Filtration

b)

Feacal coliforms   0
Turbidity   <5 T.U
Conductivity   278μS
pH   6.8

Filtration

Mud bank

Stem of banana plant

Bucket

c)

Feacal coliforms   3
Turbidity   <5 T.U
Conductivity   239μS
pH   6.7

Water collected with scoop

Figure 7.3   Innovations in water supply at Gorongosa: a) open ended oil drum in river bed; b) plant stem inserted into mud bank; c) use of two water levels

international aid (AIM 1995).

Conclusion

This chapter has shown that whilst incidence of cholera and dysentery is affected by local environmental factors and differences in adaptation of disease pathogens, changes in infrastructure and the wider development process remain important underlying influences. It confirms the need for a comprehensive approach to health and disease, as called for by Hughes and Hunter (1970) and Stock (1986), illustrating some of the mechanisms whereby the development process in Mozambique has been influential.

Changes in the physical infrastructure and in local administration of services have been identified in the field sites. One key issue is that the infrastructure and policies of the past have clashed with present initiatives with implications for preventative health, local empowerment and the environment. Increasing heterogeneity in the quality of the built environment and accentuated inequality, particularly well reflected in conditions at Beira, represent a barrier to reducing overall disease risk. The emphasis on marketing the water supply is problematical because, although it aims to implement a 'communal system', it does so without encouraging a sense of community. Ability to pay for improved services is low, suggesting that limited improvements can be made using market orientated solutions. The World Bank has interpreted this type of situation rather as one where *willingness* to pay for improved services is low, and responds as follows: 'For those communities that believe the government should provide water services free-of-charge, once government paternalism ceases, the communities may become more willing to pay' (World Bank Research Observer 1993; Briscoe 1993).

Changes in the health service in effect represent an extension of the principle of health care as a form of social control, present in former systems in Mozambique. Despite using terminology such as 'participation', the effect of structural adjustment in health care in practice is more synonymous with a return to a top down approach. A lessening of the importance of community involvement and proactive policies accompanied by an increase in commodification contributes to behaviour which affects well-being and health. There are likely to be further implications for health emanating from environmental change associated with large scale impacts on Mozambique's natural resources.

Though much common rhetoric is used amongst global institutions, there remain fundamental differences in interpretation and emphasis. For example, a report of WHO Expert Committee (1991a) on 'environmental health in urban development' largely addresses the disease burden in terms of population expansion, environmental constraints, community organisation and management. Meanwhile the main thrust of The World Bank (1993) report on 'investing in health' addresses health problems in developing countries almost exclusively in terms of finance, economic development and health care. Structural adjustment aimed at creating economic recovery in Third World countries directly and indirectly affects the health of people in vulnerable regions. Whilst the full impact has not yet developed, it is becoming clearer that globalisation of policy fails to assist affected people who are closest to their own difficulties and appropriate remedies. The success of future environmental health policy will depend on the extent to which it enables people to gain effective control of their local community resources. Overall, there remains great potential in encouraging community empowerment in environmental health issues as this will further enable the emergence of solutions which are sensitive to local environments, historical contexts, and culture. The diversity produced by this approach will limit the extent to which evolving diseases can gain an advantage in local environments and communities.

8 Emergent Ecology of Disease and Health in Mozambique: Implications and Applications of a Geo-holistic Perspective

This chapter seeks to draw together the research detailed in this book and consider its wider policy implications through an up to date understanding of diarrhoeal disease ecology. Previous chapters have identified influences on health resulting from different disease ecologies, as well as the broader role of socio-economic factors. As such, changes in health phenomena are seen as being guided both by evolutionary processes in the natural world and less deterministic processes associated with human development and behaviour. Disease distributions are altered by human impacts on their immediate ecology and by changes in susceptibility to infection. Meanwhile, wider structural changes and policy influence the context within which a health disaster can emerge.

The contents of this book illustrate that the physical environmental and societal influences on diarrhoeal disease incidence are dependent on the nature of the disease and individual locales. It is further maintained that major disease events can be identified as, not just a product of interaction between a complex of influences but, an outcome of coinciding windows of opportunity presented by pathogen ecology, environmental change and the human condition. Some of the complexity of the disease events at the field sites has been unravelled through fieldwork, enabling specific recommendations for prevention. Policy issues include avoiding areas and environmental transformations conducive to greater survivability of the pathogen, improving defences against infection through community based initiatives in primary subsistence, limiting structural adjustments which disrupt the continuity of local perspectives, and maintaining a more public approach to health care.

The Ecology of Cholera and Bacillary Dysentery at Quelimane, Beira and Gorongosa: Theoretical Issues

The specific objectives of the research described in this book were achieved through extensive primary field research in central Mozambique. New knowledge included the conclusion that physical environmental factors, identified through existing laboratory work to favour the survival of *Vibrio cholerae* 01, influenced the distribution of incidence of cholera caused by the Ogawa serotype at Quelimane. This result was reinforced by the contrasting distribution of incidence of bacillary dysentery, a further resurgent and evolving diarrhoeal disease with a different ecology to that of cholera. By way of contrast with Quelimane, the conclusion that the distributions of the two diseases at Beira were similar is consistent with a more general association of diarrhoeal disease with infrastructural conditions in that city. This explanation was supported by the conclusion that the serotype of *Vibrio cholerae* responsible for cholera at Beira is associated with a more recent epidemic strain and as such was responsible for a distribution of infection with greater similarity to that of epidemic bacillary dysentery.

The results suggest that the nature of the bacilli of different diarrhoeal diseases is associated with different environmental and human terrains and that inappropriate changes to these encourage epidemic outbreaks of disease. However, in determining influential processes on emergent disease some key issues remain open to debate. For example, though the conditions that can influence patterns of disease emergence in Mozambique have been examined, it is not known to what extent microbial evolution may have occurred, and if so, whether this has been primarily a response to environmental changes. Though it has been possible to explore environmental, socio-economic and behavioural associations with respect to different types of diarrhoeal disease, it remains unproven whether spatial changes in the prevalence of a specific serotype occurs via genetic adaptation of an existing pathogen or through being displaced by an incoming strain.

Whichever is more accurate a representation of the biological processes underlying emergence and re-emergence of infectious disease, the consequence has been varying distributions of incidence which are to a large extent reflective of specific disease ecologies and varying locales. For example, the more endemic strain of *Vibrio cholerae* was responsible for cholera in Quelimane because of favourable physical environmental conditions and the less dynamic development context of that city.

Defences against ill-health have improved throughout the last century and some diseases have been eradicated. However progress in disease eradication is not a linear development. Rather, diminution, emergence and re-emergence of pathogens has been determined by decreases and increases in environmental and human susceptibility. In the case of cholera, the changing physiological status of local environments can provide the opportunity for a dormant endemic strain to cause an epidemic. In the case of less environmentally endemic diseases, such as dysentery, similar principles of adaptation and opportunism apply to the pathogen in the human host. For example, dysentery is an invasive infection where *bacilli* penetrate the walls of the intestines. As such the disease has adapted a means of using the human body for longer term survival. The disease develops resistance to new antibiotic drugs to remain viable in a human reservoir. Meanwhile cholera *vibrios* are non-invasive and do not penetrate the walls of the intestines, instead irritating the small intestine to the point of causing extreme diarrhoea which evacuates them back into the external environment. This would explain in evolutionary terms why cholera *vibrios* have become more adapted to their occupation of the external environment. Although there has been some success in suppressing infection by these diseases through treating the symptoms, the adaptive ability of pathogens is an ongoing global concern, as indicated by the constantly changing spatial and temporal distributions of cases.

Whilst earlier research on health and population displacement had focused on specific refugee populations amongst whom there has been elevated incidence of diarrhoeal disease, a distinct lack of research focused on the health circumstances of forcibly displaced people who resettle in urban areas. A combination of previous studies and preliminary field work in Mozambique suggested that the role of population displacement in influencing health might operate through changes in exposure to local disease environments, increased susceptibility, and through the impacts of resettlement on the environment. After detailed research the health implications of population displacement observed in three urban areas of central Mozambique were found to be less a function of mobility *per se* than the nature of the physical and social environment into which people resettle. The epidemicity and endemicity of different pathogens which affected all groups of residents was a function of locational circumstances rather than importation and diffusion of pathogens through relocation from one area to another. As such it was the underlying terrain that has guided incidence of diarrhoeal disease. Further to establishing the importance of different locales, migration has 'caused' a worsening of health conditions for some forced migrants, because of their exposure to a deteriorated environment at the place of relocation.

In the case of elevated incidence of cholera caused by an endemic pathogen at Quelimane, it is suggested that population pressures exacerbated by migration had an influence on the environment favouring the survivability and virulence of *Vibrio cholerae*. Overall, an emphasis on the role of an interplay between pathogen ecology and local changes in environmental and societal terrain is reinforced. The results and analyses presented in this book are also of interest in that, additional to confirming the role of place specific factors affecting diarrhoeal disease incidence in these specific locations, they contrast with many earlier accounts of the health of refugees and forcibly displaced people in Africa. As reviewed in Chapter 2, existing accounts typically record significantly higher than expected rates of incidence of severe diarrhoea amongst refugees when compared with host populations.

In as much as the patterns of disease incidence have been shown to be a function of spatial variation in environment and society, it proved essential to consider underlying structural influences affecting the field locations. For example, Mozambique's colonial past, pro-active administration following Independence, and recent period of structural adjustment have had implications for health through associated changes in habitation, water supply, sanitation, health care and the local economy. Also, different social circumstances at Beira were reflected by higher rates of dysentery and greater susceptibility of the forcibly displaced. It is argued that this was associated with the greater loss of community co-operation and disenfranchisement of the population that accompanied the city's development.

The above assessment indicates that changes in infrastructure and the wider development process are influencing the nature of local environments and sustainability with implications for health. One mechanism by which this occurs is through weakening of existing survival strategies and defences against ill-health. The negative impact of structural adjustment on local well-being can extend to include disruption of a local sense of commitment to assist in combating ill-health. One irony is that in the post Independence years government policy was theoretically that of a centralised system, but in practice accommodated local representation and participation through its Dynamizing Groups, establishment of local heads of *Bairros*, and recruitment of *grass roots* primary health care personnel. Though the rhetoric of the 1990s encouraged by international institutions is one of decentralisation, in reality people have often ended up with less control over and representation in local health decisions than before.

The dominant socio-economic trend in recent years has been dictated by the struggle to generate foreign currency that is increasingly needed to pay off international debt and repair damage done during the war. The IMF recognises some of the problems that have ensued in such a weak economy and accepts the necessity to reschedule Mozambique's foreign debt. However, the IMF also insisted that this must be accompanied by the implementation of a further strong economic adjustment programme to bring in higher revenue (AIM 1996a). As such most other development perspectives are being restrained. For example, although environmental protection is increasingly included in the rhetoric of international finance organizations and in government policy since the Rio summit of 1992, there is little real evidence of it having much effect whilst economic demands on resources prevail. Further to this there are genuine difficulties in implementing such an approach, which is primarily based on perceptions of the environment from the post-industrial nations. Ecological principles rooted in indigenous perceptions are currently on the side lines, mainly because they are perceived as less relevant to economic development by the dominant local, national and international institutions. However, it can be argued that amongst the poorest parts of the world aspirations for better standards of living are more likely to be met by adhering to the essential guidelines for development that a local ecological awareness can provide.

There are grounds to suggest that an underlying weakness in combating ill-health occurs when control, power and self-determination of local communities are not enhanced. This shortcoming occurs despite an increase in awareness at senior administrative level of its effectiveness in correcting negative changes to local environmental health issues (WHO 1991b). Community action is far from a new concept in Mozambique but has arguably been suppressed, through conflict and structural changes. One example of community action, which represented a degree of local empowerment was the Dynamizing Groups. These provided a forum for local residents to voice opinions and were amongst other things used to organise cleaning brigades to improve levels of hygiene.

The Implications of Macro-scale Environmental Change for Incidence of Cholera and Bacillary Dysentery

The complex nature of the world's climate and ocean circulation and the unpredictability of change caused by human inputs mean that prediction of the full implications of the changing distribution of associated bacteria remains difficult. However, further effects of climate change on cholera in some countries may result from sea level rise, reduction of rainfall, and decreases in crop yields. Rising sea levels could change the balance between salt and fresh water in the low lying estuarine environments of cholera prone regions such as parts of India, Bangladesh, Pakistan, Indonesia, Thailand, Egypt, Nigeria and Mozambique. In the event of further rising sea-levels, pumping stations would have to be located further inland and coastal well water would become subject to more frequent incursions of brackish ground water. Flooding by sea water would also leave more inland lagoons of water with physical conditions favourable to the longevity of *Vibrio cholerae*. This would be intensified by the spread of unprotected sewage in flood waters.

Reduction of rainfall in the interiors of continents, another possible outcome of change to the global atmosphere-hydrosphere-cryosphere balance, could also increase incidence of inland brackish environments. The processes involved are twofold; firstly, through a shift in the fresh water and salt water margin in coastal zones and secondly, through increased evaporation and capillary rise of saline groundwater. A warning of the effects of change in the margin where fresh and saline water meet was experienced in the estuarine cities of Beira and Quelimane during the drought of 1992 where water sources were turned off on the grounds of being too saline to drink or because they dried up altogether. Desalination plants are generally expensive to maintain and are therefore only usually considered by countries with the combination of extreme fresh water shortages and extensive financial resources, such as Saudi Arabia.

Salinization and alkalinization, both of which favour *Vibrio cholerae*, are increasingly brought about by human activity. For example, the high density of people without access to an urban water network in Jakarta, Indonesia meant that large numbers of private wells were sunk. This caused heavy overpumping of the local aquifer and a fall in the water table to the extent that in northern Jakarta, sea water has contaminated the groundwater in a 5 to 10 kilometre-wide continuous belt along the coastal plain (Briscoe 1993). According to the Council on Environmental Quality

(1981), about half the world's irrigated lands have been damaged to some extent by salinization or alkalinization. Kovda (1972) estimated that about 60-70 per cent of all irrigated land was gradually being transformed into 'saline deserts'.

A further factor, which has serious implication for predisposing some communities to infection by diarrhoeal diseases and which is influenced by environmental change, is nutrition. Quantitative estimates of the effects of climate change on the amount of food produced, world food prices, and people at risk from hunger in developing countries made by the Goddard Institute for Space Studies and the Environmental Change Unit in Oxford (Rosenzweig *et al.* 1992) indicated that crop yields are likely to decline in low latitude regions but could increase at mid-high latitudes. Greatest declines in world cereal production were predicted in the developing countries where there could be an average estimated reduction of between 8 per cent and 12 per cent due to changes in rainfall. The number of people at risk from hunger was estimated to increase between 5 per cent and 50 per cent with the greatest absolute increase predicted to be in Africa (Haines and Parry 1993). Additionally, less rainfall in some countries causes a reduction in availability of drinking water. More people are likely to use inappropriate water sources in these circumstances. The outcome of these environmental pressures consistently occurring in the same parts of the world, such as during the series of droughts and famines that occurred in the Horn of Africa and Mozambique throughout the 1980s, is likely to be further displacement of populations. Congestion of these people into fewer viable resettlement locations with often poor water and sanitation would further enhance the probability of communicable disease epidemics.

Macro scale environmental and demographic differences are likely to explain the changing distribution of non-01 *Vibrio cholerae* that has recently taken on massive proportions in India and Bangladesh. This first recorded epidemic caused by a non-01 *Vibrio cholerae* accounted for over 15,000 cases and 230 deaths in Calcutta in its initial stages alone (Sarkar *et al.* 1993). In Bangladesh the epidemic began in December, 1992, in the south and spread throughout the country with a total of 107,297 cases and 1,473 deaths by the end of March 1992 (ICDDR,B 1993). The first report of the dispersion of *Vibrio cholerae* 0139 outside the region was to Bangkok (Chongsa-nguan *et al.* 1993). Chongsa-nguan *et al.* point out that whilst the seventh pandemic strain of cholera, the El Tor, took three years to spread from Celebres island in Indonesia through Bangkok to India from its first isolation in 1961, the 0139 strain of *Vibrio cholerae* is disseminating much faster. The organism is reported as causing local outbreaks in geographically distant sites and of having the potential of pandemic spread and of virtually replacing *Vibrio cholerae* 01, as happened in India and Bangladesh (Jesudason *et al.* 1993, 1994; Islam *et al.* 1993). Although the latest reports indicate that the epidemic due to serotype 0139 may be on the wane, and that high incidence in Bangladesh is again attributable to the 01 serotype (Faruque *et al.* 1996), the unpredictable appearance of new pathogenic serotypes remains an ongoing concern.

Cholera in the early 1990s became so widespread that there arose the possibility of more general climatic differences between zones north and south of the equator providing a continuum of favourable background conditions the whole year round, such as between the affected zones stretching the length of South and Central America or Africa. Variation of strains between regions and relative lack of serotype immunity of the people occupying one area against that of the other might be subject to a seasonal dimension if one *Vibrio* type maintains a different environmental sensitivity to that of the other. A hint of this occurring is presented by the reciprocal pattern in prevalence of *Vibrio cholerae* 0139 with *Vibrio cholerae* 01 in Bangladesh reported by Jesudason and John (1993).

The low level of immunity to the new strain of the disease is demonstrated by the fact that the first few years of *Vibrio cholerae* 0139 affected more adults than children. Once widespread immunity has developed, most adults are protected and more cases are found in young children (Swerdlow and Ries 1993). Since specific immunity to the 01 serotype did not provide immunity to the 0139 serotype, greater virulence of the organism during an age of increased travel and large population movements has seriously threatened to produce further large scale disease events. The phenomenon of forced population displacement, experienced by millions in recent times, leads to concentrations of people who are not only economically and biologically vulnerable but who have moved away from zones of relative immunity into areas where exposure to new disease pathogens is heightened.

The spontaneity of occurrences of cholera and dysentery epidemics in modern times suggests a possible globalisation of opportunity for those diseases to develop. Loss of diversity between regions carries the risk of a loss of protection against location specific disease. Heterogeneity as a form of protection against disease that attacks non-human species is well understood by agriculturists, agronomists and horticulturists. It remains to be investigated the extent to which similar principles apply to the current status of infectious diseases in the environment and in communities of people. In the past cholera was also a disease of temperate regions. The relative ease with which it was removed from those regions through changes to the human environment is mirrored by the relative ease with which new strains with a slightly different ecological range can return to the same regions in epidemic proportions. This is demonstrated by the disappearance of cholera from South America in 1867 and its dramatic reappearance in January 1991. It is a reminder of the fragile balance between health, ill-health, and a changing environment.

The existence of new serogroups of *Vibrio cholerae*, such as 0139, amongst the predisposing conditions of poor sanitation, continued lack of clean water provision, and a deteriorating physical environment in many parts of the Third world will ensure that large scale epidemics of cholera are likely to continue. Where there exists suitable environmental reservoirs for its survival, the long term results will be the creation of further endemic zones and a new geography of cholera.

Human Conflict as Enhancer of Cholera and Dysentery

Human conflict provides communicable disease with some of the greatest opportunities for increase. Poignant demonstrations of this are the increased prevalence of cholera and dysentery epidemics in refugee camps, as detailed by Mulholland (1985), Moren and Stefanagge *et al.* (1991), Shears and Lusty (1987), and Sørensen and Dissler (1986). Further examples are the cholera and dysentery outbreaks that accompanied the aftermath of the Iraq war and amongst the survivors of the Rwandese genocide. Khan *et al.* (1979) warned of further effects noting that, not only did the number of *Shigella dysenteriae* 1 isolations increase dramatically during the period which covered the liberation war in Bangladesh, but also a higher proportion of strains became multiply resistant during that period.

During the concentration of hundreds of thousands of Rwandan war refugees into zones across the border in Zaire and Tanzania there was immense disruption of survival mechanisms, widespread environmental degradation and extensive disease. The largest epidemics were in Goma, Zaire where almost 50,000 refugees died, due to diarrhoeal disease, first caused by *Vibrio cholerae* 01 serotype Ogawa and subsequently by *Shigella dysenteriae* 1 (Goma Epidemiology Group 1995). The catastrophic nature of this event was that 25,000 people a day arrived in

Zaire from Rwanda (over 1 million in four days) and that 6,000 cases of severe diarrhoea were reported in just one day of the epidemic (The Goma Epidemiology Group 1995, p341). Médicins Sans Frontières employed its largest ever contingent in the Goma region (Byrne 1994) but were unable to prevent the disaster developing (The Times, August 1994). Conditions were so bad that it caused a return movement back across the border despite continued security concerns. Large quantities of people returning remained infected with cholera.

Some important observations can be made about the epidemics. Firstly, both cholera and dysentery were already endemic in the region. A clue to the endemicity of cholera there was that serotype Ogawa rather than Inaba was isolated, consistent with other accounts of endemicity in Africa already outlined in this book. Also of interest is that the two main river sources in that area were reported as being heavily alkaline by technical teams struggling to neutralise it for drinking purposes (Byrne 1994). On the basis of recent micro-biological details it is not unreasonable to suggest that *Vibrios* survived in this environmental reservoir prior to refugee arrivals. The association of contaminated lake water, which was the common drinking water source, was recognised as a major reason for the rapid transmission (Goma Epidemiology Group 1995, p342), but it is possible that *Vibrio cholerae* was also autochthenous to that environment. Indication of the endemicity of *Shigella dysenteriae* 1 in the community prior to the disaster are that there had already been severe attacks in recent years (Ries and Wells *et al.* 1994), with estimated cases of 50,000 in Burundi (WHO personal communication 1993), and that there was resistance to similar antibiotics in both present and past epidemics (Ries and Wells *et al.* 1994, p1035; Goma Epidemiology Group 1995, p341).

The sequence of cholera followed by dysentery may be related to differential endemicity of the pathogens in the physical environment and the community, cholera having the more immediate impact as the people drank the water and dysentery resurgent in existing carriers as resistance diminished. In both cases lowered nutritional status will have played a role in increasing the odds of infection, poor sanitation and congestion increasing the opportunity for secondary transmission. Meanwhile back in Rwanda there was a potentially good harvest, one of the best years for some time. In Angola, potentially one of the richest countries in Africa, harvests for 1994 would also have been good, but ongoing intensive fighting and displacement of people caused widespread malnutrition. Cholera and other communicable diseases abounded in contrast to the decline of cholera in Mozambique where a successful peace accord was achieved in October 1992.

Determinism and Possibilism in Environmental Health: Methodological Issues and a Geographical Research Strategy

Existing research has emphasised the importance of epidemiological surveillance for communicable disease monitoring. Toole and Waldman (1988) have indicated its potential relevance amongst refugees in Somalia, Sudan and Thailand and Moren and Bitar *et al.* (1991) amongst Mozambican refugees in Malawi. Siddique and Zaman *et al.* (1992) outline the absence of reliable surveillance as one of the factors responsible for excess deaths during the cholera epidemics in Bangladesh between 1985 and 1991. They call for 'effective simple and representative surveillance in the country which could provide early warning signals for impending outbreaks' (p79). Though still in its infancy, some of the technological tools for turning this aspiration into reality are already available as computer workstations for famine early warning and food security (Marsh and Hutchinson *et al.* 1994). Babille and Colombani *et al.* (1994), who monitored health trends amongst 25,000 displaced Kurds, called for international agencies and NGOs in the field to extend their use of available technology to monitor health and disease amongst refugees, returnees and the permanently displaced. Whilst recognising some limitation in mistakenly assessing the proportion of risk attributable to the disaster rather than the post-disaster experience, they point out that 'Comparative data and data on trends from cross-sectional and prospective studies ... can help to identify and solve specific health problems when the international donors begin to lose interest' (p73).

Labonte (1992) has drawn attention to the potential of community based approaches in describing local surveillance of the spread of cholera in South America in 1991. Referring to the same events in the Amazon region, Quick and Vargas *et al.* (1993) suggest a long-term strategy which includes 'an effort to provide health training to residents of every village, and to develop a co-ordinated system of communication to provide a means of disseminating information rapidly' (p600).

Recent research indicating that zooplankton can be associated with the aquatic reservoir of *Vibrio cholerae* also provides opportunity for monitoring areas at risk from cholera. Using satellite telemetry of phytoplankton in coastal zones, which precedes the zooplankton bloom, it has been suggested that it may be possible to forecast outbreaks of cholera in endemic regions (Huq and Colwell *et al.* 1995). However, although this macro-scale approach may be a contribution, the results of this research suggest that more interactive and closely sensed information systems are needed to address the local complexity of the human disease environment. Conant (1994) points out in more general terms that human ecology and 'space age technology' will be around for a long time to come, with an increased involvement of anthropology in interpreting the results. Clearly, there will be more opportunity for detailed ecological studies with the future launch of satellites carrying sensors with a spatial resolution as low as one metre (Oppenheimer 1994), although such a resolution is not necessary for detecting algal blooms.

Surveillance and the Role of Geographical Health Information Systems in Third World Disease Epidemics

Whilst it is maintained that the results and implications of the research described in this book go beyond that attainable from GIS, limited by its intrinsic concern with physical space, there are some useful aspects of GIS as a tool for assisting in health research and management at a local level. In addition to the well-established capacity of GIS to store and output large quantities of data for cross-sectional associative analysis by use of different 'coverages' of areal, line and point data, three further uses were identified. As initially pointed out in Chapter 3, rather than being associated with the cutting edge of GIS technology in the industrialised world, these are considered as being of use in the circumstances of less developed areas and deserve some mention.

Firstly, where there was only very poor cartographic representation available, it was a relatively simple procedure to combine the best aspects of different maps plotted at different scales. It was also possible to add geographical co-ordinates where these were missing, and update missing detail such as roads and boundaries, using GPS's whilst in the field. Secondly, as was demonstrated in the sampling of field sites for the environmental tests, it was possible to interactively use the local knowledge of informants in identifying the current and heavily used water sources, since these were indicated and positioned in 'real time'. This can reduce error of interpretation or perception caused by unrepresentative pre-research cartographic material. It is a well-established phenomenon that cartographic representation unconsciously assigns subjective visual meaning and importance to the items is represents (Robinson and Sale *et al.* 1978, p281, Gould and White 1992). This is a strong point in the case of Third World cities using maps produced in the colonial period. These tended to perceive and uniformly cross-hatch large areas of suburb as 'spontaneous indigenous areas', whilst indicating intricate infrastructural detail for neighbouring European areas. Being able to identify locations interactively amidst the congested urban expansion of Third World countries, such as the position of initial isolated cases in a disease epidemic, in itself represents a useful application of GPS.

Thirdly, it became apparent that should a Geographical Health Information System (GHIS) be set up for use by the heterogeneous groups of policy makers in central and local government, this may assist in developing more integrated environmental health management through being a catalyst for co-operation. In this sense the application of GHIS extends beyond integrating the information to integrating the authors of the information.

These aspects of GIS and GPS can become useful for organisational assistance programmes dealing with emergency environmental health situations, when combined with improved understanding of the ecology and spatial epidemiology of communicable diseases. For example, understanding new patterns of cholera as they emerge may be particularly relevant in planning risk reduction strategies through determining the availability of more favourable zones or areas of avoidance for communities that suffer from recurring epidemics and in the resettlement of refugees and displaced populations. Surveillance can also benefit by monitoring levels of *Vibrio cholerae* in the physical environment using improved methods of detection, which allow for the identification of *vibrios* maintained in a temporary state of dormancy. This has the capacity to assist in delineating the distribution of possible zones of primary transmission. Also, deriving patterns of secondary transmission may be assisted by more rapid techniques for detecting *Vibrio cholerae* in cholera patients by use of coagglutination assay (Abbott and Janda 1993) and rapid diagnostic kits (Andersson and Morales *et al.* 1992; Carillo and Gilman *et al.* 1994).

The importance of applying advanced surveillance and early warning systems to emergence and re-emergence of diseases is not only important in terms of how much incidence or where it will occur, but also in terms of who and why? This requires understanding the defences and policies that best reduce the risk of increased vulnerability amongst different population sectors. The corollary of early warning of disease epidemics is that the best interventions can be applied at the right time. The need for this is crucial to all relief and development exercises but is rarely achieved. Frerks and Kliest *et al.* (1995) identify the consequences of mis-timing in relief and development as not only having a negative outcome for mitigation of initial periods of high mortality, but also in the devaluing of local coping mechanisms through over-application of aid during the subsequent recovery periods. Locally based information systems which draw on indigenous knowledge, and represent the integration of local needs, are best placed in guiding resource allocation and relief.

Further Comments on Field Methods

The soil density survey of the sites did not produce any clear results, despite some clear observations being made about different surface environments. Nonetheless, this part of the research deserves some mention here in that it serves as an example of how a plural approach to data collection can sometimes be more informative than over-simplified quantitative assessments.

Soil density tests to measure compaction were carried out in an attempt to confirm an association of population density with geophysical surface environments. However, the variation in the results was insufficient to draw any significant conclusions through this method. This could be due to the limitations of the soil-density technique in detecting relevant geomorphologic differences in areas with a high sand content. However, whilst experimentation with quantitative measures aimed at determining compaction turned out to have limited application, the presence of black alkali soils in the devegetated areas was in itself an indication of a changed surface environment, since they are not the natural local soils. This was confirmed by comparing the black alkalis found in the heavily populated areas with no vegetation with the nearby soils of areas that remain more vegetated. As might be expected the black alkali soils have a similar distribution to areas of higher alkalinity determined by the water analysis and are frequently found in the areas of high cholera incidence. They were never observed in the well-vegetated areas, which had low incidence of cholera.

Explanations for the existence of black alkali soils were considered partly to be related to the influence of frequent flooding and rapid evaporation due to there being little shade. Further contributing factors were a build up of ash from household fires (confirmed by close observation of the constituent parts of soil samples), and the deposition of soap laden waste water after washing in densely inhabited areas. These are further factors which suggest that environmental change conducive to favouring environmentally endemic cholera could result from a combination of geophysical processes and population pressure. Though the research has not ultimately needed to rely on detailed assessment of the geophysical processes which have been involved in changing surface environments, and indeed this would have been beyond the scope of this book, these results represent useful additional observations.

Further Comments on Epistemology

The research described in this book is also relevant to some epistemological issues. Rather than distracting from the specific objectives of the research, it was considered that a theoretical view of health contributes insights of potential relevance to tackling incidence of disease. Despite a dearth of applied investigations which integrate recent microbiological advances with contextual analysis, new information on pathogen ecology generated in laboratory conditions and used in this research, has proved to be important in understanding disease incidence in different field contexts. Further to this it is suggested in this book that the use of systems approaches to understand disease ecology is applicable to both the natural and social science perspectives. Principles of complexity in dynamic systems, where the whole is greater than its parts, and where dynamic order emerges, are common concepts relevant to both pathogen evolution and change in human society.

The overall disease system can be considered as having a highly intricate microstructure, but with emergent macrodynamics, a concept which is consistent with notions of complexity referred to in Chapter 3. A relevant theoretical aspect of identifying disease emergence as part of a complex system is that ultimately outcomes can become self constraining. Thus, it is reasonable to suggest that complex physical environmental and human terrains, supporting variable incidence of a disease, can periodically revert to being free of disease once an equilibrium of immunity has been re-established throughout the community.

Theoretically, devising strategies to intervene in the chaotic origins of disease emergence presents a greater challenge than intervening through creation of further defences against infection. However, by identifying emergent macrodynamics, trends in disease emergence can become easier to discern. This is assisted by observing the spatial and temporal coincidence of the predisposing aspects of nature and society that result in incidence of ill-health. For example, some advance warning of the likelihood of emergent infectious disease in an area can be gained by assessing ecosystem diversity, rapid environmental change, and human poverty. More intuitive approaches to health and disease, as characterised by many indigenous perceptions, have often proved to be an effective resource and may be evidence of the strength of this approach. Overall, it is suggested here that it is the indication of collective emergent phenomena in geographical areas or sectors of society that enables the identification of critical risk regions. Consistent with this perspective it is argued that there is considerable methodological value in using applied research, empirically based on the health consequences of environment and population displacement, as a framework for analysing the health implications of changes to local areas.

A further implication of the approach that has been used in this research is that understanding of the efficacy of different intervention strategies can be best gained by combining awareness of the deterministic aspects of disease, such as environmental and genetic adaptation, with awareness of underlying influences in decision making and administration. However, whereas identification of some deterministic aspects, such as inherent chaos and complexity in disease emphasise uncertainty, it is added here that identification of potentially negative aspects of policy may provide a more predictive capability.

In summary, this book has presented an essentially geographical and holistic outline of incidence of cholera and dysentery through discussion of the organism, its physical and human environment, and links to infrastructure and the wider development process. This perspective on health is valuable in that it provides understanding of the issues borne out of a multifaceted research strategy with due attention to circumstances unique in place and time. It provides a framework for empirical investigations of patterns and processes associated with cholera and dysentery, whilst it is also able to combine contextual understanding of the wider issues involved.

Policy Issues in Environmental Health Management

The results generated by this research apply to environmental health management issues in several ways. One immediate practical application is that guidelines for helping to reduce the incidence of cholera should take into account the nature of the physical environment in which vulnerable communities are located, and more specifically, that consideration should be given to risks posed by environmental reservoirs of *Vibrio cholerae*. The identification of risk areas is important for planning purposes, in determining whether or not there are more favourable zones for resettlement or areas which can be avoided by communities suffering from recurring epidemics. For example resettlement of large numbers of potentially susceptible people to less environmentally vulnerable areas at Quelimane would have reduced the tendency to exacerbate the emergence of more favourable environmental conditions for an endemic pathogen.

A factor in preventing the primary transmission and subsequent persistence of cholera in areas of established settlement would be in limiting processes of environmental change which could lead to the creation of physical conditions favourable to *Vibrio cholerae*, such as salinization and alkalinization. Theoretically, revegetation could revert alkalinised areas to becoming more acidic. However, it is recognised that this may be difficult given that the ground quality is already so poor, and it is unclear to what extent, if any, such action would have in reverting the incursion of saline water. Clearly, the possibilities for improving individual areas would need to be individually assessed. For the case of the worst areas of Quelimane described in this book, such as Manhawa, it would be reasonable to suggest that the occupants be offered better more elevated land in the north-eastern part of the municipality.[1] These areas would have been preferable as they would have become less congested and have used groundwater which is free from saline incursions and acidic. Further to this, more could be made of encouraging people to use simple water purification techniques, such as lowering the pH of drinking water by adding citrus juice.

---

[1] The theme of avoiding certain physiochemical factors may extend to include other additional influences on *Vibrio cholerae* which have been suggested since carrying out this research such as iron content (Patel and Isaäcson *et al.* 1995). Though this is unlikely to have been of specific relevance to the conditions at the field sites used in this research, the implication of its influence through corroding metal pipes and industrial effluents needs to be investigated.

This book has also suggested that monitoring the disease ecology of different habitats includes understanding how local communities develop their own defences against ill-health, and the health consequences of structural change. Generation of appropriate policy through awareness of the specific nature of different diseases, and the context within which they occur has the potential to be effective. It can be argued that economically intense interventionism, which has been the hallmark of structural adjustment, has failed to improve the standards of living of the worlds poorest communities (UNDP 1996). This was witnessed first hand in Mozambique between the period 1987 (the initiation of structural adjustment in Mozambique) to the mid 1990s. Such an approach has left the country with an unsustainable foreign debt of about $US5.5 thousand million that it did not have 10 years ago (AIM 1996b). A large percentage of international financial assistance for Mozambique is now associated with tending to this problem. For example, out of $881 million worth of funding pledged by donors at the World Bank's Consultative Group meeting on Mozambique in Paris on 20th April, 1996, $314 million (35.6%) was for debt relief, $295.2 million (33.5%) for economic investments (largely aimed at paying off more debt), and $181 million (20.6%) for balance of payments support (to facilitate the mechanisms for paying of debt). A further $56.9 million (6.5%) is tied up in food aid, leaving only $34.4 million (3.8%) for all 'other programmes'. Sadly it is from the smallest 'other programmes' proportion of this financing that there may be some trickling down of finance for environmental health issues. Also, if levels of incidence of the 'old diseases' of poverty and underdevelopment, such as cholera and dysentery, are to be used as a yardstick of well-being, there is further evidence that structural adjustment has failed in other Third World countries. The example of Peru, presented in Chapter 2, is a particularly clear case.

In so much as the environment can be socially constructed and therefore its interpretation subject to the idiosyncrasies of culture (Blaikie 1995), influences on policy in Mozambique, as elsewhere, reflect a complex of interests within which the most powerful set the agenda. At present this constitutes the now global perspective of economic development based on competition, commodification and financial borrowing. This has had an underlying effect of delinking economic decisions from their social consequences and largely explains the emerging trend of increasing intra-urban disparities in wealth and rise in related crime. Negative behavioural responses have resulted from a devaluation of local community perception of improvement in basic subsistence whilst economic initiatives expand at medium and macro level. This dichotomy of development has most recently been underwritten by manifestations of sectoral disenfranchisement, such as several major strikes by government employees and demonstrations by demobilised soldiers (AIM 1996c). Further disenfranchisement looms if the amendments to land policy, that have been debated amidst a widespread rush to acquire and 'develop', do not genuinely work in favour of protecting the rights of local communities (AIM 1996d; Meldrum 1996). Ironically, this threat has become greater at a time when local farming communities were producing one of their best grain harvests ever (AIM 1996d, p4).

Restoring confidence and co-operation in local administrations will require the creation of security in primary subsistence, namely water, sanitation, nutrition and fuel, and re-empowerment of local communities. This will hopefully form a central theme in the implementation of the Local Government Reform Project (PROL) for the cities of Mozambique. To be successful the programme will require avoiding 'public and corporate policy standardised to the global monoculture and deprived of ethics' (Bellamy and McIntosh 1996). The limitations of some humanitarian developmentalist perspectives relates to perceptions of the underlying nature of the situation which is being assisted. As such Myers (1994, p202) pointed out how Eurocentric perception of urban planning failed to recognise the 'disorderly order' of the 'spontaneous' urban settlements of 'Zanzibar's other side' (p195). It is suggested that the approaches to environmental health management advocated by a fully holistic understanding of disease in the environment and community, with an emphasis on information and awareness rather than intervention and restructuring, can avoid much of this shortcoming. In a practical sense this means further developing the concept of information systems which are based on local knowledge and perception of the issues concerned. Implementation of policies for avoiding areas, impacts on areas, and institutional mechanisms, conducive to ill-health will be a more feasible proposition if decision making is based within the communities concerned.

The most appropriate role of any assistance programme in such an approach would be in enhancing local skills and aspirations and/or in sharing any tried and tested approaches from similar situations elsewhere, rather than intervention *per se*. One suggested way in which this could be facilitated is through area resource centres for dealing with environmental health issues and community action plans in urban areas. Such an approach could be complimented by existing planning departments putting more emphasis on their role as an information service, and reducing their role as a legislative body. Community based initiatives grounded in local information may soon be recognised as the only way of appeasing some of the limitations of intervention and assistance perspectives. For example, Slim (1995) suggests that the western humanitarian perspective is already under threat of not being tolerated in some developing areas, and consequently predicts the demise of the role of the foreign 'expert'.

In conclusion, it is suggested by this book that it is possible to be non-presumptive about the complex nature of emerging health problems whilst gaining clear guidelines about preferred approaches in damage limitation. This is particularly the case in confirming or negating the independent or synergistic role of changing environmental, socio-economic, and contextual circumstances in disease affected zones. The extent to which the constitutive character of society-nature relations can be identified through the pattern of emergence of disease is important to understanding these phenomena and increasingly vital to environmental health management.

Research based on geographical perspectives has much still to offer in understanding the emerging ecology of disease. This book has indicated some of the methods and applications that are incorporated by such a perspective and has included some specific results that contribute to the study of cholera and dysentery. Whilst comparison between urban areas in central Mozambique has been achieved, further research is required to assess these and similar emergent health problems in different regions. This is important to understanding the spatial differences in ecology and processes of environmental change that predispose to disease epidemics, and because institutional frameworks for prevention have developed differently. Understanding the changes that enhance local disease ecologies and human vulnerability, hitherto only encountered in the context of one region, can assist in identifying more effective developments in prevention policy between different locations. This represents a bottom up approach to environmental health concerns and is of major relevance to understanding wider issues of development.

Many aspects of health ecology are crucially important to environmental management concepts and practices. This book has demonstrated why changing disease ecologies require individual research in changing locales and has indicated some of the ways in which this can be approached and achieved. It is maintained that there is much to be gained from exploring health ecology principles in the light of wider perspectives in environmental management and sustainable development. To have addressed this last point more extensively in this book would have greatly increased its size and detracted from its pathogenic and regional focus. I will therefore concentrate on this theme further elsewhere.

Bibliography

Abbott, S.L. and Janda, J.M. (1993), 'Rapid detection of acute cholera in airline passengers by coagglutination assay', *Journal of Infectious diseases*, vol. 168, pp. 797-9.

Abler, R.F. (1993), 'Everything in its place: GPS, GIS, and Geography in the 1990s', *Professional Geographer*, vol. 45:2, pp. 131-9.

Acra, A., Jurdi, M., Mu'Allem, H., Karahagopian, Y. and Raffoul, Z. (1989), 'Sunlight as disinfectant', *The Lancet*, vol. 1989,i, p. 280.

Adesina, H.O. (1987), 'The temporal and spatial analysis of cholera diffusion within Ibadan, Nigeria 1971 -1974', in R. Akhtar (ed), *Health and Disease in Tropical Africa: Geographical and Medical Viewpoints*, Univ. of Zambia 1987 and Harwood Academic Publishers, London, pp. 167-92.

Administração do Distrito de Gorongosa (1994), Posto Administrativo-Sede. 'Mapa estatístico da população do posto administrativo-sede'.

AFRICARE (1994), Unpublished data. 'Resultados do inquerito realizado na Cidade da Beira em Dezembro de 1993, Resultados Globais'.

Aguas da Beira (1992), in *Boletim Estatístico, Província de Sofala 1992*, Serviço Provincial de Estatística, Comissão Provincial do Plano de Sofala, República de Moçambique.

Ahmed, F., Clemens, J.D., Rao, M.R. and Sack, D.A. et al. (1992), 'Community-based evaluation of the effect of breast-feeding on the risk of microbiologically confirmed or clinically presumptive shigillosis in Bangladeshi children', *Pediatrics*, vol. 90:3, pp. 406-11.

Ahmed, F., Clemens, J.D., Rao, M.R. and Khan, M.R. et al. (1993), 'Initiation of food supplements and stopping of breast-feeding as determinants of weanling shigellosis', *Bulletin of the World Health Organization*, vol. 71:5, pp. 571-8.

Ahmed, F., Clemens, J.D., Rao, M.R. and Banik, A.K. (1994), 'Family latrines and paediatric shigellosis in rural Bangladesh: benefit or risk?', *International Journal of Epidemiology*, vol. 23:4, pp. 856-62.

AHRTAG (1993), 'Appropriate Health Resources and Technologies Action Group', *Dialogue on Diarrhoea*, vol. 53.

AIM (Agência de Informação de Moçambique) (1994), 'First offical election results', No 45 8th November, 1994.

AIM (Agência de Informação de Moçambique) (1995), 'Nation must seek internal solutions to compliment international aid', No 62 13th July, 1995.

AIM (Agência de Informação de Moçambique) (1996a), 'IMF plans to reschedule Mozambique's debt', No 80 21st March, 1996.

AIM (Agência de Informação de Moçambique) (1996b), 'Strong donor support for Mozambican development plans', No 83 2nd May, 1996.

AIM (Agência de Informação de Moçambique) (1996c), 'AMODEG calls for peaceful demonstrations', No 81 4th April, 1996.

AIM (Agência de Informação de Moçambique) (1996d), 'Major conference debates future of land policy', No 86 14th June, 1996.

Akogun, O.B (1992), 'The effect of selected health education schemes on knowledge and attitude of the Kanuri towards certain parasitic diseases', *Journal of the Royal Society of Health*, December 1992, pp. 180-285.

Al-Qarawi, S., Fontaine, R.E. and Al-Qahtani, M.S. (1995), 'An outbreak of Hemolytic Uremic Syndrome associated with antibiotic treatment of hospital inpatients for dysentery', *Emerging Infectious Diseases*, vol. 1:4, pp. 138-40.

Amin, S., Chitala, D. and Mandaza, T. (eds)(1987), *SADCC: Prospects for Disengagement and Development in Southern Africa*, The United Nations/Third World Forum. Studies in African Political Economy. Zed Books, London.

Anand, J.K. (1995), 'Cholera treatment in Goma' (Letter), *The Lancet* vol. 345, p. 1568.

Andersson, N., Morales, A. and Gillespie, S.H. (1992), 'Cholera: getting the message across', *British Medical Journal*, vol. 304, pp. 1243-4.

Anyinam, C.A. (1989), 'The social costs of the International Monetary Fund's adjustment programs for poverty: the case of health care development in Ghana', *International Journal of Health Services*, vol. 19:3, pp. 531-47.

Aragon, M. and Chambule, J. et al. (1993), 'Cólera em Moçambique, 1992', *Noticiário Epidemiológico*, vol. 3:12, pp. 15-32.

Aragon, M., Barreto, A., Tabbard, P., Chambule, J., Santos, C. and Noya, A. (1994), 'Epidemiologia da cólera em Moçambique no período de 1973-1992', *Revista da Saúde Pública*, vol. 28:5, pp. 332-6.

Aragon, M., Barreto, A., Chambule, J., Noya, A. and Tallarico, M. (1995), 'Shigellosis in Mozambique: the 1993 outbreak rehabilitation - a follow up study', *Tropical Doctor*, vol. 25, pp. 159-62.

Arnold, D. (1993), 'Social crisis and epidemic disease in the famines of nineteenth-century India', *Social History of Medicine*, vol. 6:3, pp. 385-404.

Asthana, S. (1994), 'Economic crisis, adjustment and the impact on health', in D.R. Phillips, and Y. Verhasselt (eds), *Health and Development*, Routledge, London.

Atlas, R.M. and Bartha, R. (1993), *Microbial Ecology Fundamentals and Applications*, Third edition, The Benjamin/Cummings Publishing Company, Inc. California, USA.

Awad El Karim, M.A., El Hassan, B.M. and Hussien, K.K. (1985), 'Social and public health implications of water supply in arid zones in the Sudan', *Social Science and Medicine*, vol. 20, pp. 393-8.

Azeveo, M. (1992), *Historical Dictionary of Mozambique*, Africa Book Centre Ltd. London.

Aziz, K.M.A., Hoque, B.A., Hasan, K.Z. and Patwary, M.J. (1990), 'Reduction in diarrhoeal diseases in children in rural Bangladesh by environmental and behavioural modifications', *Transactions of the Royal Society of Tropical Medicine and Hygiene*, vol. 84, pp. 433-8.

Babille, M., Colombani, P.De., Guerra, R., Zagaria, N. and Zanetti, C. (1994), 'Post-emergency epidemiological surveillance in Iraqi-Kurdish refugee camps in Iran', *Disasters*, vol. 18:1, pp. 58-75.

Baine, W.B., Zampieri, A., Mazzotti, M. et al. (1974), 'Epidemiology of cholera in Italy in 1973', *The Lancet*, vol. 2, pp. 1370-4.

Baltazar, J.C., Tiglao, T.V. and Tempongko, S.B. (1993), 'Hygiene behaviour and hospitalized severe childhood diarrhoea: a case-control study', *Bulletin of the World Health Organization*, vol. 71:3/4, pp. 323-8.

Baqui, A.H., Black, R.E., Yunus, M.D. and Azimul Hoque, A.R. et al. (1991), 'Methodological issues in diarrhoeal diseases epidemiology: Definition of diarrhoeal episodes', *International Journal of Epidemiology*, vol. 20:4, pp. 1057-63.

Barker, C. (1984), 'Are 300 drugs too many?' in G. Walt and A. Melamed (eds), *Mozambique: Towards a Peoples Health Service*, Zed Books, London.

Barrell, R.A.E. and Rowland, M.G.M. (1979), 'The relationship between rainfall and well water pollution in a West African (Gambian) village', *Journal of Hygiene* (Cambridge), vol. 83, p. 143.

Barreto, J. (1993), 'Cólera, prevenção e mortalidade', *Revista Médica de Moçambique*, vol. 4:4, p. 1.

Bartram, J. (1990), *Drinking Water Supply Surveillance*, The Robens Institute, Guildford, England.

Barua, D. and Greenough 111, W.B. (1992), *Cholera*, Plenum Medical Book Company, New York.

BBC World Service for Africa, Focus on Africa news reports, 1994, London.

Bellamy, D. and McIntosh, A. (1996), 'Getting away from the science of Dr Strangelove', *The Guardian* Education Suppliment, 9th April, 1996.

Bergstrom, S.K.D. and Ramalingaswami, V. (1992), 'Health', in J.C.I. Dooge, G.T. Goodman, J.W.M. la Rivière and J. Marton-Lefèvre, et al.(eds), *An Agenda of Science for Environment and Development into the 21st Century* based on a conference held in Vienna, Austria in November 1991, Cambridge University Press, Cambridge, pp. 119-24.

Bernardino, L., Espirito Santo, V. and Santos, R.P. (1993), 'Haemorrhagic colitis epidemic in Africa', *The Lancet*, vol. 342, pp. 495-6.

Bhardwaj, S.M. and Rao, M.N. (1988), 'Regional development and seasonality of communicable diseases in rural Andhra Pradesh, India', *Social Science and Medicine*, vol. 26:1, pp. 15-24.

Bhattacharya, S.K., Bhattacharya, M.K., Ramamurthy, T., Datta, D. et al. (1992), 'Cholera in young children in an endemic area', *The Lancet*, vol. 340, p. 1549.

Bhattacharya, S.K., Bhattacharya, M.K., Balakrish Nair, G. and Dutta, D. et al. (1993), 'Clinical profile of acute diarrhoea cases infected with the new epidemic strain of *Vibrio cholerae* 0139: designation of the desease as cholera', *Journal of Infection*, vol. 27, pp. 11-5.

Bhattacharya, M.K., Bhattacharya, S.K., Paul, M. and Dutta, D. et al. (1994), 'Shigellosis in Calcutta during 1990-1992: Antibiotic susceptibility pattern and clinical features', *Journal of Diarrhoeal Disease Research*, vol. 12:2, pp. 121-4.

Bin Saeed, A.A., El Bushra, H.E. and Al-Hamdan, N.A. (1995), 'Does treatment of bloody diarrhea due to *Shigella dysenteriae* type 1 with Ampicillin precipitate Hemolytic Uremic Syndrome?', *Emerging Infectious Diseases*, vol. 1:4, pp. 134-7.

Black, R. (1990), *Marginalisation and Agrarian Change in the Sierra do Alvão, Northern Portugal*, University of London PhD Thesis.

Black, R. (1994a), *Refugees and Environmental Change: Global Issues*, Report prepared for ODA Population and Environment Research Programme, University of Bradford, UK.

Black, R. (1994b), 'Environmental change in refugee-affected areas of the Third World: The role of policy and research', *Disasters*, vol. 18:2, pp. 107-16.

Blacker, J. G. C. (1991), 'Infant and child mortality: Development, Environment, and Custom', in R.G. Feachem and D.T. Jamison (eds)(1991), *Disease and Mortality in Sub-Saharan Africa*, Oxford University Press for the World Bank, Oxford.

Blaikie, P. (1995), 'Changing environments or changing views? A political ecology for developing countries', *Geography*, vol. 80:3, pp. 203-14.

Blaser, M.J. and Newman, L.S. (1982), 'A review of human salmonellosis. 1. Infective dose', *Review of Infectious Diseases*, vol. 4, pp. 1096-106.

Blaser, M.J., Miotto, K. and Hopkins, J.A. (1992), 'Molecular probe analysis of *Shigella dysenteriae* type 1 isolates from 1940 to 1987', *International Journal of Epidemiology*, vol. 21:3, pp. 594-8.

Boletim da Assistencia Mêdica aos Indegenas (1928), in M.F. Shapiro, (1983) *Medicine in the Service of Colonialism: Medical Care in Portuguese Africa 1885-1974*, Doctoral Thesis, UCLA, USA.

Bradford, D. and Gessner, M.D. (1994), 'Mortality rates, causes of death, and health status among displaced and resident populations of Kabul, Afghanistan', *Journal of the American Medical Association*, vol. 272:5, pp. 382-5.

Bradley, D. (1977), 'Health aspects of water supplies in tropical countries', in R. Feachem, M. McGarry and D. Mara (eds), *Water, Wastes and Health in Hot Climates*, John Wiley, Chichester.

Bratoeva, M.P and John, J.F Jr. (1994), '*In vivo* R-plasmid transfer in a patient with a mixed infection of shigella dysentery', *Epidemiology and Infection*, vol. 112, pp. 247-52.

Brinkmann, U.K. (1994), 'Economic development and tropical disease', *Annals of the New York Acadamy of Sciences*, vol. 740, pp. 303-11.

Briscoe, J. (1993), 'When the cup is half full. Improving water and sanitation services in the developing world', *Environment*, vol. 35:4, pp. 7-37.

Bryant, R.L. (1991), 'Putting politics first: the political ecology of sustainable development', *Global Ecology and Biogeography Letters*, vol. 1, pp. 164-6.

Bryant, R.L. (1992), 'Political ecology: an emerging research agenda in Third World Studies', *Political Geography Quarterly*, vol. 11:1, pp. 12-36.

Byrne, L. (1994), 'Doctors battle to contain cholera in Rwandan camps', *British Medical Journal*, vol. 309, p. 289.

Cairncross, A.M. and Feachem, R.G. (1983), *Environmental Health Engineering in the Tropics: An Introductory Text*, John Wiley, Chichester.

Carillo, L., Gilman, R.H., Mantle, R.E., Nunez, N. et al. (1994), 'Rapid detection of *Vibrio cholerae* 01 in stools of Peruvian cholera patients by using monoclonal, immunodiagnostic kits', *Journal of Clinical Microbiology*, vol. 32:3, pp. 856-7.

Cash, R.A., Music, S.I., Libonati, J.P. and Snyder, R.P. (1974), Response of man to infection with *Vibrio cholerae*. Clinical, serologic, and bacteriologic responses to a known inoculum', *Journal of Infectious Diseases*, vol. 129, pp. 45-52.

CDD (Programme for Control of Diarrhoeal Diseases)(1994), *Ninth Programme Report 1992-1993*, WHO/CDD/94.46.

Chambers, R., Longhurst, R. and Arnold, P. (eds) (1981), *Seasonal Dimensions to Rural Poverty*, Francis Pinter, Exeter.

Chapman, D. (ed) (1992), *Water Quality Assessments: A Guide to the Use of Biota, Sediments and Water in Environmental Monitoring*, Chapman and Hall, London on behalf of UNESCO, WHO and UNEP 1992.

Chaudhary, V. (1992), 'Argentina waits for summer and cholera', *British Medical Journal*, vol. 305, pp. 542-3.

Chisholm, M. (1967), *Transactions of the Institute of British Geographers*, pp. 45-52.

Chongsa-nguan, M., Chaicumpa, W., Moolasart, P., Kandhasingha, P. et al. (1993), '*Vibrio cholerae* 0139 Bengal in Bankok', *The Lancet*, vol. 342, pp. 430-1.

Clark, J., Modgil, C. and Modgil, S. (eds)(1990), *Anthony Giddens. Consensus and Controversy*, The Falmer Press, London.

Clemens, J.D., Sack, D.A., Harris, J.R., Khan, M.R. et al. (1990), 'Breastfeeding and the risk of severe cholera in rural Bangladesh children', *American Journal of Epidemiology*, vol. 3, pp. 400-11.

Clemens, J.D., Van Loon, F., Sack, D.A. and Rao, M.R. et al. (1991), 'Biotype as determinant of natural immunizing effect of cholera', *Lancet*, vol. 337, pp. 883-4.

Cliff, J. and Noormahomed, A.R. (1988), 'Health as a target: South Africa's destabilization of Mozambique' *Social Science and Medicine*, vol. 27:7, pp. 717-22.

Cohen, D., Green, M., Block, C. and Slepon, R. et al. (1991), 'Reduction of transmission of shigellosis by control of houseflies *(Musca domestica)'*, *The Lancet*, vol. 337, pp. 993-7.

Collins, A.E. (1991), 'Um estudo de verificação de possível conexção entre fatores físico no meio ambiente e a distribuição dos casos da cólera na cidade de Quelimane', Report prepared for the Ministry of Health, Maputo, Mozambique.

Collins, A.E. (1992), *Environmental Influences on the Distribution of Incidence of Cholera: A Case Study in Quelimane, Mozambique*, BSc(Hons) final year project/dissertation. Kingston University, Surrey.

Collins, A.E. (1993a), 'Environmental influences on the distribution of incidence of cholera: a case study in Quelimane, Mozambique', *Disasters*, vol. 17:4, pp. 321-40.

Collins, A.E. (1993b), 'Environment and cholera in Quelimane, Mozambique: a spatial study', *King's College Department of Geography Occasional Paper No.39*.

Collins, A.E (1996a), 'The geography of cholera', in B.S. Drasar, and B.D. Forrest (eds), *Cholera and the Ecology of Vibrio cholerae*, Chapman and Hall, London, pp. 255-94.

Collins, A.E. (1996b), 'Environment, health, population displacement and sustainable development', paper presented to the International Seminar on Environment, Sustainable Development and Human Health at Varanasi, India February 11-15, 1995. Revised for *Journal of Environment, Disease and Health Care Planning*, APH Publishing Corporation, New Delhi. 17pages.

Colombo, M.M., Francisco, M., Ferreira, B.D., Rubino, S. and Cappuccinelli, P. (1993), 'The early stage of the recurrent cholera epidemic in Luanda, Angola', *European Journal of Epidemiology*, vol. 9:5, pp. 563-5.

Colwell, R.R., Brayton, P., Grimes, D.J., Roszak, D.R., Huq, S.A. and Palmer, L.M. (1985), 'Viable, but non-culturable *Vibrio cholerae* and related pathogens in the environment: implications for release of genetically engineered micro-organisms', *Bio/Technology*, vol. 3, pp. 17-820.

Colwell, R.R. and Spira, W.M. (1992), 'The ecology of *Vibrio cholerae*' in D. Barua, and W.B. Greenough 111 (eds)(1992), *Cholera*, Plenum Medical Book Company, New York, pp. 107-27.

Colwell, R.R. and Huq, A. (1994), 'Environmental reservoir of *Vibrio cholerae*: The causative agent of cholera', *Annals of The New York Acadamy of Sciences*, vol. 740, pp. 44-54.

Comissão do Plano de Conselho Executive de Cidade da Beira (1994), Posto Administrativo No 2, Bairro No. 9 Inquerito, CECB, Beira.

Comissão Provincial do Plano de Sofala (1992), *Boletim Estatístico, Província de Sofala*, Serviço Provincial de Estatística, Beira.

Comissão Provincial do Plano de Zambézia (1991), *Resumo de Apuramento da Contagem da População da Cidade de Quelimane*, Quelimane.

Conant, F.P. (1994), 'Human ecology and space age technology: some predictions', *Human Ecology*, vol. 22:3, pp. 405-13.

Conteh, A., David, P.H. and Bauni, E.K. (1990), 'Environmental risk factors of childhood mortality in Liberia: Evidence and policy implications', in A.G. Hill (ed)(1990), *Determinants of Health and Mortality in Africa*, The Population Council, Institute for Resource Development/Macro Systems Inc.

Cook (1973) Quoted in R. Ellen (1982), *Environment, Subsistence and System. The Ecology of Small-scale Social Formations*, C.U.P.

Cooper Weil, D.E., Alicbusan, A.P., Wilson, J.F., Reich, M.R. and Bradley, D.J. (1990), *The Impact of Development Policies on Health: A Review of the Literature*, World Health Organization, Geneva.

Costello, A. and Woodward, D. (1993), 'World Bank's development report', *The Lancet*, vol. 342, pp. 440-1.

Council on Environmental Quality (C.E.Q) (1981), Speth, G. (ed), *Global Future - Time to Act*, Government Printing Office, Washington D.C.

Craig, M. (1988), 'Time-space clustering of *Vibrio cholerae* 01 in Matlab, Bangladesh, 1970-1982', *Social Science and Medicine*, vol. 26:1, pp. 5-13.

Cruz, J.R., Cano, F., Bartlett, A.V. and Mendez, H. (1994), 'Infection, diarrhoea, and dysentery caused by *Shigella* species and *Campylobacter jejuni* among Guatemalan rural children', *The Pediatric Infectious Disease Journal*, vol. 13:3, pp. 216-23.

Cunguara, A. (1991), 'Surto de Cólera na Cidade da Beira', *Noticiário Epidemiológico*, vol. 3:9, pp. 21-8.

Cutts, F.T. (1988), 'The use of WHO cluster survey method for evaluating the impact of the expanded programme on immunization on target disease incidence', *Journal of Tropical Medicine and Hygiene*, vol. 91, pp. 231-9.

Daniels, D.L., Cousens, S.N., Makoae, L.N. and Feachem, R.G. (1990), 'A case control study of the impact of improved sanitation on diarrhoea morbidity in Leotho', *Bulletin of the World Health Organization*, vol. 68:4, pp. 455-63.

Dargent-Molina, P., James, S.A., Strogatz, D.S. and Savitz, D.A. (1994), 'Association between maternal education and infant diarrhea in different household and community environments of Cebu, Philippines', *Social Science and Medicine*, vol. 38:2, pp. 343-50.

Dawkins, R. (1996), *Climbing Mount Improbable*, Viking, England.

Delgado, J.M., Azevedo, A. D., Mapor, M and Inroga, M.B. (1992), 'Alguns pontos epidemiologicos sobre a epidemia de cólera na Cidade de Quelimane Janeiro/Junho de 1991', *Noticiário Epidemiológico*, vol. 3:11, pp. 3-13.

Dick, B. (1984), 'Diseases of refugees - causes, effects and control', *Transactions of the Royal Society of Tropical Medicine and Hygiene*, vol. 78, pp. 734-41.

Dick, B. (1985), 'The impact of refugees on the health status and health services of host communities: Compounding bad with worse?', *Disasters*, vol. 9:4, pp. 259-69.

Direccao Nacional de Aguas (DNA)(1991), 'Estudo de avaliação das possibilidades de captação de agua subterranea na zona costeira de Quelimane', *Relatorio 19/91*, June 1991.

Dodge, C.P., Mohamed, A. and Kuch, P.J. (1987), 'Profile of the displaced in Khartoum', *Disasters*, vol. 11:4, pp. 243-50.

Donovan, P. (1991), 'Collateral Damage', *South Magazine*, Aug 1991, p. 28.

Doran, M., Shillan, P., Hoffman, R.E., MacFarland, L.M. (1989), 'Toxigenic Vibrio Cholerae 01 infection acquired in Colorado', *Morbidity and Mortality Weekly Report*, vol. 38:2, pp. 19-20.

Dorn, M. and Laws, G. (1994), 'Social theory, body politics, and Medical Geography: Extending Kearns's invitation', *Professional Geographer*, vol. 46:1, pp. 106-10.

Drasar, B.S. (1992), 'Pathogenesis and ecology: the case of cholera', *Journal of Tropical Medicine and Hygiene*, vol. 95, pp. 365-72.

Drasar, B.S. and Forrest, B.D. (eds) (1996), *Cholera and the Ecology of Vibrio cholerae*, Chapman and Hall, London.

Dunn, C.E., Woodhouse, J., Bhopal, R.S. and Acquilla, S.D. (1995), 'Asthma and factory emissions in northern England: addressing public concern by combining geographical and epidemiological methods', *Journal of Epidemiology and Community Health*, vol. 49, pp. 395-400.

DuPont, H.L. (1990), 'Shigella species (bacillary dysentery)', in G.L. Mandell, R.G. Douglas and J.E. Bennett (eds), *Principles and Practice of Infectious Diseases*, Third edition.

DuPont, H.L., Levine, M.M., Hornick, R.B. and Formal, S.B. (1989), 'Inoculum size in shigellosis and implications for expected mode of transmission', *The Journal of Infectious Diseases*, vol. 159:6, pp. 1126-8.

Ebright, J.R., Moore, E.C., Sanborn, W.R. and Schaberg, D. et al. (1984), 'Epidemic shiga bacillus dysentery in central Africa', *American Journal of Tropical Medicine and Hygiene*, vol. 33:6, pp. 1192-7.

Economist The (1994), 'Africa: a flicker of light', *The Economist*, March 5th, pp. 23-8.

Egunjobi, L. (1994), 'Spatial distribution of mortality from leading notifiable diseases in Nigeria', *Social Science and Medicine*, vol. 36:10, pp. 1267-72.

Eko, F.O. and Utsalo, J. (1991), 'Antimicrobial resistance trends of shigellae isolates from Calabar, Nigeria', *Journal of Tropical Medicine and Hygiene*, vol. 94, pp. 407-10.

El Samani, E.F., Willett, W.C. and Ware, J.H. (1988), 'Association of malnutrition and diarrhea in children aged under five years', *American Journal of Epidemiology*, vol. 128:1, pp. 93-105.

Ellen R. (1982), *Environment, Subsistence and System. The Ecology of Small-scale Social Formations*, C.U.P., Cambridge.

Epstein, P.R. (1992), 'Cholera and the environment' *The Lancet*, vol. 339, pp. 1167-8.

Epstein, P.R., Rogers, D.J. and Sloof, R. (1993), 'Satellite imaging and vector-borne disease', *The Lancet*, vol. 341, pp. 1404-6.

Epstein, P.R., Ford, T.E., Puccia, C. and De A Possas, C. (1994), 'Marine ecosystem health: Implications for public health', *Annals of the New York Academy of Sciences*, vol. 740, pp. 13-23.

Esrey, S.A., Feachem, R.G. and Hughes, J.M. (1985), 'Interventions for the control of diarrhoeal diseases among young children: improving water supplies and excreta disposal facilities', *Bulletin of the World Health Organization*, vol. 63, pp. 757-72.

Esrey, S.A. and Habitch, J.P. (1986), 'Epidemiologic evidence for health benefits from improved water and sanitation in developing countries', *Epidemiologic Review*, vol. 8, pp. 117-28.

Eyles, J. (1985), *Senses of Place*, Warrington, Silverbrook Press.

Eyles, J. and Wood, K.J. (1983), *The Social Geography of Medicine and Health*, Croom Helm, London and Canberra, St. Martins Press, New York.

Fabricant, S.J. and Harpham, T. (1993), 'Assessing response reliability of health interview surveys using reinterviews', *Bulletin of the World Health Organization*, vol. 71:3/4, pp. 341-8.

Farr, W. (1885), Facsimile reprint of ed. published by the Office of the Sanitary Institute, London, 1885 in *Vital Statistics: A Memorial Volume of Selections from the Reports and Writings of William Farr*, Scarecrow Press, London, 1975.

Faruque, A.S.G., Fuchs, G.J. and Albert, M.J. (1996), 'Changing epidemiology of cholera due to *Vibrio cholerae* 01 and 0139 Bengal in Dhaka, Bangladesh', *Epidemiology and Infection*, vol. 116, pp. 275-8.

Fauveau, V., Yunus, M., Zaman, K. and Chakraborty, J. et al. (1991), 'Diarrhoea mortality in rural Bangladeshi children', *Journal of Tropical Pediatrics*, vol. 37, pp. 31-6.

Feachem, R.G. (1977), 'Water supplies for low-income communities: resource allocation, planning and design for a crisis situation', in R. Feachem, M. McGarry and D. Mara (eds), *Water, Wastes and Health in Hot Climates*, Wiley, Chichester.

Feachem, R.G. (1981), 'Environmental aspects of cholera epidemiology. A review of selected reports of endemic and epidemic situations during 1961-80', *Tropical Diseases Bulletin*, vol. 78, pp. 675-98.

Feachem, R.G., Bradley, D.J., Garelick, H. and Mara, D.D. (1983), *Sanitation and Disease. Health Aspects of Excreta and Wastewater Management*, John Wiley, Chichester.

Feachem R.G., Graham, W.J. and Timæus, I.M (1989), 'Identifying health problems and health research priorities in developing countries', *Journal of Tropical Medicine and Hygiene*, vol. 92, pp. 133-91.

Feachem, R.G. and Jamison, D.T. (eds)(1991), *Disease and Mortality in Sub-Saharan Africa*, World Bank, O.U.P.

Ferguson, A.G. (1977), 'Probability mapping of the 1975 Cholera epidemic in Kisumu District, Kenya', *Journal of Tropical Geography*, vol. 44, pp. 23-32.

Ferreccio, C., Prado, V., Ojeda, A. and Cayyazo, M. et al. (1991), 'Epidemiologic patterns of acute diarrhoea and endemic shigella infections in children in a poor periurban setting in Santiago, Chile', *American Journal of Epidemiology*, vol. 134, pp. 614-27.

Foley, R. and Frost, P. (1996) 'Caring for the carers; GIS and respite care planning in East Sussex', paper presented at *VIIth International Symposium in Medical Geography* at University of Portsmouth, 30th July - 2nd August, 1996.

Folgosa, E., Valdivia, J.A. and Hung, M. (1994), 'Cólera na Cidade e Província de Maputo: Resultados laboratorias das amostras analisadas no período de Junho de 1991 a Junho de 1992', *Revista Médica de Moçambique*, vol. 5:3, pp. 9-12.

Forsberg, B.C., Van Ginneken, J.K. and Nagelkerke, N.J.D. (1993), 'Cross-sectional household surveys of diarrhoeal diseases: A comparison of data from the Control of Diarrhoeal Diseases and Demographic and Health Surveys Programmes', *International Journal of Epidemiology*, vol. 22:6, pp. 1137-45.

Frerks, G.E., Kliest, T.J., Kirkby, S.J., Emmel, N.D., O'Keefe, P. and Convery, I. (1995), 'A 'disaster' continuum?', *Disasters*, vol. 19:4, pp. 362-6.

Gabinete de Epidemiologia, Ministério da Saúde (1993), 'Cólera em Moçambique', *Noticiário Epidemiológico*, vol. 3:12, pp. 15-32.

Gangarosa, E.J., Perera, D.J., Mata, L.J. and Mendizábal-Morris, C. et al. (1970), 'Epidemic shiga bacillus dysentery in Central America. II. Epidemiologic studies in 1969', *The Journal of Infectious Diseases*, vol. 122:3, pp. 181-90.

Garcia, R.V. and Escudero, J.C. (eds) (1972), *The Constant Catastrophe: Malnutrition, Famines and Drought*, Pergamon, Oxford.

Garfield, R. and Williams, G. (1989), *Health and Revolution: the Nicaraguan Experience*, Oxfam, Oxford.

Gatrell, A.C. (1993), Presentation given at conference *Spatial Analysis in ARC/INFO*, Lancaster University 28-30 June 1993.

Gatrell, A.C., Dunn, C.E. and Boyle, P.J. (1991), 'The relative utility of the Central Postcode Directory and Pinpoint Address Code in applications of geographical information systems', *Environment and Planning A*, vol. 23, pp. 1447-58.

Gibb, R. (1987), 'The effect on the countries of SADCC of economic sanctions against the Republic of South Africa', *Transactions of the Institute of British Geographers*, vol. 12:4, pp. 398-412.

Giggs, J., Ebdon, D.S. and Bourke, J.B. (1980), 'The epidemiology of acute pancreatitis in the Nottingham Defined Population Area', *Transantions of The Institute of British Geographers*, vol. 5, pp. 229-42.

Glass, R.I., Holmgren, J., Haley, C. et al. (1985), 'Predisposition for cholera of individuals with O blood group: possible evolutionary significance', *American Journal of Epidemiology*, vol. 121, pp. 791-6.

Glass, R.I., Claeson, M., Blake, P.A., Waldman, R.J. and Pierce, N.F. (1991), 'Cholera in Africa: lessons on transmission and control for Latin America' *The Lancet*, vol. 338, pp. 791-5.

Glass, R.I., Libel, M. and Brandling-Bennett, A.D. (1992), 'Epidemic cholera in the Americas', *Science*, vol. 256, pp. 1524-5.

Goma Epidemiology Group (1995), 'Public health impact of Rwandan refugee crisis: what happened in Goma, Zaire, in July, 1994?', *Lancet*, vol. 345, pp. 339-44.

Gorden, J. and Small, P.L.C. (1993), 'Acid resistance in enteric bacteria', *Infection and Immunity*, vol. 61:1, pp. 364-7.

Gorter, A.C., Sandiford, P., Smith G.D. and Pauw, J.P. (1991), 'Water supply, sanitation and diarrhoeal disease in Nicaragua: results from a case-control study', *International Journal of Epidemiology*, vol. 20:2, pp. 527-39.

Gould, P. and White, R. (1992), *Mental Maps*, Second edition, Routeledge, London.

Grant, J.P (1993), 'World Bank's development report', *The Lancet*, vol. 342, p. 440.

Green, R.H. (1992), 'The four horsemen ride together: Scorched fields of war in Southern Africa', Paper presented at Refugees Studies Programme, Oxford 11th Novermber 1992.

Gregory, D. (1985), 'People, places and practices: the future of human geography', in King, R. (ed), *Geographical Futures*, Geographical Association, Sheffield.

Guglielmetti, P., Bartolini, A., Roselli, M. and Gamboa, H. et al. (1992), 'Population movements and cholera spread in Cordillera Province, Santa Cruz Department, Bolivia', *The Lancet*, vol. 340, p. 113.

Haider, K., Kay, B.A., Talukder, K.A. and Huq, M.I. (1988), 'Plasmid analysis of *Shigella dysenteriae* type 1 isolates obtained from widely scattered geographical locations', *Journal of Clinical Microbiology*, vol. 26:10, pp. 2083-6.

Haila, Y. and Levins, R. (1992), *Humanity and Nature: Ecology, Science and Society*, Pluto Press, London.

Haines, A. and Parry, M. (1993), 'Climate change and human health', *Journal of the Royal Society of Medicine*, vol. 86, pp. 707-11.

Hanlon, J. (1983), *Mozambique: The Revolution Under Fire*, Zed Books, London.

Hanlon, J. (1991), *Mozambique: Who Calls the Shots*, James Currey, London.

Hardoy, J., Cairncross, S. and Satterthwaite, D. (eds) (1990), *The Poor Die Young: Housing and Health in Third World Cities*, Earthscan, London.

Hardoy, J.E. and Satterthwaite, D. (1991), 'Environmental problems of Third World cities: a global issue ignored?', *Public Administration and Development*, vol. 11, pp. 341-61.

Harpham, T. (1994), 'Cities and health in the Third World', in D.R. Phillips, and Y. Verhasselt (eds), *Health and Development*, Routledge, London.

Harpham, T., Lusty, T. and Vaughan, P. (eds)(1988), *In the Shadow of the City: Community Health and the Urban Poor*, Oxford University Press, Oxford.

Harpham, T. and Tanner, M. (eds)(1995), *Urban Health in Developing Countries: Progress and Prospects*, Earthscan, London.

Harris, J. C. (1982), 'Environmental decline in North Arcot, India', in P. Blaikie (1985), *The Political Economy of Soil Erosion*, Longman.

Hatch, D.L., Waldman, R.J., Lungu, G.W. and Piri, C. (1994), 'Epidemic cholera during refugee resettlement in Malawi', *International Journal of Epidemiology*, vol. 23:6, pp. 1292-9.

Heikens, G.T., Schofield, W.N., Christie, C.D.C. and Gernay, J. et al. (1993), 'The Kingston Project. III. The effects of high energy supplement and metronidazole on malnourished children rehabilitated in the community: morbidity and growth', *European Journal of Clinical Nutrition*, vol. 47, pp. 174-91.

Henry, F.J. (1991), 'The epidemiologic importance of dysentery in communities', *Review of Infectious Diseases*, vol. 13(suppl 4) S. pp. 238-44.

Higa, N., Honma, Y., Albert, M.J. and Iwanaga, M. (1993), 'Characterization of *Vibrio cholerae* 0139 synonym Bengal isolated from patients with cholera-like disease in Bangladesh', *Microbiol. Immunol*, vol. 37:12, pp. 971-4.

Hoile, D. (1989), *Mozambique a Nation in Crisis*, Claridge Press, London.

Holt-Jensen, A. (1988), *Geography History and Concepts*, Second edition, Paul Chapman Publishing, London.

Hospedales, C.J. (1992), 'Cholera in Belize', *West Indian Medical Journal*, vol. 41, pp. 88-9.

Hossain, M.D.A., Albert, J.M. and Hasan, Z.K.H. (1990), 'Epidemiology of shigellosis in Teknat, a coastal area of Bangladesh', *Epidemiology and Infection*, vol. 105, pp. 41-9.

Howe, G.M.(1982), 'Disease and environment', in A.R. Rees and H.J. Purcell (eds), *Disease and the Environment: Proceedings of the Inaugural Conference of the Society for Environmental Therapy, held in Oxford 21-23 March 1981*, Wiley, Chichester, pp. 1-9.

Howe, G.M. & Phillips, D.R. (1983), 'Medical Geography in the United Kingdom 1945-1982', in N. McGlashan and J.R. Blunden (eds), *Geographical Aspects of Health*, Academic Press, 1983.

Howe, G.M. (1972), *Man Environment and Disease in Britain*, David and Charles, Newton Abbot.

Howe, G.M. (1986), 'Disease Mapping', in M. Pacione (ed)(1986), *Medical Geography - Progress and Prospect*, Croom Helm, London.

Hugget, R.J. (1980), *Systems Analysis in Geography*, Open University Press, Oxford.

Hughes, C.C. and Hunter, J.M. (1970), 'Disease and 'development' in Africa', *Social Science and Medicine*, vol. 3, pp. 443-93.

Hughes, J.M., Boyce, J.M., Levine, R.J., Moslemuddin, K. et al. (1982), 'Epidemiology of El Tor cholera in rural Bangladesh: importance of surface water in transmission' *Bull. World Health Organization*, vol. 60, pp. 395-404.

Huq, A., Colwell, R.R., Chowdhury, M.A.R. and Xu, B. et al. (1995), 'Coexistence of *Vibrio cholerae* 01 and 0139 Bengal in plankton in Bangladesh', *The Lancet*, vol. 345, p. 1249.

Huskins, W.C., Griffiths, J.K., Faruque, A.S.G. and Bennish, M.L. (1994), 'Shigellosis in neonates and young infants', *The Journal of Pediatrics*, vol. 125:1, pp. 14-22.

HWGNRD (1995), (Harvard Working Group in New and Resurgent Diseases) 'New and resurgent diseases: The failure of attempted eradication', *The Ecologist*, vol. 25:1, pp. 21-6.

ICDDR,B (1993), International Centre for Diarrhoeal Diseases Research, Bangladesh. 'Large epidemic of cholera-like disease in Bangladesh caused by *Vibrio cholerae* 0139 synonym Bengal', *The Lancet*, vol. 342, pp. 387-90.

Islam, D. and Lindberg, A.A. (1992), 'Detection of *Shigella dysenteriae* Type 1 and *Shigella flexneri* in faeces by Immunomagnetic Isolation and Polymerase Chain Reaction', *Journal of Clinical Microbiology*, vol. 30:11, pp. 2801-6.

Islam, M.S., Hasan, M.K., Miah, M.A. and Sur, G.C. et al. (1993a), 'Use of the Polymerase Chain Reaction and Flourescent-Antibody methods for detecting viable but nonculturable *Shigella dysenteriae* Type 1 in laboratory microcosms', *Applied and Environmental Microbiology*, vol. 59:2, pp. 536-40.

Islam, M.S., Hasan, M.K., Miah, M.A., Qadri, F. et al. (1993b), 'Isolation of *Vibrio cholerae* 0139 Bengal from water in Bangladesh', *The Lancet*, vol. 342, p. 430.

Islam, M.S., Miah, M.A., Hasan, M.K. and Sack, R.B. et al. (1994), 'Detection of non-culturable *Vibrio cholerae* 01 associated with a cyanobacterium from aquatic environment in Bangladesh', *Transactions of the Royal Society of Medical Hygiene*, vol. 88, pp.298-9.

Jesudason, M.V. (1994), 'The appearance and spread of *Vibrio cholerae* 0139 in India', *Indian Journal of Medical Research*, vol. 99, pp. 97-100.

Jesudason, M.V. and Jacob John, T. (1993), 'Major shift in prevalence of non-01 and El Tor *Vibrio cholerae*', *The Lancet*, vol. 341, pp. 1090-1.

Johnston, R.J. (1986), *Philosophy and Human Geography*, Second edition, Arnold, London.

Johnston, R.J., Gregory, D. and Smith, D.M. (1986), *The Dictionary of Human Geography*, Second edition, Blackwell Reference, Oxford.

Jones, H.R. (1981), *A Population Geography*, Paul Chapman, Suffolk.

Jones, K. and Moon, G. (1987), *Health, Disease and Society: An Introduction to Medical Geography*, Routledge and Kegan, London.

Jones, K. and Moon, G. (1993), 'Medical geography: taking space seriously', *Progress in Human Geography*, vol. 17:4, pp. 515-24.

José, A. (1989), 'Beira: Lembranças da cidade colonial', *Boletim do Arquivo Histórico de Moçambique*, No.6 Especial, 181-200.

Kahn, H.A. and Sempos, C. T. (1989), *Statistical Methods in Epidemiology*, Monographs in Epidemiology and Biostatistics Volume 12, Oxford University Press, Oxford.

Kasl, S.V. (1979), 'Mortality and the business cycle: some questions about research strategies when utilizing macro-social and ecological data', *American Journal of Public Health*, vol. 69, pp. 784-8.

Kauffman, S. (1995), *At Home in the Universe: the Search for Laws of Complexity*, Viking, London.

Kaysner, C.A., Abeyta, C. Jr., Wekell, M.M., De Paola, A. Jr., Stott, R.F. and Leitch, J.M. (1987), 'Incidence of *Vibrio cholerae* from esturies of the United States West Coast', *Applied and Environmental Microbiology*, vol. 53:6, pp. 1344-8.

Kearns, R.A. (1993), 'Place and health: Towards a reformed Medical Geography', *Professional Geographer*, vol. 45:1, pp. 39-47.

Kearns, R.A. (1994), 'Putting health and health care into place: An invitation accepted and declined', *Professional Geographer*, vol. 46:1, pp. 111-5.

Kennedy, B.A. (1979), 'A naughty world', *Transactions of the Institute of British Geographers*, New series vol. 4, p. 550.

Keusch, G.T. and Bennish, M.L. (1989), 'Shigellosis: recent progress, persisting problems and research issues', *The Pediatric Infectious Disease Journal*, vol. 8:10, pp. 713-9.

Khan, M.U. (1982), 'Interruption of shigellosis by hand washing', *Transactions of the Royal Society of Tropical Medicine and Hygiene*, vol. 76:2, pp. 164-8.

Khan, M.U., Curlin, G.T. and Huq, M.I. (1979), 'Epidemiology of *Shigella dysenteriae* type 1 infections in Dacca urban area', *Trop. Geogr. Med.*, vol. 31, pp. 213-23.

Koo, D., Aragon, A., Moscoso, V. and Gudiel, M. et al. (1996), 'Epidemic cholera in Guatemala, 1993: transmission of a newly introduced epidemic strain by steet vendors', *Epidemiology and Infection*, vol. 116, pp. 121-6.

Kovda, V.A. (1972), 'Soil preservation', in N. Polunin (ed)(1972), *The Environmental Future*, Macmillan, London.

Krebs, J. (1995), 'Brass without muck', *The Times Higher*, Aug 18th.

Kunstadter, P. (1991), 'Social and behavioural factors in transmission and response to shigellosis', *Reviews of Infectious Diseases*, vol. 13(suppl 4), Spp. 272-8.

Labonte, R. (1992), 'South America's cholera pandemic provides lesson in public health, politics', *Can Med Assoc J.*, vol. 147:7, pp. 1052-6.

LaMont-Gregory, E. (1995), 'The environment, cooking fuel and UN Resolution 46/182', *Refugee Participation Network*, No. 18, Refugee Studies Programme, Oxford.

Langton, J. (1972), 'Potentialities and problems of adopting a systems approach to the study of change in human geography', *Progress in Geography*, vol. 4, pp. 125-79.

Lappé, F.M. and Beccar-Varela, A.N. (1980), *Mozambique and Tanzania: Asking the Big Questions*, Institute for Food and Development Policy, San Francisco, USA.

Lasch, E.E., Abed, Y., Marcus, Y and Sheibeir, M et al. (1984), 'Cholera in Gaza in 1981: epidemiological characteristics of an outbreak', *Transactions of the Royal Society of Tropical Medicine and Hygiene*, vol. 78, pp. 554-7.

Leach, M. and Mearns, R. (1988), *Beyond the Woodfuel Crisis: People, Land and Trees in Africa*, Earthscan, London.

Leach, M. (1991), 'Refugees and the environment: environmental impact of liberian refugees in Sierra Leone', *Refugee Participation Network* no. 11, pp. 20-4.

Learmonth, A. (1988), *Disease Ecology*, Blackwell, Oxford.

Le Sueur, D., Ngxongo, S., Martin, C. and Sharp, B. (1996) 'Using a geographic information system to investigate the epidemiology of malaria in South Africa and assist in health care planning', paper presented at *VIIth International Symposium in Medical Geography* at University of Portsmouth, 30th July - 2nd August, 1996.

Levine, M.M., Black, R. E., Clements, M.L and Cisneros, L. (1981), 'The quality and duration of infection-derived immunity to cholera', *Journal of Infectious Diseases*, vol. 143, pp. 818-20.

Levine, O.S. and Levine, M.M. (1991), 'Houseflies *(Musca domestica)* as mechanical vectors of shigellosis', *Reviews of Infectious Diseases*, vol. 13, pp. 688-96.

Lewis, R. (1993), *Complexity*, Phenix, London.

Lida, T., Shrestha, J., Yamamoto, K. and Honda, T. (1993) Letter, *The Lancet*, vol. 342, p. 926.

Lijima, Y., Oundo, J.O., Taga, K and Saidi, S.M (1995), 'Simultaneous outbreak due to *Vibrio cholerae* and *Shigella dysenteriae* in Kenya', *The Lancet*, vol. 345, pp. 69-70.

Lima, A.A.M. and Lima, N.L. (1993), 'Epidemiology, therapy, and prevention of infedtion with *Shigella* organisms and *Clostridium difficile*'. *Current Opinion in Infectious Diseases* vol. 6, pp. 63-71.

Lindskog, R.U.M., and Lindskog, P.A. (1988), 'Bacteriological contamination of water in rural areas: an intervention study from Malawi', *Journal of Tropical Medicine and Hygiene*, vol. 91, pp. 1-7.

Loewenson, R. (1993), 'Structural adjustment and health policy in Africa', *International Journal of Health Services*, vol. 23:4, pp. 717-30.

MacKenzie, D.T., Ellison, III, R.T. and Mostow, S.R. (1992), 'Sunlight and cholera', *The Lancet*, vol. 340, p. 367.

Mackereth, F.J.H., Heron, J. and Talling, J.F. (1978), 'Water analysis, some revised methods for limnologists', *1978 Ambleside, Freshwater Biological Association, Scientific Publications* No. 36.

Mahalanabis, D., Faruque, M.J., Albert, M.A., Salam, M.A. and Hoque, S.S. (1994), 'An epidemic of cholera due to *Vibrio cholerae* 0139 in Dhaka, Bangladesh: clinical and epidemiological features', *Epidemiology and Infection*, vol. 112, pp. 463-71.

Mandal, B.K. (1993), 'Epidemic cholera due to a novel strain of *Vibrio cholerae* non-01: the beginning of a new pandemic', *Journal of Infection*, vol. 27, pp. 115-7.

Marfin, A.A., Moore, J., Collins, C. and Biellik, R. et al. (1994), 'Infectious disease surveillance during emergency relief to bhutanese refugees in Nepal', *Journal of the American Medical Association*, vol. 272:5, pp. 377-81.

Marsden, P.D. (1992), 'Cholera', *British Medical Journal*, vol. 304, pp. 1170-1.

Marsh, S.E., Hutchinson, C.F., Pfirman, E.E., Des Rosiers, S.A. and Van der Harten, C. (1994), 'Development of a computer workstation for famine early warning and food security', *Disasters*, vol. 18:2, pp. 117-29.

Martin, D. (1991), *Geographic Information Systems and their Socioeconomic Applications*, Routledge, London.

Martin, D. and Bracken, I. (1993), 'The integration of socioeconomic and physical resource data for applied land management information systems', *Applied Geography*, vol. 13, pp. 45-53.

Martins, M.T., Sanchez, P.S., Sato, M.I.Z., Brayton, P.R. and Colwell, R.R. (1993), 'Detection of *Vibrio cholerae* 01 in the aquatic environment in Brazil employing direct immunofluorescence microscopy', *World Journal of Microbiology and Biotechnology*, vol. 9, pp. 390-2.

Mata, L.J., Gangarosa, E.J., Cáceres, A and Perera, D.R et al. (1970), 'Epidemic shiga bacillus dysentery in Central America. I. Etiologic investigations in Guatemala, 1969', *Journal of Infectious Diseases*, vol. 122:3, pp. 170-80.

May, J.M. (1950), 'Medical Geography: its methods and objectives', *Geographical Review*, vol. 40, pp. 9-41; reprinted *Social Science and Medicine*, vol. 11, pp. 715-30.

May, J.M. (1958), *The Ecology of Human Disease*, M.D Publications, New York.

May, J.M. (1960), *Disease Ecology*, Hafner, New York.

May, J.M. and McLellan, D.L. (1970), *The Ecology of Malnutrition in Eastern Africa and Four Countries of Western Africa*, Studies in Medical Geography, Hafner Publishing Company, New York.

Mayer, J.D. (1982), 'Relations between two traditions of Medical Geography: Health systems planning and geographical epidemiology', *Progress in Human Geography*, vol. 6:2, pp. 16-30.

Mayer, J.D. (1993), 'The political ecology of disease: A new focus for Medical Geography?', Presentation made to IBG Medical Geography Study Group and the IGU Commission on Health, Environment and Development 13th-15th July 1993, Exeter.

Mayer, J.D. and Meade, M.S. (1994), 'A reformed Medical Geography reconsidered', *Professional Geographer*, vol. 46:1, pp. 103-6.

Mbwette, T.S.A. (1987), 'Cholera outbreaks in Tanzania', *Journal of the Royal Society of Health*, vol. 4, pp. 134-6.

McCormack, W.M., Mosley, W.H., Fahimuddin, M. and Benenson, A.S. (1969), Endemic cholera in rural East Pakistan, *American Journal of Clinical Nutrition*, vol. 25, pp. 1236-42.

McGregor, J. (1993), 'Refugees and the environment', in R. Black, and V. Robinson (eds), *Geography and Refugees: Patterns and Processes of Change*, Belhaven, London.

McPake, B., Hanson, K. and Mills, A. (1992), *Implimenting the Bamako Initiative in Africa: A Review and Five Case Studies*, PHP Departmental Publication No.8, London School of Hygiene and Tropical Medicine.

Meade, M.S. (1977), 'Medical geography as human ecology: The dimension of population movement', *The Geographical Review*, vol. 67:4, pp. 377-99.

Meade, M.S. (1979), 'Cardiovascular mortality in the South Eastern United States: the coastal plain enigma', *Social Science and Medicine*, vol. 13D, pp. 257-65.

Meade, M.S, Florin, J. and Gesher, W. (1988), *Medical Geography*, The Guildford Press, London and New York.

Medecins Sans Frontieres (MSF) (1992a), *Célula Inter Secções. Moçambique*, November issue.

Medecins Sans Frontieres (MSF) (1992b), *Célula Inter Secções. Moçambique*, December issue.

Medecins Sans Frontieres (MSF) (1993a), *Célula Inter Secções. Moçambique*, September issue.

Medecins Sans Frontieres (MSF) (1993b), *Célula Inter Secções. Moçambique*, October issue.

Medecins Sans Frontieres (MSF) (1993c), *Célula Inter Secções. Moçambique*, June issue.

Medecins Sans Frontieres (MSF) (1993d), *Célula Inter Secções. Moçambique*, February issue.

Medecins Sans Frontieres (MSF) (1994a), *Célula Inter Secções. Moçambique*, February issue.

Medecins Sans Frontieres (MSF) (1994b), *Célula Inter Secções. Moçambique*, October issue.

Medecins Sans Frontieres (MSF) (1994c), *Célula Inter Secções. Moçambique*, January issue.

Medecins Sans Frontieres (MSF) (1994d), *Célula Inter Secções. Moçambique*, March issue.

Medecins Sans Frontieres (MSF) (1995), *Célula Inter Secções. Moçambique*, July issue.

Medecins Sans Frontieres (MSF) (1997), *Célula Inter Secções. Moçambique*, March issue.

Melamed, A. and Walt, G. (1984), 'Postscript', in G. Walt and A. Melamed (eds) *Mozambique: Towards a Peoples Health Service*, Zed Books, London.

Meldrum, A. (1996), 'Land rush crushes peasants who survived so much', *The Guardian*, June 11, p. 12.

Merson, M.H., Black, R.E., Moslemuddin, K. and Huq, I. (1980), 'Epidemiology of Cholera and Enterotoxigenic *Escherichia coli* Diarrhoea', in *Cholera and Related Diarrhoea, 43rd Nobel symp., Stockholm 1978*, Karger, Basel, pp. 34-45.

MGSG (RGS-IBG Medical Geography Study Group) (1995), Newsletter 26, Spring.

Miller, C.J., Drasar, B.S. and Feachem, R.G., (1982), 'Cholera and estuarine salinity in Calcutta and London', *The Lancet*, vol. 29, pp. 1216-18.

Miller, C.J., Drasar, B.S. and Feachem, R.G. (1984), 'Response of toxigenic *Vibrio cholerae 01* to stresses in aquatic environments', *Journal of Hygiene Camb.* vol. 93, pp. 475-95.

Miller, C.J., Feachem, R.G. and Drasar, B.S. (1985), 'Cholera epidemiology in developed and developing countries: new thoughts of transmission, seasonality, and control', *The Lancet*, vol. 2, pp. 261-3.

Miller, C.J., Feachem, R.G. and Drasar, B.S. (1986), 'The impact of physio-chemical stress on the toxigenicity of *Vibrio cholerae*', *Journal of Hygiene Camb*, vol. 96, pp. 49-57.

Miyaki, K., Iwahara, S., Sato, K., Fujimoto, S. and Aibara, K. (1967), 'Basic studies on the viability of El Tor Vibrios', *Bulletin of the World Health Organization*, vol. 37, pp. 773-8.

MMWR (Morbidity and Mortality Weekly Report)(1995), 'Update: *Vibrio cholerae* 01-Western hemisphere, 1991-1994, and *Vibrio cholerae* 0139-Asia, 1994', *Journal of the American Medical Association*, vol. 273:15, p. 1169.

Moe, C.L., Sobsey, M.D., Samsa, G.P. and Mesolo, V. (1991), 'Bacterial indicators of risk of diarrhoeal disease from drinking-water in the Philippines', *Bulletim of the World Health Organization*, vol. 69:3, pp. 305-17.

Mole, P.N (1994), 'O impacto social do Programa de Ajustamento Económico', in Castel-Branco (ed) *Moçambique: Perspectivas económicas*, Universidade Eduardo Mondlane em associação com Fundação Fredrich Ebert, Maputo. 158-74.

Moore, H.A., de la Cruz, E. and Vargas-Mendez, O. (1965), 'Diarrhoeal disease studies in Costa Rica', *American Journal of Epidemiology*, vol. 82, pp. 162-4.

Moore, P.S., Marfin, A.A., Quenemoen, L.E. and Gessner, B.D. et al. (1993), 'Mortality rates in displaced and resident populations of central Somalia during 1992 famine', *The Lancet*, vol. 341, pp. 935-8.

Moren, A., Bitar, D., Navarre, I. and Gastellu, M. et al. (1991), 'Epidemiological surveillance among mozambican refugees in Malawi, 1987-1989', *Disasters*, vol. 15:4, pp. 363-72.

Moren, A., Stefanagge, S., Antona, D. and Bitar, D. et al. (1991), 'Practical field epidemiology to investigate a cholera outbreak in a Mozambican refugee camp in Malawi, 1988', *Journal of Tropical Medicine and Hygiene*, vol. 94, pp. 1-7.

Morgan, L.M. (1993), *Community Participation in Health*, Cambridge University Press.

Morgan, R.K. (1981), 'Systems analysis: a problem of methodology?', *Area*, vol. 13, pp. 219-23.

Morris, R.D. and Munasinghe, R.L. (1993), 'Aggregation of existing geographic regions to diminish spurious variability of disease rates', *Statistics in Medicine*, vol. 12, pp. 1915-29.

Mosley, W.H. and Chen, L. C. (1984), 'An analytical framework for the study of child survival in developing countries', *Population and Development Review*, vol. 10 (supplement), pp. 25-45.

Mozambique Information Office (1991), *News Review*, No. 193, January. MIO, London.

Muchangos, Aniceto dos (1989), 'Aspectos geográficos da cidade da Beira', in *Boletim do Arquivo Histórico de Moçambique*, 6 (especial), pp. 239-96.

Mujica, O. J., Quick, R.E., Palacios, A.M. and Beingolea, L. et al. (1994), 'Epidemic cholera in the Amazon: the role of produce in disease risk and prevention', *The Journal of Infectious Diseases*, vol. 169, pp. 1381-4.

Mulholland, K. (1985), 'Cholera in Sudan: An account of an epidemic in a refugee camp in Eastern Sudan, May-June 1985', *Disasters*, vol. 9:4, pp. 247-58.

Munslow, B. (1983), *Mozambique: The Revolution and its Origins*, Zed Press, London.

Munslow, B. (1985), *Samora Machel: An African Revolutionary*, Zed Press, London.

Munslow, B. et al. (1988), *The Fuelwood Trap: A Study of the SADCC Region*, Earthscan, London.

Myers, G.A. (1994), 'Eurocentrism and African urbanisation: the case of Zanzibar's other side', *Antipode*, vol. 26:33, 195-215.

Nalin, D.R. (1994), 'Cholera and severe toxigenic diarrhoeas', *Gut*, vol. 35, pp. 145-7.

Nalin, D.R., Levine, R.S., Levine, M.M. and Hoover, D. et al. (1978), 'Cholera non-vibrio cholera and stomach acid', *The Lancet*, vol. 2, pp. 856-9.

Newby, H. (1993), 'Geographical Information Systems: their social and economic aspects. Paper presented to conference organized by the Royal Geographical Society', *Progress in Geographical Information Handling*, 4th-5th February, 1993.

Nichter, M. (1991) 'Use of social science research to improve epidemiologic studies of and interventions for diarrhea and dysentery', *Reviews of Infectious Diseases*, vol. 13(suppl 4), 265-71.

Noticias (1993), 'Movimentação de populações também pode agravar problema da malária', 6th May 1993, p.3.

O'Connor, A. (1991), *Poverty in Africa: A Geographical Approach*, Belhaven, London.

O'Keefe, P., Kirkby, J. and Cherrett, I. (1991), 'Mozambican environmental problems: myths and realities', *Public Administration and Development*, vol. 11, pp. 307-24.

Openshaw, S. (1977), 'A geographical study of scale and aggregation problems in region-building, partitioning, and spatial modelling', *Transactions of the Institute of British Geographers*, vol. 2, pp. 459-72.

Openshaw, S. (1984), *The Modifiable Areal Unit Problem*, CATMOG 38, Geo Books, Norwich.

Oppenheimer, C. (1994), 'Discussion Meeting on Natural Hazard Assessment and Mitigation: The Unique Role of Remote Sensing'. The Royal Society, London, 8-9 March, 1994', *Disasters*, vol. 18:3, pp. 294-7.

Owen, M., Headworth, H.G. and Morgan-Jones, M. (1991), 'Groundwater in basin management', in R.A. Downing and W.B. Wilkinson (eds), *Applied Groundwater Hydrology: A British Perspective*, Oxford Science Publications, Clarendon Press, Oxford, pp. 16-34.

Pacey A. (1980), *Rural Sanitation: Planning and appraisal*, Oxfam/ Intermediate Technology Publications Ltd., London.

Pan American Health Organization (1991), 'Cholera situation in the Americas', *Epidemiological Bulletin*, vol. 12:2.

Pandit, C.G., Pal, S.C., Murti, G.V.S., Misra, B.S., Murty, D.K., and Shivastav, J.B. (1967), 'Survival of *Vibrio Cholerae* Biotype El Tor in well water', *Bulletin of The World Health Organization*, vol. 37, pp. 681-5.

Paquet, C. (1992), 'Outbreak of bloody diarrhoea in Lisungwi Refugee Camps, Malawi', Unpublished investigation report for Epicentre, France.

Patel, M., Issaäcson, M. and Gouws, E. (1995), 'Effect of iron and pH on the survival of *Vibrio cholerae* in water', *Transactions of the Royal Society of Tropical Medicine and Hygiene*, vol. 89, pp. 175-7.

Pavlovskiy, E.N., Petrishcheva, P.A., Zasukhin, D.N. and Olsofiev, N.G. (eds) (1955), *Natural Nidi of Human Diseases and Regional Epidemiology*. Medgiz, Leningrad. Translation appears in Levine, N.D.(1966), *The Natural Nidality of Transmissible Diseases*, Univ. of Illinois Press, Urbana, 1966.

Pearce, D.W. and Turner, R.K. (1990), *Economics of Natural Resources and the Environment*.

Pellegrino, C. (1994), *Return to Sodom and Gomorrah: Bible Stories from Archaeologists*, Random House Inc., New York.

Pelto, G.H. (1991), 'The role of behavioural research in the prevention and management of invasive diarrheas', *Reviews of Infectious Diseases*, vol. 13(Suppl 4), pp.255-8.

Phillips, D.R. (1990), *Health and Health Care in the Third World*, Longman Development studies, U.K.

Phillips, D.R. and Verhasselt, Y. (1994a), 'Introduction: health and development', in D.R. Phillips, and Y. Verhasselt (eds), *Health and Development*, Routledge, London, pp. 3-32.

Phillips, D.R. and Verhasselt, Y. (1994b), 'Health and development: retrospect and prospect', in D.R. Phillips and Y. Verhasselt (eds) *Health and Development*, Routledge, London, pp. 301-18.

Poore, P. (1993), 'World Bank's development report', *The Lancet*, vol. 342, p. 441.

Popper, K. (1968), *The Logic of Scientific Discovery*, Revised Edition.

Prescott, L.M. and Bhattacharjee, N.K. (1969), *Bulletin of The World Health Organization*, vol. 40, pp. 980-2.

Preston, N.W. (1993), 'Cholera isolates in relation to the "eighth pandemic"', *The Lancet*, vol. 342, pp. 925-6.

Prothero, R.M.(1977), 'Disease and human mobility: a neglected factor in epidemiology', *International Journal of Epidemiology* vol. 6, pp. 259-67.

Prothero, R.M. (1994), 'Forced movements of population and health hazards in tropical Africa', *International Journal of Epidemiology*, vol. 23:4, pp. 657-64.

Quick, R.E., Vargas, R., Moreno, D., Mujica, O. et al. (1993), 'Epidemic cholera in the Amazon: the challenge of preventing death', *American Journal of Tropical Medicine and Hygiene*, vol. 48:5, pp. 597-602.

Rahman, M.M., Kabir, I., Mahalanabis, D. and Malek, M.A. (1992), 'Decreased food intake in children with severe dysentery due to *Shigella dysenteriae* 1 infection', *European Journal of Clinical Nutrition*, vol. 46, pp. 833-8.

Reed, D. (ed)(1993), *Structural Adjustment and the Environment*, Earthscan, London.

Refugees Policy Group (1992), *Internally Displaced Persons in Africa: Assistance Challenges and Opportunities*, Washington D.C.

Rich, B. (1994), *Morgaging the Earth. The World Bank, Environmental Impoverishment and the Crisis of Development*, Earthscan, London.

Ries, A.A., Wells, J.G., Olivola, D. and Ntakibirora, M. et al. (1994), 'Epidemic *Shigella dysenteriae* type 1 in Burundi: Panresistance and implications for prevention', *The Journal of Infectious Diseases*, vol. 169, pp. 1035-41.

Roberts, D.F., Fujiki, N. and Torizuka, K. (eds)(1992), 'Isolation, Migration and Health', *Society for the Study of Human Biology Symposium Series* 33, Cambridge University Press.

Robinson, A.H., Sale, R.D., Morrison, J.L. (1978), *Elements in Cartography*, Fourth edition, Wiley, Chichester.

Robinson, E. (1991), 'Peru battles 12,600 cases of cholera', *The Washington Post*, Feb. 14th.

Rogers, D.J. and Randolph, S.E. (1991), 'Mortality rates and population density of tsetse flies correlated with satellite imagery', *Nature*, vol. 351, pp. 739-41.

Rogers, D.J. and Williams, B.G. (1993), 'Monitoring trypanosomiasis in space and time', *Parasitology*, vol. 106, pp. S77-S92.

Roy, S.K., Akramuzzaman, S.M., Haider, R., Khatun, M. et al. (1994), 'Persistent diarrhoea: efficacy of a rice-based diet and role of nutritional status in recovery and nutrient absorption', *British Journal of Nutrition*, vol. 71, pp. 123-34.

Rozenzweig, C., Parry, M., Fischer, G. and Frohberg, K. (1992), *Climate Change and World Food Supply - a Preliminary Report*, Environmental change unit, University of Oxford.

Rutherford, G.W. and Mahanjane, A.E. (1985), 'Morbidity and mortality in the Mozambican famine of 1983: Prevalence of malnutrition and causes and rates of death and illness among dislocated persons in Gaza and Inhambane provinces', *Journal of Tropical Pediatrics*, vol. 31, pp. 143-9.

Salazar-Lindo, E. (1993), 'Recent developments in gastrointestinal infections with a focus on cholera', *Current Opinion in Infectious Diseases*, vol. 6, pp. 41-7.

Sandiford, P., Gorter, A.C., Davey Smith, G. and Pauw, J.P.C. (1989), 'Determinants of drinking water quality in rural Nicaragua', *Epidemiology and Infection*, vol. 102, pp. 429-38.

Sandiford, P., Gorter, A.C., Orozco, J.G. and Pauw, J.P. (1990), 'Determinants of domestic water use in rural Nicaragua', *Journal of Tropical Medicine and Hygiene*, vol. 93, pp. 383-9.

Sarkar, B.L., De, S.P., Sircar, B.K., Garg, S. et al. (1993), 'Polymyxim B sensitive strains of *Vibrio cholerae* non-01 from recent epidemic in India', *The Lancet*, vol. 341, p. 1090.

Saul, J.S. (ed)(1985), *A Difficult Road: The Transition to Socialism in Mozambique*, Monthly Review Press, New York.

Sazawal, S., Bhan, M.K., Bhandari, N. and Clemens, J. et al. (1991), 'Evidence for recent diarrhoeal morbidity as a risk factor for persistent diarrhoea: a case-control study', *International Journal of Epidemiology*, vol. 20:2, pp. 540-5.

Schwartz, S. (1994), 'The fallacy of the ecological fallacy: The potential misuse of a concept and the consequences', *American Journal of Public Health*, vol. 84:5, pp. 819-24.

Scrimshaw, N.S., Taylor, C.E. and Gordon, J.E. (1968), 'Interactions of nutrition and infection', *WHO monograph series* no.57, Geneva: WHO 1968.

Sepulveda, J., Gomes-Dantes, H. and Bronfman, M. (1992), 'Cholera in the Americas: An overview', *Infection*, vol. 20:5, pp. 243-8.

Serviço Provincial de Estatística (SPE)(1993), *Boletim Estatístico, Província de Sofala 1992*, Serviço Provincial de Estatística, Comissão Provincial do Plano de Sofala, República de Moçambique.

Shapiro, M.F. (1983), 'Medicine in the service of colonialism: medical care in Portuguese Africa 1885-1974', PhD Thesis, University of California, Los Angeles, USA.

Shears, P. (1994), 'Cholera', *Annals of Tropical Medicine and Parasitology*, vol. 88:2, pp. 109-22.

Shears, P. and Lusty, T. (1987), 'Communicable disease epidemiology following migration: Studies from the African famine', *International Migration Review*, vol. 21:3, pp. 783-95.

Siddique, A.K., Baqui, A.H., Eusof, A., Haider, K. et al. (1991), 'Survival of classic cholera in Bangladesh', *The Lancet*, vol. 337, pp. 1125-7.

Siddique, A.K., Zaman, K., Baqui, A.H., Akram, K. et al. (1992), 'Cholera epidemics in Bangladesh: 1985-1991', *Journal of Diarrhoeal Disease Research*, vol. 10:2, pp. 79-86.

Siddique, A.K., Zaman, K., Akram, K. and Mutsuddy, A. et al. (1994), 'Emergence of a new epidemic strain of *Vibrio cholerae* in Bangladesh: an epidemiological study', *Tropical and Geographical Medicine*, vol. 46:3, pp. 147-50.

Singleton, F.L., Attwell, R.W., Jangi, M.S. and Colwell, R.R. (1982), 'Influence of salinity and nutrient concentration on survival and growth of *Vibrio cholerae 01* in aquatic microcosms', *Applied Environmental Microbiology*, vol. 43, pp. 1080-5.

Slim, H. (1995), 'The continuing metamorphosis of the humanitarian practitioner: some new colours for and endangered chameleon', *Disasters*, vol. 19:2, pp. 110-26.

Smith, J.A. (1988), 'The Beira Corridor Project', *Geography*, vol. 73:320, pp. 258-61.

Smith, P.D. and Thomasson, A.J. (1974), 'Density and water-release characteristics', in B.W. Avery, and C.L. Bascomb (eds), *Soil Survey Laboratory Methods*, Technical Monograph No. 6, Harpenden, England.

Snow, J. (1855), *On the Mode of Communication of Cholera*, 1855 London.

Snow, R.W., Schellenberg, J.R.M., Peshu, N., Forster, D. et al. (1993), 'Periodicity and space-time clustering of severe childhood malaria on the coast of Kenya', *Transactions of the Royal Society of Tropical Medicine and Hygiene*, vol. 87, pp. 386-90.

Snyder, J.D. and Black, P.A. (1982), 'Is cholera a problem for US travellers?', *Journal of the American Medical Association*, vol. 247, pp. 1495-9.

Sørensen and Dissler (1986), 'Practical experience with the management of a cholera outbreak in a refugee camp in Eastern Sudan, 1985', *Disasters*, vol. 12:3, pp. 274-81.

St Louis, M.E., Porter, J.D., Helai, A., Drame, K. et al. (1990), 'Epidemic cholera in West Africa: the role of food handling and high-risk foods', *American Journal of Epidemiology*, vol. 131, pp. 719-28.

Stephens, C. and Harpham, T. (1992), 'Health and environment in urban areas of developing countries', *Third World Planning Review*, vol. 14:3, pp. 267-82.

Stock, R. (1986), '"Disease and development" or "The underdevelopment of health": A critical review of geographical perspectives on African health problems', *Social Science and Medicine*, vol. 23:7, pp. 689-700.

Stock, R. (1995), *Africa South of the Sahara: A Geographical Interpretation*, The Guildford Press, New York and London.

Strockbine, N.A., Parsonnet, J., Greene, K. and Kiehlbauch, J.A. et al. (1991), 'Molecular epidemiologic techniques in analysis of epidemic and endemic *Shigella dysenteriae* type 1 strains', *The Journal of Infectious Diseases*, vol. 163, pp. 406-9.

Struelens, M.J., Mondal, G., Roberts, M. and Williams, P.H. (1990), 'Role of bacterial and host factors in the pathogenesis of *Shigella* septicemia',

European Journal of Clinical Microbiology and Infectious Disease, vol. 9:5, pp. 337-44.

Susser, M. (1973), *Causal Thinking in the Health Sciences: Concepts and Strategies of Epidemiology.*

Swerdlow, D.L., Mintz, E.D., Rodriguez, M., Tejada, E. et al. (1992), 'Waterborne transmission of epidemic cholera in Trujillo, Peru: lessons for a continent at risk', *The Lancet*, vol. 340, pp. 28-32.

Swerdlow, D.L. and Ries, A.A. (1993), '*Vibrio cholerae* non-01: The eighth pandemic?', *The Lancet*, vol. 342, pp. 382-3.

Swerdlow, D.L., Mintz, E.D., Rodriguez, M. and Tejada, E., et al. (1994), 'Severe life-threatening cholera associated with blood group O in Peru: implications for the Latin American epidemic', *Journal of Infectious Diseases*, vol. 170, pp. 468-72.

Talsma, T. and Philip, J.R. (eds) (1971), *Salinity and Water Use: A Practical Symposium on Hydrology, Sponsered by the Australian Acadamy of Science 2-4 November, 1971*, Macmillan, London.

Tamplin, M.L., Gauzens, A.L., Huq, A. and Sack, D.A. et al. (1990), 'Attatchment of *Vibrio cholerae* serotype 01 to zooplankton and phytoplankton of Bangladesh waters', *Applied Environmental Microbiology*, vol. 56, pp. 1977-80.

Tamplin, M.L. and Parodi, C.C. (1991), 'Environmental spread of *Vibrio cholerae* in Peru', *The Lancet*, vol. 338, pp. 1216-7.

Tanner, M. and Harpham, T. (1995), 'Features and determinants of urban health status', in T. Harpham, and M. Tanner, (eds), *Urban Health in Developing Countries: Progress and Prospects*, Earthscan, London.

Taylor, D.N., Bodhidatta, L., Brown, J.E. et al. (1989), 'Introduction and spread of multiresistant *Shigella dysenteriae* 1 in Thailand', *American Journal of Tropical Medicine and Hygiene*, vol. 40, pp. 77-85.

Taylor, D.N., Bodhidatta, L. and Echeverria, P. (1991), 'Epidemiologic aspects of shigellosis and other causes of dysentery in Thailand', *Review of Infectious Diseases*, vol. 1:13(Suppl 4), pp. S226-30.

Tempo (1993), 'Diarreia sanguinolenta', 9th May 1993, Maputo.

Thomason, H., Burke, V. and Gracey, M. (1981), 'Impaired gastric function in experimental malnutrition', *American Journal of Clinical Nutrition* vol. 34, pp. 1278-80.

Thompson, R.D., Mannion, A.M., Mitchel, C.W. and Parry, M. and Townsend, J.R.G. (1986), *Processes in Physical Geography*, Longman, London and New York.

Thrift, N. (1983), 'On the determination of social action in space and time', *Environment and Planning D*, vol. 1, pp. 23-57.

Timberlake, L. (1985), *Africa in Crisis*, Earthscan, London.

Times Newspaper (1994a), '2,000 refugees a day die of cholera in Rwanda camps', July 25th 1994.

Times Newspaper (1994b), 'Drug-resistant dysentery sweeps Goma camps', August 9th 1994.

Tivy, J. and O'Hare', G. (1989), *Human Impact on the Ecosystem*, Oliver and Boyd, Edinburgh.

Toole, M.J. (1995), 'Mass population displacement. A global public health challenge', *Infectious Disease Clinics of North America*, vol. 9:2, pp. 353-66.

Toole, M.J. and Waldman, R.J. (1988), 'An analysis of mortality trends among refugee populations in Somalia, Sudan, and Thailand', *Bulletin of the World Health Organization*, vol. 66:2, pp. 237-47.

Toole, M.J. and Waldman, R.J. (1993), 'Refugees and displaced persons. War, hunger and public health', *Journal of the American Medical Association*, vol. 270:5, pp. 600-5.

Traoré, E., Cousens, S., Curtis, V., Mertens, T. and Tall, F. (1994), 'Child defecation behaviour, stool disposal practices, and childhood diarrhoea in Burkina Faso: results from a case-control study', *Journal of Epidemiology and Community Health*, vol. 48, pp. 270-5.

Tumwine, J.K. (1992), 'Zimbabwe's success story in education and health: will it weather economic structural adjustment?', *Journal of the Royal Society of Health*, December 1992, pp. 286-90.

UNDP (United Nations Development Programme)(1996), *Human Development Report*, Oxford University Press.

UNEP (United Nations Environment Programme)(1993), *Environmental Data Report 1993-1994*, Blackwell, Oxford.

UNHCR (United Nations High Commissioner for Refugees) (1992), 'Focus: emergency', *Refugees*, vol. 91, pp. 4-35.

UNICEF (United Nations Children's Fund)(1989a), *Towards the 1990's: The Water and Sanitation Sector Workplan for 1990-1995*, New York, UNICEF, WET/567/89.

UNICEF (1989b), in UNICEF/Government of Zimbabwe, *Situation of Women and Children in Zimbabwe 1985-1990*, Jongwe Printers, Harare.

UNICEF (1991), *The State of The World's Children 1991*, Oxford University Press.

UNICEF (1995), *The State of The World's Children 1991*, Oxford University Press.

UNOHAC (1993), 'Mozambique Report. Humanitarian Activities in a Post-war Mozambique', *Monthly Bulletin*, 6.

US Committee for Refugees (1993), *World Refugee Survey, 1993*, Washington D.C.

Utsalo, S.J., Eko, F.O. and Antia-Obong, E.O. (1992), 'Features of cholera and *Vibrio parahaemolyticus* diarrhoea endemicity in Calabar, Nigeria', *European Journal of Epidemiology*, vol. 8:6, pp. 856-60.

Vail, L. and White, L. (1980), *Capitalism and Colonialism in Mozambique: A study of Quelimane District*, Heinemann, London, Nairobi, Ibadan.

Van Damme, W. (1995), 'Do refugees belong in camps? Experiences from Goma and Guinea', *The Lancet*, vol. 346, pp. 360-2.

Van Demark, P. (1992), 'Exhibits redux: What I saw at GIS/LIS '91', URISA News, vol. 119, pp. 5-6.

Van Loon, F.P.L. (1993), 'Cholera: developments in prevention and cure', *Tropical and Geographic Medicine*, vol. 45:6, pp. 269-73.

Ventura, G., Roberts, L. and Gilman, R. (1992), '*Vibrio cholerae* non-01 in sewage lagoons and seasonality in Peru cholera epidemic', *The Lancet*, vol. 339, pp. 937-8.

Vogel, F. (1992), 'Break-up of isolates', in Roberts, D.F., Fujiki, N. and Torizuka, K. (eds), 'Isolation, Migration and Health', *Society for the Study of Human Biology Symposium Series 33*, Cambridge University Press.

Vugia, D.J., Rodriguez, M., Vargas, R. and Ricse, C. et al. (1994), 'Epidemic cholera in Trujillo, Peru 1992: utility of a clinical case definition and shift in *Vibrio cholerae* 01 serotype', *American Journal of Tropical Medicine and Hygiene*, vol. 50:5, pp. 566-9.

Wachsmuth, I.K., Evins, G.M., Fields, P.I., Olsvik, O. et al. (1993), 'The molecular epidemiology of cholera in Latin America', *The Journal of Infectious Diseases*, vol. 167, pp. 621-6.

Waldor, M.K. and Mekalanos, J.J. (1994a), 'ToxR regulates virulence gene expression in non-01 strains of *Vibrio cholerae* that cause epidemic cholera'.

Waldor, M.K. and Mekalanos, J.J. (1994b), 'Emergence of a new cholera pandemic: analysis of virulence determinants in *Vibrio cholerae* 0139 and development of a live vaccine prototype', *Journal of Infectious Deseases*, vol. 170, pp. 278-83.

Waller, L.A. and Turnbull, B.W. (1993), 'The effects of scale on tests for disease clustering', *Statistics in Medicine*, vol. 12, pp. 1869-84.

Walt, G. (1984), 'The evolution of health policy', in G. Walt, and A. Melamed (eds), *Mozambique: Towards a Peoples Health Service*, Zed Books, London.

Walt, G. and Melamed, A. (eds)(1984), *Mozambique: Towards a Peoples Health Service*, Zed Books, London.

Webb, C. (1984), 'Changing attitudes in nurse training', in G. Walt, and A. Melamed (eds), *Mozambique: Towards a Peoples Health Service*, Zed Books, London.

White, G., Bradley, D. and White, A. (1972), *Drawers of Water*, Chicago University Press, Chicago. pp 162-76.

WHO (1948), *The Constitution*, Geneva, WHO.

WHO (1970), *Principles and Practice of Cholera Control*, Geneva, WHO.

WHO (1983), *Minimum Evaluation Procedure (MEP) for Water Supply and Sanitation Projects*, CDD/OPR/83.1 Geneva.

WHO (1985), *Guidelines for Drinking-water Quality. Vol. 3. Drinking-water Quality Control in Small-community Supplies*, WHO, Geneva.

WHO (1986), *Guidelines for Cholera Control*, WHO/CDD/SER/80.4RE.1.

WHO (1988), *Guidelines for the Control of Epidemics due to Shigella dysenteriae 1*, Programme for Control of Diarrhoeal Diseases, WHO/CDD/SER/88.12, Geneva.

WHO (1989), *The Work of WHO in the African Region 1987-1988. Biennial Report of the Regional Director*, WHO Regional Office for Africa, Brazzaville, AFR/RC.

WHO (1990), 'Cholera today', *WHO Features 1990*.

WHO (1991a), *Environmental Health in Urban Development, Report of a WHO Expert Committee*, WHO Technical Report Series 807, Geneva.

WHO (1991b), *Community Involvement in Health Development: Challenging Health Services, Report of a WHO Study Group*, WHO Technical Report Series 809, Geneva.

WHO (1991c), *Weekly Epidemiological Record*, No. 19.

WHO (1991d), *The Work of WHO in the African region 1989-1990. Biennial Report of the Regional Director*, WHO Regional Office for Africa, Brazzaville, AFR/RC41/3.

WHO (1992a), 'Choléra, 1991 - Viel ennemi, nouveau visage', *World Health Statistics Quarterly*, vol. 45, pp. 208-19.

WHO (1992b), *The International Drinking Water Supply and Sanitation Decade: End of Decade Review*, WHO/CWS/92.12, WHO, Geneva.

WHO (1993a), *Weekly Epidemiological Record*, No. 21.

WHO (1993b), (Personal communication August) Phone call to Ronald Waldman, Coordinator of the Global Task Force on Cholera Control.

WHO (1994a), *Weekly Epidemiological Record*, No. 28.

WHO (1994b), *Weekly Epidemiological Record*, No. 7.

WHO (1995), *The World Health Report: Bridging the Gaps*, Geneva.

Wildt, Gilles de., Sogge, D., Peters, A., Kemkes J., Hansma, G. and Bannenberg W. (1993), 'World Bank's development report', *The Lancet*, vol. 342, p. 440.

Williams, R. (1983), *Keywords*, Fontana, London.

Wilson, A.L. (1974), *The Chemical Analysis of Water: General Principles and Techniques*.

Wilson, K.B. (1992), (unpublished paper) 'The implications of health and educational service infrastructure in Renamo-held areas of Western Zambezia, An independent study', Refugees Studies Programme, Oxford University.

Wilson, M.E., Levins, R. and Spielman, A. (eds)(1994), 'Disease in evolution: global changes and emergence of infectious diseases', *Annals of The New York Acadamy of Sciences*, vol. 740, pp. 1-503.

Winblad, U. and Kilama, W. (1986), *Sanitation Without Water*, Macmillan, Basingstoke, England.

Woodward, W.E. and Mosley, W.H. (1971), 'The spectrum of cholera in rural Bangladesh. Comparison of El Tor, Ogawa and classical Inaba infection', *American Journal of Epidemiology*, vol. 96, p. 342.

World Bank (1992), *The World Bank Development Report 1992: Development and the Environment*, World Bank, Washington D.C.

World Bank (1993), *The World Bank Development Report 1993: Investing in Health*, World Bank, Washington D.C.

World Bank Water Demand Research Team (1993), 'The demand for water in rural areas: Determinants and policy implications', *World Bank Research Observer*, vol. 8:1.

Wright, R.C. (1986), 'The seasonality of bacterial quality of water in a tropical developing country (Sierra Leone)', *Journal of Hygiene (Cambridge)*, vol. 96, p. 75.

Xu H.S., Roberts, N., Singleton, F.L., Attwell, R.W., Grimes, D.J., Colwell, R.R. (1982), 'Survival and viability of non-culturable *Escherichia coli* and *Vibrio cholerae* in the estuarine and marine environment', *Microb Ecol*, vol. 8, pp. 313-23.

Yip, R. and Sharp, T.W. (1993), 'Acute malnutrition and high childhood mortality related to diarrhea. Lessons from the 1991 kurdish refugee crisis', *Journal of the American Medical Association*, vol. 270:5, pp. 587-90.

Young, L. (1985), 'A general assessment of the environmental impact of refugees in Somalia with attention to the refugee agricultural programme', *Disasters*, vol. 9:2, pp. 122-33.

Zeitlyn, S. and Islam, F. (1991), 'The use of soap and water in two Bangladeshi communities: implications for the transmission of diarrhea', *Reviews of Infectious Diseases*, vol. 13(suppl 4), pp. 259-64.

Index

References from Notes indicated by 'n' after page preference